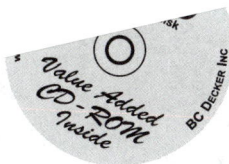

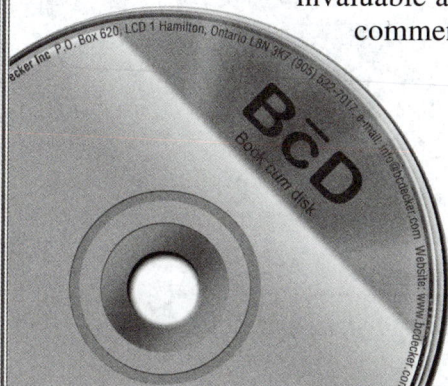

*PDQ** SERIES

ACKERMANN
PDQ PHYSIOLOGY

BAKER, MURRAY
PDQ BIOCHEMISTRY

CORMACK
PDQ HISTOLOGY

DAVIDSON
PDQ MEDICAL GENETICS

JOHNSON
PDQ PHARMACOLOGY, 2/e

McKIBBON

PDQ EVIDENCE-BASED PRINCIPLES AND PRACTICE

NORMAN, STREINER
PDQ STATISTICS, 2/e

STREINER, NORMAN
PDQ EPIDEMIOLOGY, 2/e

---

*PDQ (Pretty Darned Quick)

PDQ HEMATOLOGY

William F. Kern, MD

Department of Pathology
University of Oklahoma Health Sciences Center
OU Medical Center
Oklahoma City, Oklahoma

2002

BC Decker Inc

Hamilton • London

BC Decker Inc
20 Hughson Street South
P.O. Box 620, LCD 1
Hamilton, Ontario L8N 3K7
Tel: 905-522-7017; 1-800-568-7281
Fax: 905-522-7839; 1-888-311-4987
E-mail: info@bcdecker.com
Web site: www.bcdecker.com

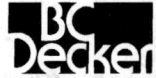

02 03 04 05 / CP/ 9 8 7 6 5 4 3 2 1

ISBN 1-55009-176-X

Printed in Canada

Sales and Distribution

United States
BC Decker Inc
P.O. Box 785
Lewiston, NY 14092-0785
Tel: 905-522-7017; 1-800-568-7281
Fax: 905-522-7839; 1-888-311-4987
E-mail: info@bcdecker.com
Web site: www.bcdecker.com

Canada
BC Decker Inc
20 Hughson Street South
P.O. Box 620, L.C.D. 1
Hamilton, Ontario L8N 3K7
Tel: 905-522-7017; 1-800-568-7281
Fax: 905-522-7839; 1-888-311-4987
E-mail: info@bcdecker.com
Web site: www.bcdecker.com

Japan
Igaku-Shoin Ltd.
Foreign Publications Department
3-24-17 Hongo, Bunkyo-ku
Tokyo 113-8719, Japan
Tel: 81 3 3817 5680
Fax: 81 3 3815 6776
E-mail: fd@igaku-shoin.co.jp

U.K., Europe, Scandinavia, Middle East
Elsevier Science
Customer Service Department
Foots Cray High Street
Sidcup, Kent DA14 5HP, UK
Tel: 44 (0) 208 308 5760
Fax: 44 (0) 181 308 5702
E-mail: cservice@harcourt_brace.com

Singapore, Malaysia, Thailand, Philippines, Indonesia, Vietnam, Pacific Rim, Korea
Elsevier Science Asia
583 Orchard Road
#09/01, Forum
Singapore 238884
Tel: 65-737-3593
Fax: 65-753-2145

Australia, New Zealand
Elsevier Science Australia
Customer Service Department
STM Division
Locked Bag 16
St. Peters, New South Wales, 2044
Australia
Tel: 61 02 9517-8999
Fax: 61 02 9517-2249
E-mail: stmp@harcourt.com.au
Web site: www.harcourt.com.au

Foreign Rights
John Scott & Company
International Publishers' Agency
P.O. Box 878
Kimberton, PA 19442
Tel: 610-827-1640
Fax: 610-827-1671
E-mail: jsco@voicenet.com

Mexico and Central America
Rafael Sainz
ETM SA de CV
Calle de Tula 59
Colonia Condesa
061 40 Mexico DF, Mexico
Tel: 52-5-5553-6657
Fax: 52-5-5211-8468
E-mail: editoresdetextosmex@prodigy.net.mx

Preface

Hematology is the study of blood, the bone marrow where blood is produced, and the hemostasis system. Disorders of lymph nodes and related tissues are also often included in the field of hematology. Hematology includes a wide variety of diseases, including genetic diseases (such as the hemoglobinopathies and thalassemias), immune diseases (such as immune hemolytic anemia), and malignancies (such as leukemias and lymphomas). Historically, hematology has been important in many ways: in studying blood and its disorders, we learned much about gene structure and function, the importance of chromosomal abnormalities in malignancies, the molecular biology of neoplasia, and many other things. Some of our first successes in the treatment of neoplasia occurred in hematologic malignancies. (Personally, I feel that it is the most fascinating field in all of medicine, though I must admit that I am a little biased about it.)

PDQ *Hematology* is intended to be a quick and practical introduction to hematology. It covers the most important aspects of the field, with an emphasis on clinical features, diagnosis, and treatment. Several reference books on hematology are available and should be consulted for details that could not be covered in PDQ *Hematology*. I have tried to emphasize those conditions that the average physician is likely to encounter on a frequent basis in his clinical practice. The field of hematology is evolving with bewildering speed, with new developments in diagnosis and treatment appearing almost on a daily basis. Therefore, discussion of treatment for more unusual or complicated diseases has been limited to general principles rather than specific details (for example, drug doses for treatment of acute leukemia). Please confirm the treatment recommendations and doses contained here by consulting current sources.

The two comprehensive references that I depended on for specific details are *Hematology: Basic Principles and Practice*[1] and *Wintrobe's Clinical Hematology*[2]; I used both heavily. *Red Cell Manual*[3] is a concise, readable discussion of red cells and their disorders. For those interested in the laboratory aspects of hematology, I would recommend *Diagnostic Hematology*[4] and *Clinical Hematology and Fundamentals of Hemostasis*.[5] *Hemostasis and Thrombosis*[6] is a quick, pocket-sized introduction to coagulation and hemostasis, whereas *Hemostasis and Thrombosis: Basic Principles and Clinical Practice*[7] is the primary comprehensive coagulation reference.

Acknowledgments

Special acknowledgments go to Drs. Jim George, Tom Carter, and Joan Parkhurst for reviewing and critiquing portions of PDQ Hematology.

References

1. Hoffman R, Benz EJ Jr, Shattil SJ, et al, editors. Hematology: basic principles and practice. 3rd ed. New York: Churchill Livingstone; 2000.
2. Lee GR, Foerster J, Lukens J, et al, editors. Wintrobe's clinical hematology. 10th ed. Baltimore: Williams & Wilkins; 1999.
3. Hillman RS, Finch CA. Red cell manual. 7th ed. Philadelphia: FA Davis; 1996.
4. Rodak BF, editor. Diagnostic hematology. Philadelphia: WB Saunders; 1995.
5. Harmening DM, editor. Clinical hematology and fundamentals of hemostasis. 3rd ed. Philadelphia: FA Davis; 1997.
6. DeLoughery TG. Hemostasis and thrombosis. Austin (TX): Landes Bioscience; 1999.
7. Colman RW, Hirsh J, Marder VJ, Clowes AW, George JN, editors. Hemostasis and thrombosis: basic principles and clinical practice. 4th ed. Philadelphia: Lippincott Williams & Wilkins; 2001.

William F. Kern, MD
Oklahoma City, Oklahoma
February 2002

*This book is dedicated to my teachers in hematology,
Drs. Lewis Glasser, Thomas Grogan, and Catherine Spier;
to my colleagues in Pathology and Hematology–Oncology at the
University of Arizona and the University of Oklahoma Health
Sciences Center; to the residents in Pathology at Arizona and
Oklahoma; to the technologists in Hematology, Special Hematology, and Flow Cytometry at Oklahoma; to Dr. Fred Silva, for his
constant support; and to my wife, Kathleen Duncan, for
her inspiration and encouragement.*

Contents

Cells and Composition of the Peripheral Blood

The average person has approximately 70 mL of blood per kilogram body weight (70 mL/kg), or ~5 L total for a 70-kg man. Approximately 50 to 60% of the blood volume is liquid; the remainder is cells. The liquid component, called **plasma**, is nearly 90% water. The remaining 10% includes ions, glucose, amino acids and other metabolites, hormones, and various proteins. The proteins of interest are the coagulation proteins, which will be described in detail in Chapter 20. **Serum** is the liquid remaining after blood clots; it is essentially the same as plasma, except that the clotting factors and fibrinogen have been removed. The cells of the blood can be divided into **erythrocytes** (*red blood cells*), **leukocytes** (*white blood cells*) of various types, and **platelets**.

ERYTHROCYTES (RED BLOOD CELLS)

The primary function of **erythrocytes** is gas exchange. They carry oxygen from the lungs to the tissues and return carbon dioxide (CO_2) from the tissues to the lungs to be exhaled. Erythrocytes are anucleate cells containing few organelles; a large proportion of their cytoplasm consists of the iron-containing oxygen transport molecule **hemoglobin**. Erythrocytes are shaped like biconcave disks approximately 7 to 8 μm in diameter. The biconcave disk shape gives red blood cells (RBCs) the flexibility to squeeze their way through capillaries and other small blood vessels. Viewed under the microscope, RBCs look like a circle with a central hole, or **central pallor**, which is approximately one-third the diameter of the cell (Figure 1–1).

Erythrocytes are the most common cells in blood. The normal RBC count is approximately 4.5 to 6 million cells per microliter. The parameters by which erythrocytes are usually measured are the blood **hemoglobin** (**Hgb**) in grams per deciliter (g/dL), the **hematocrit** (**Hct**) or **packed cell volume** (volume of RBCs as a percent of total blood volume), and the RBC

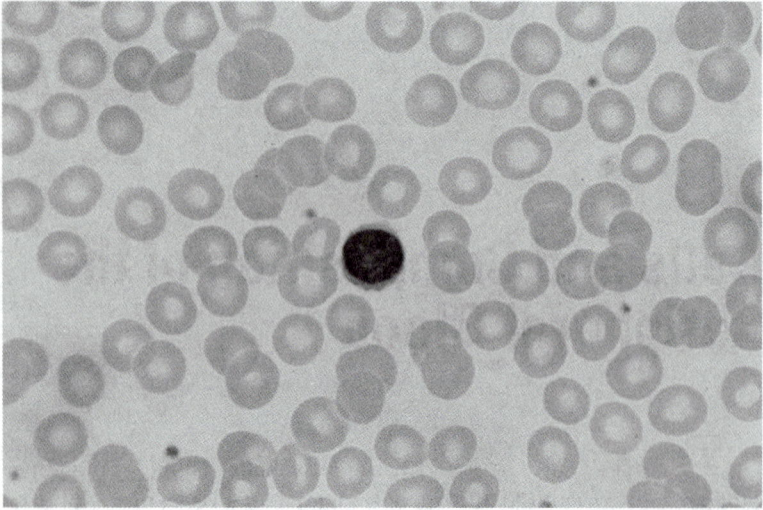

Figure 1–1 Erythrocytes. Note that the size of the erythrocytes is about the same as the nucleus of the small resting lymphocyte.

count (millions of cells per μL) (Table 1–1). The size of red cells is measured as the **mean corpuscular volume** (**MCV**), reported in femtoliters (fL; 1 fL = 10^{-15} L). The normal MCV is ~80 to 100 fL. Red blood cells that are smaller than 80 fL are called **microcytic**; those that are larger than 100 fL are called **macrocytic**.

Red cells have a life span of approximately 120 days; therefore, approximately 1% of red cells are replaced each day. Young red cells can be identified because they contain ribonucleic acid (RNA). With special stains such as new methylene blue, the RNA aggregates as visible particles called **reticulin**. Young RBCs containing RNA are designated as **reticulocytes**, and the number of reticulocytes in the peripheral blood (**reticulocyte count**) is the

Table 1–1
Approximate Normal Blood Values

Value*	Male	Female
Hemoglobin (g/dL)	14–18	12–16
Hematocrit (%)	42–52	37–47
RBC count (10^6/μL)	4.7–6.1	4.2–5.4
WBC count (10^3/μL)	4.0–10.0	4.0–10.0
Platelet count (10^3/μL)	150–400	150–400

*Values vary between different laboratories and different instruments.

best estimate of RBC production. Reticulocytes cannot be specifically identified on the usual blood smear stains, but they stain slightly more blue (an appearance that is designated **polychromasia**) than older RBCs.

LEUKOCYTES (WHITE BLOOD CELLS)

Several types of leukocytes, or white blood cells (WBCs), are found in the blood. The normal WBC count is ~4,000 to 10,000/μL (4.0–10.0 $\times$ 10^3/μL) (see Table 1–1). Leukocytes are usually divided into **granulocytes**, which have specific granules, and **agranulocytes**, which lack specific granules. Granulocytes are divided into **neutrophils** (with faintly staining granules), **eosinophils** (with large reddish or eosinophilic granules), and **basophils** (with large dark blue or basophilic granules). Agranulocytes are divided into **lymphocytes** and **monocytes**.

Although they are called white *blood* cells, leukocytes predominantly function in tissues. They are only in the blood transiently, while they travel to their site of action.

Neutrophils

Neutrophils are the most common type of WBCs in adults. Two types are described: **segmented neutrophils** and **band neutrophils**:

- **Segmented neutrophils** ("segs," also called **polymorphonuclear neutrophil leukocytes** [PMNs or "polys"]) have a nucleus divided into multiple distinct lobes connected by thin strands of chromatin. The cytoplasm has fine granules that stain lightly with the usual blood stains. Polys normally comprise ~50 to 70% of total WBCs (Figure 1–2).
- **Band neutrophils** ("bands," sometimes called "stabs") have a horseshoe-shaped nucleus, without the distinct lobes of polys. They are an earlier stage than segmented neutrophils but are fully functional. Bands normally represent ~2 to 6% of all WBCs; the number of bands increases with acute stress or infection (Figure 1–3).

The primary function of neutrophils is phagocytosis, predominantly of bacteria; **neutrophils are the primary defense against bacterial infection**. Bacteria are killed by antimicrobial agents contained or generated within neutrophil granules.

Neutrophils circulate in the blood for ~10 hours and may live 1 to 4 days in the extravascular space. The trip is one way; once neutrophils leave the blood to enter tissues, they cannot return. A significant number of neutrophils are rolling along the endothelial surface of blood vessels (the *marginating pool*). This population can be rapidly mobilized with acute stress or infection.

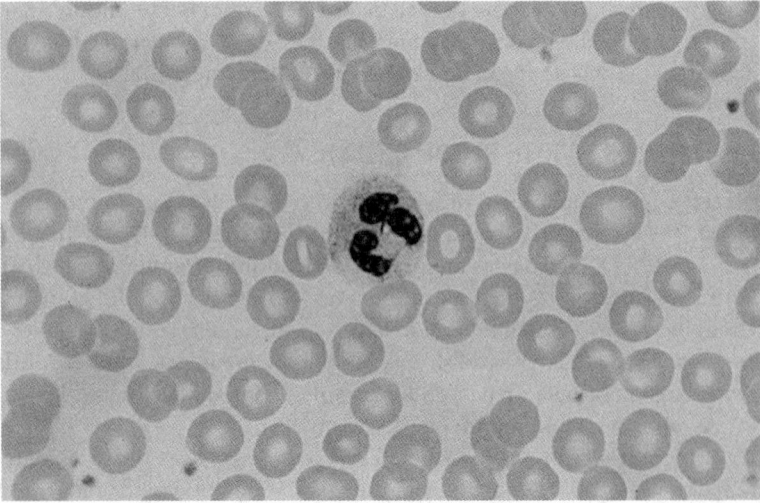

Figure 1–2 Mature segmented neutrophil. Note the thin strand of chromatin connecting the distinct nuclear lobes.

Eosinophils ("Eos")

Eosinophils contain large granules that stain reddish-orange (eosinophilic) with usual blood smear stains. The nucleus is segmented (often bilobed). Functions of eosinophils include phagocytosis of antigen-antibody complexes and defense against parasitic infection. The normal eosinophil count

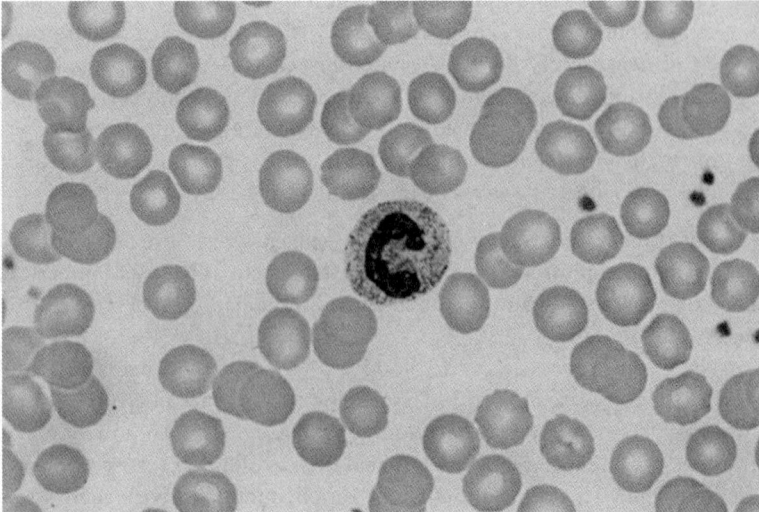

Figure 1–3 Band neutrophil. Note the unsegmented horseshoe-shaped nucleus.

is ~2 to 4% of total WBC. The number of eosinophils increases with allergic reactions and parasitic infections (Figure 1–4).

Basophils ("Basos")

Basophils contain large dark blue or purple (basophilic) granules, which often obscure the nucleus. The nucleus is segmented. Basophils are the least common type of leukocytes, normally ≤1% of total WBCs. The basophil granules contain heparin (an anticoagulant), histamine (a fast vasodilator), the slow-reacting substance of anaphylaxis (a slow vasodilator), and other compounds. Basophils appear to be involved in immediate hypersensitivity reactions related to immunoglobulin class E (IgE) (Figure 1–5).

Lymphocytes ("Lymphs")

Lymphocytes are the second most common type of leukocytes in adults (~20–40% of WBC). The lymphocyte number is higher in children and also increases with viral infections.

- **Resting lymphocytes:** Resting lymphocytes are usually small (7–10 μm), with a dark round to oval nucleus and scant amounts of pale blue cytoplasm (Figure 1–6).
  - ⇨ The nucleus of a small, resting lymphocyte is about the same diameter as a normal erythrocyte.

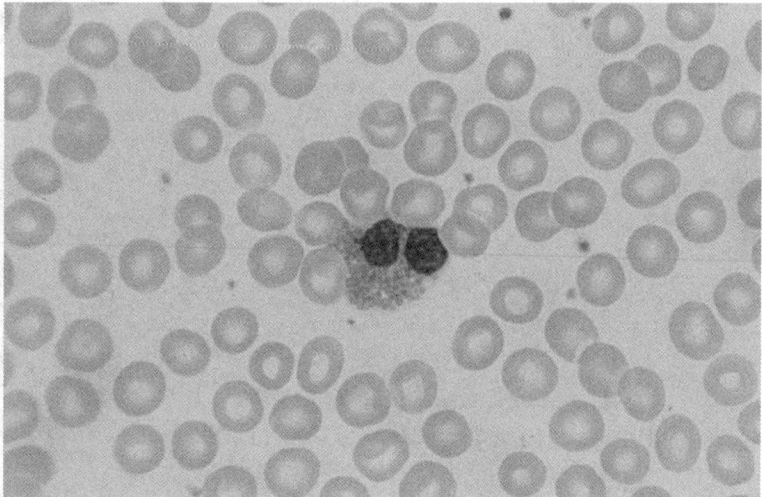

Figure 1–4   **Eosinophil.** Note the bilobed nucleus and the large granules.

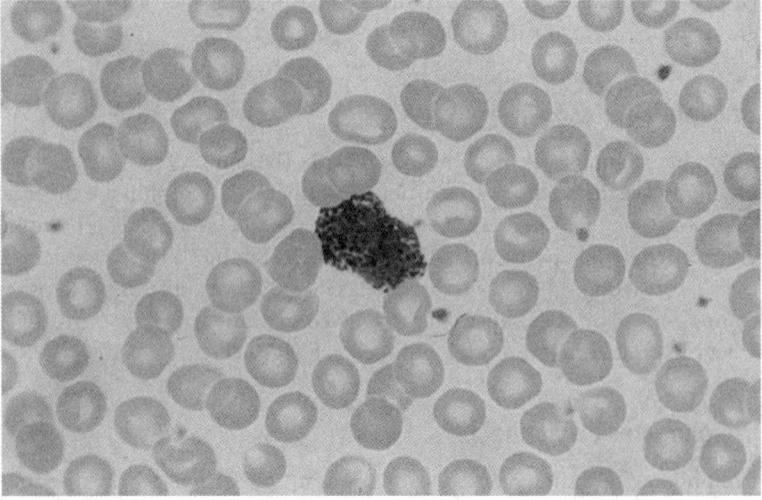

Figure 1–5 Basophil. Note the dark granules that obscure the nucleus.

- **Reactive ("*atypical*") lymphocytes:** A minority of lymphocytes are larger, with more abundant pale blue cytoplasm and larger nuclei with less condensed chromatin, and perhaps a nucleolus. These are designated reactive or atypical lymphocytes. The number of large lymphocytes may be increased in viral infections such as infectious mononucleosis (Figure 1–7).

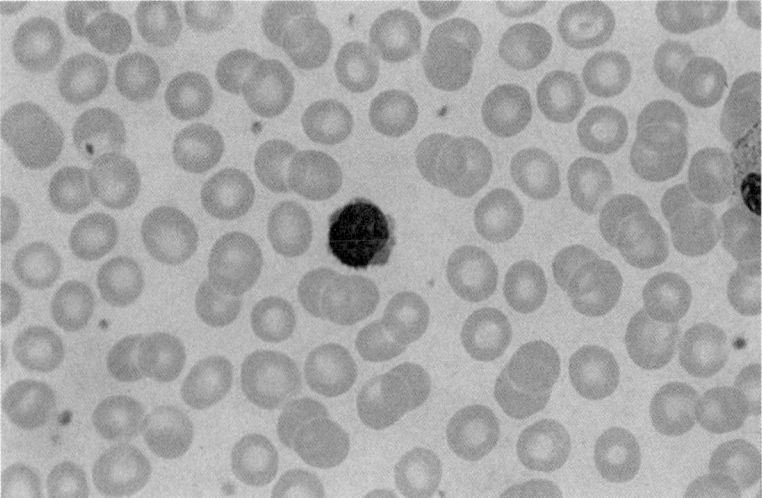

Figure 1–6 Resting lymphocyte. Note the small round nucleus and scant cytoplasm.

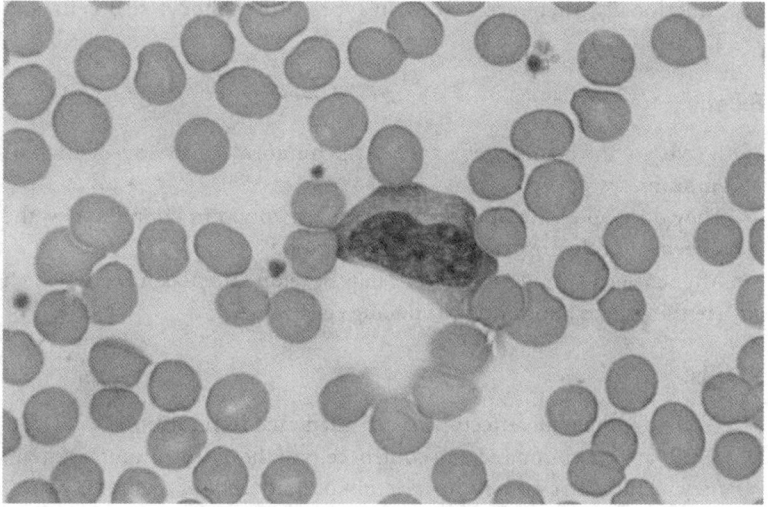

Figure 1–7 Reactive lymphocyte. Note the abundant cytoplasm that "hugs" erythrocytes.

- **Large granular lymphocytes:** A small number of lymphocytes in normal blood are slightly larger than resting lymphocytes, with reddish-purple (azurophilic) granules. This appearance generally corresponds to **natural killer** (**NK**) cells (Figure 1–8).

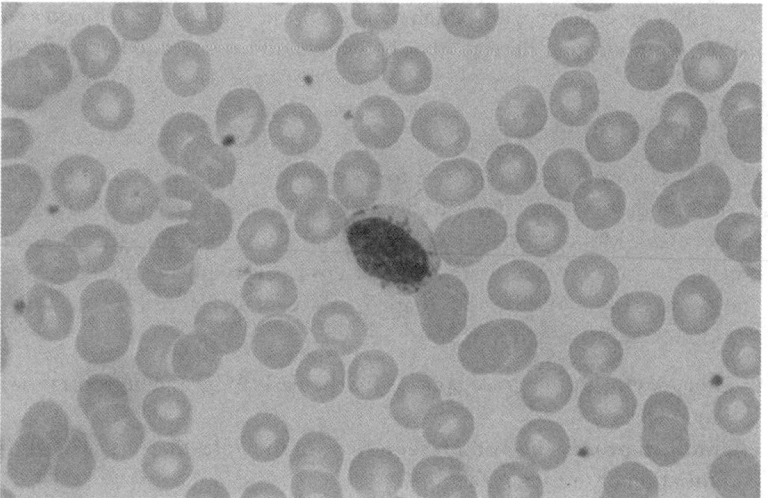

Figure 1–8 Large granular lymphocyte.

Functionally, there are two main types of lymphocytes: **B cells** and **T cells**.

B Cells:

- B cells are the primary effectors of the **humoral** (**antibody-mediated**) **immune system**.
- They develop in the bone marrow and are found in lymph nodes, the spleen and other organs, as well as the blood.
- After antigen stimulation, B cells may develop into **plasma cells**, which are the primary antibody-producing cells.

T Cells:

- T cells are the main effectors of **cell-mediated immunity**.
- T cells are the command and control cells of the entire immune system: they stimulate or inhibit the function of other cells of the immune system, including B cells, monocytes and macrophages, and other T cells.
- T cell precursors originate in the bone marrow but develop and mature in the thymus (T = thymic dependent).
- Normally, the majority of circulating lymphocytes are T cells.
- T cells are divided into two main subtypes:
    - **T helper cells**, which are the major regulatory cells of the immune system, usually express a surface antigen designated **CD4**.
    - **T suppressor/cytotoxic cells** are involved in the destruction of virally infected cells and rejection of transplanted organs. They usually express the **CD8** surface antigen.

Unlike other leukocytes, which make a one-way trip between blood and tissues, lymphocytes can recirculate between blood, tissue, and lymph fluid.

Monocytes ("Monos")

Monocytes normally comprise ~3 to 8% of leukocytes. After 8 to 14 hours in the blood, they enter tissue to become **tissue macrophages** (also called **histiocytes**). Monocytes are large cells, with abundant light gray to light blue finely granular cytoplasm. The nucleus has very finely granular chromatin and is often folded, bean shaped, or irregular (Figure 1–9).

Monocytes have two functions:

- **Phagocytosis** of microorganisms (particularly fungi and mycobacteria) and debris
- **Antigen processing and presentation**. In this role, they are critical in initiation of immune reactions.

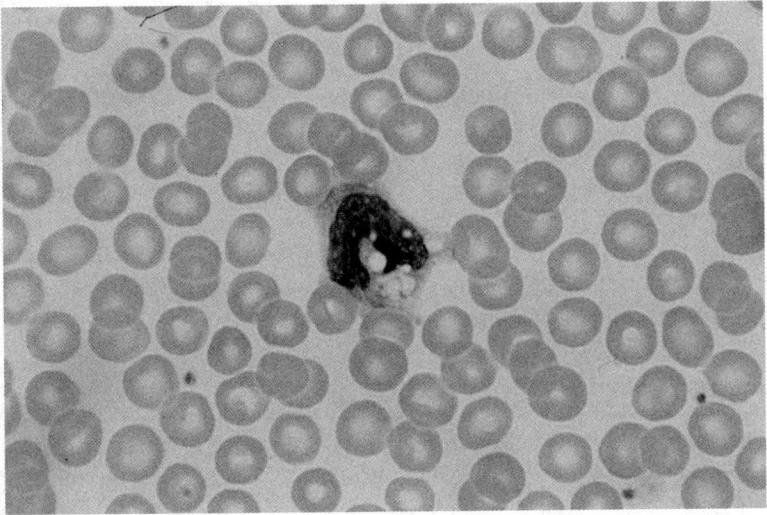

Figure 1–9   Monocyte. Note the large size, folded nucleus, and cytoplasmic vacuoles.

The Leukocyte Differential

The leukocyte differential is the listing of the different WBC types by percent in the peripheral blood (Table 1–2). These were formerly done by counting 100 or 200 cells on blood smears, but currently they are usually done by automated hematology analyzers, which count thousands of cells. Sophisticated hematology analyzers produce five-part differentials (neutrophils [segs + bands], lymphocytes, monocytes, eosinophils, and basophils). Manual differentials include band neutrophils as a separate category. Examination of

Table 1–2
Normal Leukocyte Differential

Cell Type	Percent	Absolute Number (cells/μL)*
Segmented neutrophils	50–70	1,500–8,000 (1.5–8.0 × 10³)
Band neutrophils	2–6	≤1,300 (≤1.3 × 10³)
Lymphocytes	20–40	600–5,000 (0.6–5.0 × 10³)
Monocytes	2–9	100–800 (0.1–0.8 × 10³)
Eosinophils	2–4	≤700 (≤0.7 × 10³)
Basophils	≤1	≤100 (≤0.1 × 10³)

*Values given are for adults; children tend to have a higher proportion of lymphocytes. The exact ranges will vary slightly between different laboratories.

blood smears and manual differentials are done if the hematology analyzer indicates the presence of abnormal cell types or numbers.

⇨ Although we usually think of the leukocyte differential in terms of percent of total WBCs, it is actually more appropriate to think of absolute numbers of the different types. For example, the percent of lymphocytes can be increased by either an increase in total lymphocytes (**absolute lymphocytosis**) or by a decrease in the number of other cells, particularly neutrophils (**relative lymphocytosis**). In the latter case, the abnormality is not the increase in percent of lymphocytes but the decrease in total granulocytes.

PLATELETS (THROMBOCYTES)

Platelets, occasionally called thrombocytes, are involved in hemostasis. They adhere to tears in the endothelial lining of blood vessels, forming a **platelet plug**.

- Platelets are anucleate discs with a diameter of ~1 to 4 μm. They have pale blue cytoplasm with reddish-purple granules (Figure 1–10).
- They are derived from megakaryocytes in the bone marrow by release of fragments of megakaryocyte cytoplasm.
- The normal platelet number is ~150,000 to 350,000 cells/μL.
- Platelets have different types of granules, designated alpha granules and dense bodies. Platelet granules contain clotting factors, adenosine diphosphate (ADP) and adenosine triphosphate (ATP), calcium, sero-

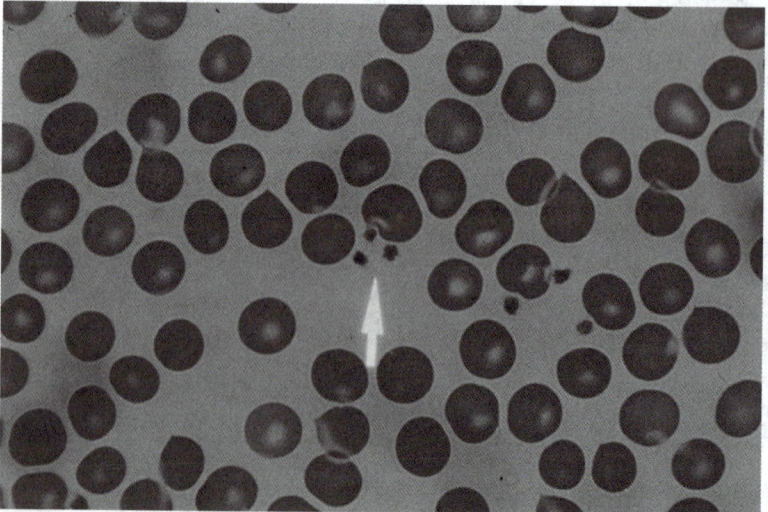

Figure 1–10 Platelets (*arrow*).

tonin, and catecholamines; many of these stimulate platelet aggregation or are important in the coagulation cascade.

- Platelets have a life span of approximately 10 days. Senescent platelets are removed by the spleen.

THE COMPLETE BLOOD COUNT (CBC)

The complete blood count (CBC) produced by automated hematology analyzers provides several results, some of which are more important than others (Table 1–3).

Erythrocytes

The most important values to consider are the **hemoglobin** and the **mean corpuscular volume** (**MCV**). These values, together with the RBC count,

Table 1–3
The Complete Blood Count (CBC)

Component	Reported Units
RBC count	10^6 cells/μL
Hemoglobin	g/dL
Hematocrit	Volumes %
Mean corpuscular volume (MCV)	fL
Mean corpuscular hemoglobin (MCH)	pg
Mean corpuscular hemoglobin concentration (MCHC)	g/dL
Red cell distribution width (RDW)	%
WBC count	10^3 cells/μL
Differential	% and 10^3 cells μL
Neutrophils (segs + bands)	
Lymphocytes	
Monocytes	
Eosinophils	
Basophils	
Platelet count	10^3 cells/μL
Mean platelet volume (MPV)	fL

The most important values of the CBC are listed in bold type.

are directly measured in most hematology instruments; the hematocrit and other parameters are calculated from these values.

The **red cell indices** include the mean corpuscular volume (MCV), the **mean corpuscular hemoglobin** (**MCH**), and the **mean corpuscular hemoglobin concentration** (**MCHC**). The MCV is important in the evaluation of erythrocyte disorders. The MCH and MCHC are generally not of great value.

The **red cell distribution width** (**RDW**) is a mathematical description of the variation in RBC sizes; a high RDW indicates greater variation in RBC size.

Leukocytes

Sophisticated hematology analyzers produce the **total WBC count** and a five-part **WBC differential** (percentages and absolute numbers of each cell type). More attention is paid to the percent of each cell type, but the absolute number is really more relevant than the percent.

Platelets

The most important value to consider is the **total platelet count**. Hematology analyzers also give a **mean platelet volume** (**MPV**), analogous to the MCV. It has been suggested that larger platelets are more effective than smaller platelets; however, the MPV has generally not proven very useful.

Commonly Used versus International Units

The units that are commonly used in the United States for reporting CBC values differ from those used in Europe (Table 1–4). It has been suggested that all laboratories should switch to international units, which are used in many journals; however, most physicians in the United States are more comfortable with the commonly used units, and most laboratories continue to use them. Fortunately, most of the numbers do not really change: a WBC count of $5 \times 10^3/\mu L$ equals 5×10^9 L; a RBC count of $5 \times 10^6/\mu L$ equals $5 \times 10^{12}/L$;

Table 1–4
Reporting CBCs: Common versus International Units

Component	Common Units	International Units
RBC count	10^6 cells/μL	10^{12} cells/L
Hemoglobin	g/dL	g/L
WBC count	10^3 cells/μL	10^9 cells/L
Platelet count	10^3 cells/μL	10^9 cells/L

$1 \times 10^6/\mu L = 1 \times 10^{12}/L$; $1 \times 10^3/\mu L = 1 \times 10^9/L$; 1 g/dL = 10 g/L.

a platelet count of $150 \times 10^3/\mu L$ equals $150 \times 10^9/L$. However, the hemoglobin does change as 15 g/dL equals 150 g/L.

Conditions That Interfere with Hematology Analyzers

There are a variety of conditions that can interfere with hematology analyzers and give spurious results (Table 1–5). A good laboratory should pick up most of these, but, occasionally, there may be difficulties in meas-

Table 1–5
Conditions That May Interfere with Hematology Analyzers

Parameter	Spurious Increase	Spurious Decrease
WBC count	Cryoglobulins Heparin Nucleated erythrocytes Unlysed erythrocytes Platelet clumping	Clotted specimen Leukemia Uremia Some immunosuppressive agents
RBC count	Cryoglobulins Giant platelets High WBC count (>50,000 cells/μL)	Autoagglutinins Clotted specimen Hemolysis (in vitro) Microcytic RBCs
Hemoglobin	Carboxyhemoglobin (>10%) Cryoglobulins Heparin Hyperbilirubinemia Lipemia High WBC count (>50,000 cells/μL)	Clotted specimen Sulfhemoglobin
Platelet count	Cryoglobulins Hemolysis (in vitro) Microcytic RBCs WBC fragments (acute leukemia)	Clotted specimen Giant platelets Heparin Platelet clumping Platelet satellitism
Mean corpuscular volume	Autoagglutination or rouleaux High WBC count (>50,000 cells/μL) Hyperglycemia Reduced RBC deformability	Cryoglobulins Giant platelets Hemolysis (in vitro)

uring and reporting CBC values. Therefore, it is useful to have an idea of the conditions that can interfere with hematology analyzers.

Examination of a Peripheral Blood Smear

Modern automated hematology analyzers usually produce accurate reliable results and, most of the time, provide all the information you need. However, it is sometimes still very useful to examine a blood smear. Getting the most information out of a blood smear requires experience and practice. It also requires a careful, systematic approach.

Three microscope objectives should be used: a low power ($10\times$), a high dry ($40\times$), and an oil immersion (50 or $100\times$). It is important to evaluate all three cell lines (erythrocytes, leukocytes, and platelets) and to not focus solely on an obvious abnormality in one cell line while possibly missing another in a second cell line.

Low-power examination (first $10\times$, then $40\times$ objectives):

- Evaluate the quality of the blood smear.
- Look for rouleaux (stacks of RBCs) or RBC agglutination.
- Estimate the WBC number (decreased, normal, or increased) and get a sense of the different types of WBCs present.
- Look for abnormal WBCs. Examine the end ("feather edge") and sides of the smear, looking for large cells or cells with a very high nucleus-to-cytoplasm ratio.
- Look for clumps of platelets.

Oil immersion (50 or $100\times$ objective):

- Find a place on the smear where RBCs are evenly spread out and have a central pale area. Most RBCs should be single, but occasional groups of two or three RBCs may be present.
- Systematically examine all three cell lines in order: first erythrocytes, then leukocytes, and, finally, platelets.
- Examine the RBCs for size (the normal RBC size is about the same as the nucleus of a mature resting lymphocyte), abnormal shape, and presence of any inclusions or organisms (Table 1–6).
- Examine the WBCs for abnormal or immature cells, any abnormalities in the nucleus or cytoplasm, and any inclusions or organisms (Table 1–7).
- Examine the platelets for number (normal, increased, or decreased), size, appearance, platelet clumping, or platelet satellitism around neutrophils. There should be approximately 7 to 25 platelets in a $100\times$ oil immersion field.

Table 1–6

Blood Cell Morphology: Morphologic Changes in Erythrocytes

Term	Meaning	Conditions or Diseases
Anisocytosis	Increased variation in RBC size; RDW increased	Various disorders
Microcytosis	Decreased RBC size (MCV < 80 fL)	Iron deficiency; thalassemia; occasionally anemia of chronic disease; sideroblastic anemia
Hypochromia	Increased central pallor (> 1/3 to 1/2 the cell diameter)	Iron deficiency
Macrocytosis	Increased RBC size (MCV > 110 fL)	Megaloblastic anemia; liver disease; reticulocytosis; myelodysplastic syndromes; alcoholism
Target cells (codocytes)	Central thick area surrounded by pale ring	Liver disease; hemoglobinopathies (thalassemia, sickle cell anemia)
Schistocytes	Fragmented RBCs	Mechanical trauma: malfunctioning prosthetic heart valve; thrombotic microangiopathy (TTP/HUS); severe burns; joggers; severe shock or acidosis; severe intravascular hemolytic anemia
Sickle cells ("drepano-cytes")	Curved RBCs with pointed ends	Sickle cell anemia and other sickle cell diseases
Burr cells ("echinocytes")	Cells with relatively even spicules around periphery; central pallor preserved	Renal failure; often seen as artifact on blood smears ("crenated cells")
Acanthocytes	Cells with irregular shape and a few long projections; no central pallor	Severe liver disease; abetalipoproteinemia; severe starvation
Spherocytes	Small round cells with no central pallor	Hereditary spherocytosis; immune hemolytic anemia
Bite cells and blister cells	Bite cells: deep rounded notch in side of RBC Blister cells: clear vacuole along one side of RBC	Unstable hemoglobins; hemolytic anemia due to RBC enzyme deficiencies (G6PD deficiency)
Teardrop cells ("dacrocytes")	RBCs shaped like teardrops, with one pointed end	Extramedullary hematopoiesis; myelophthisic anemias (myelofibrosis, space-occupying lesions in bone marrow)

Continued

Table 1–6
Morphologic Changes in Erythrocytes—Continued

Term	Meaning	Conditions or Diseases
Polychromasia	RBCs with bluish color on routine stains	Young RBCs (reticulocytes); often seen in hemolytic anemias or recovery from blood loss
Basophilic stippling	RBCs with fine to coarse bluish speckles	Lead poisoning; thalassemias; any severe stress on the bone marrow
Rouleaux	RBCs in long lines or stacks	Hypergammaglobulinemia; monoclonal gammopathies
Howell-Jolly body	Small round fragment of nuclear material in RBC	Splenectomy; sickle cell anemia; severe thalassemia
Heinz body	Blue dots in RBC; seen on supravital stains such as crystal violet (not seen on routine blood stains)	Unstable hemoglobin; severe oxidant stress

RBC = red blood cells; ROW = red cell distribution width; MCV = mean corpuscular volume;
TTP = thrombotic thrombocytopenic purpura; HUS = hemolytic-uremic syndrome;
G6PD = glucose-6-phosphate dehydrogenase.

Table 1–7
Blood Cell Morphology: Morphologic Changes in Leukocytes

Term	Meaning	Conditions or Diseases
Toxic granulation	Heavy, dark granules in neutrophils	Severe stress; sepsis or other severe infection
"Left shift"	Increased numbers of band neutrophils or other immature granulocytes	Severe stress or infection
Döhle's bodies	Pale blue inclusions in neutrophil cytoplasm	Severe stress or infection

2

Hematopoiesis and the Bone Marrow

Hematopoiesis is the process of making blood cells. The term comes from the Greek *haima* (blood) and *poiein* (to make). For the average adult, the bone marrow produces ~5 × 10^{11} cells per day. Production of blood cells is highly regulated and balanced.

HEMATOPOIESIS OF EMBRYOLOGY

Hematopoiesis begins in the yolk sac during the first month of embryogenesis but gradually shifts to the liver and, to a lesser extent, the spleen. The liver is the primary site of hematopoiesis during the second trimester; however, the bone marrow becomes the primary site of hematopoiesis after the seventh month. After birth, the bone marrow is normally the sole site of hematopoiesis (**intramedullary hematopoiesis**). Hematopoiesis may resume in the liver and spleen after birth in conditions associated with fibrosis of the bone marrow (**extramedullary hematopoiesis**).

POSTNATAL HEMATOPOIESIS

During infancy and childhood, there is active hematopoiesis in the medullary cavity of virtually every bone. With age, the hematopoietically active marrow (**red marrow**) is gradually replaced by inactive marrow (**yellow marrow**), which consists predominantly of adipose tissue. In adults, hematopoiesis is restricted to the proximal long bones and the axial skeleton (skull, vertebral bodies, ribs, sternum, and pelvis). The yellow marrow can resume active hematopoiesis under conditions of chronic hematologic stress (chronic bleeding or hemolytic anemia).

THE BONE MARROW MICROENVIRONMENT

The medullary cavities contain vascular spaces (sinuses), hematopoietic cells, and specialized stromal cells of various types. All the cells form a complex microenvironment, with numerous intricate and interdependent relationships between stromal cells and hematopoietic cells (Figure 2–1).

- **Hematopoietic Cords:** The hematopoietic cords (parenchyma) are the extravascular portions of the bone marrow and the site of blood cell production.
- **Sinuses:** The sinuses (vascular spaces) of the marrow are lined with specialized endothelial cells, which prevent the premature escape of immature cells into the peripheral blood. The basal lamina is incomplete, allowing mature cells to pass through the wall of the sinuses.
- **Stromal Cells:** The stromal cells compose the supportive tissues of the bone marrow. Some of these cells produce hematopoietic growth factors. Examples include:
  - Adventitial (reticular) cells: Modified fibroblasts that produce the reticulin framework of the bone marrow
  - Macrophages: Produce hematopoietic growth factors, store iron for hemoglobin production, and carry out phagocytosis of debris
  - Adipocytes: Store energy in the form of fat

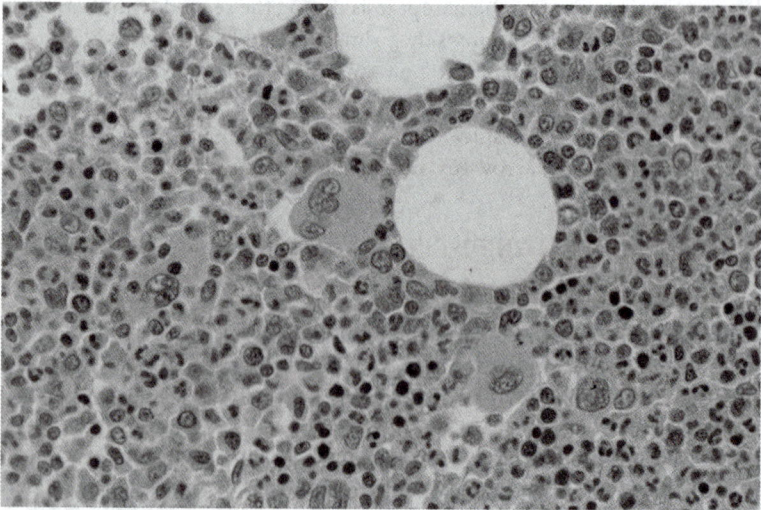

Figure 2–1 Bone marrow biopsy. The clear space is an adipocyte; the large cells with abundant pink cytoplasm and folded nuclei are megakaryocytes; the small cells with opaque dark nuclei are late-stage erythroid precursors; the cells with folded or bent nuclei are granulocytes.

STEM CELL MODEL OF HEMATOPOIESIS

All blood cells derive from **pluripotent hematopoietic stem cells** (Figure 2–2). The progeny of these cells are capable of giving rise to all the different lines of mature blood cells: erythrocytes, granulocytes, monocytes, and megakaryocytes (platelets). The pluripotent stem cells are capable of self-renewal. They are rare in the bone marrow (~1 per 1,000 to 2,000 marrow cells) and cannot be recognized morphologically. The majority of pluripotent stem cells at any given time are in the resting (G_o) phase of the cell cycle.

Expression of **CD34**, a marker of immature cells, is used as a marker for hematopoietic stem cells. However, CD34 is not specific for stem cells, and only a minority of CD34$^+$ cells (perhaps 1%) are actually pluripotent stem cells. Isolation of cells expressing CD34 can be used to enrich a bone marrow suspension for stem cells.

Low numbers of hematopoietic stem cells can be found circulating in the peripheral blood (**peripheral blood progenitor cells**). The number of circulating progenitor cells can be greatly increased by the administration of cytotoxic chemotherapy (the number of cells increases during the recovery phase) or by the administration of high doses of hematopoietic growth factors. Circulating progenitor cells can be harvested by apheresis and have now become the primary source for bone marrow transplants in many circumstances.

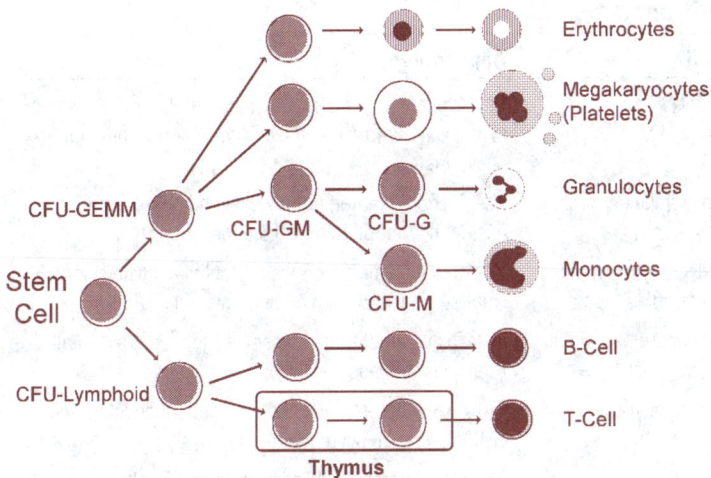

Figure 2–2 Stem cell model of hematopoiesis.

Pluripotent hematopoietic stem cells give rise to **committed progenitor cells**. This is a multistep process in which the cells become sequentially more committed to a specific lineage. These committed progenitor cells are given various names, such as **colony-forming unit** (**CFU**) or **burst-forming unit** (**BFU**). The initial differentiation step is into either **CFU-GEMM** (GEMM = granulocytes, erythrocytes, monocytes/macrophages, and megakaryocytes) or **CFU-L** (L = lymphoid). The CFU-GEMM gives rise to the **CFU-GM** (granulocyte-macrophage), **BFU-E** (erythroid), and **CFU-Mk** (megakaryocyte). Each committed progenitor cell gives rise to a thousand or more mature blood cells.

PRODUCTION OF SPECIFIC CELL LINES

Erythrocyte Production (Erythropoiesis)

The **erythron** is the sum of all erythroid cells, including circulating red blood cells (RBCs) and marrow erythroid precursors. Erythroid precursors are derived from the CFU-GEMM. The earliest progenitor committed exclusively to erythroid lineage is the burst-forming unit–erythroid (**BFU-E**); this is followed by the colony-forming unit–erythroid (**CFU-E**). The earliest recognizable RBC precursor is the **proerythroblast**, which is characterized by fine nuclear chromatin and intensely blue cytoplasm (Table 2–1). The last nucleated RBC precursor is the **orthochro-**

Table 2–1
Erythropoiesis

Cell	Appearance
Proerythroblast	14–19 μm diameter; small amount of deeply basophilic cytoplasm; large round nucleus with fine chromatin, nucleolus
Basophilic erythroblast	12–17 μm diameter; deeply basophilic cytoplasm; nuclear chromatin begins to condense
Polychromatophilic erythroblast	12–15 μm diameter; grayish cytoplasm; nucleus is smaller with increased chromatin condensation
Orthochromatophilic erythoblast	8–12 μm diameter; cytoplasm red to pale gray; small totally opaque nucleus
Reticulocyte	7–10 μm diameter; nucleus extruded; ribonucleic acid visible on reticulocyte stain
Erythrocyte	7–8 μm diameter; reddish cytoplasm; anucleate

matophilic erythroblast, which is characterized by well-hemoglobinized cytoplasm; the nucleus is then lost, producing the **reticulocyte**. Reticulocytes are identified using supravital stains such as new methylene blue; they cannot be definitively identified with routine Wright-Giemsa stains. Reticulocytes contain ribonucleic acid (RNA) for 4 days; normally, the first 3 days are spent in the marrow and fourth in the blood. However, under intense stimulation by erythropoietin, reticulocytes may be released into the blood early where they may contain RNA for 2.0 to 2.5 days (**shift reticulocytes**).

Granulocyte Production (Granulocytopoiesis)

Neutrophils, eosinophils, and basophils go through similar and parallel maturation processes. The earliest two stages of the three pathways are not distinctive (**myeloblast and promyelocyte**); the appearance of specific (secondary) granules at the myelocyte stage differentiates the three cell types (Table 2–2).

Table 2–2
Granulocytopoiesis

Cell	Appearance
Myeloblast	10–20 μm diameter; large round nucleus with fine chromatin, nucleolus; high nucleus to cytoplasm ratio; small amounts of light gray to pale blue cytoplasm without granules
Promyelocyte	Distinguished by presence of large, reddish-purple primary granules; immature nucleus with nucleolus; grayish to dark blue cytoplasm
Myelocyte	Distinguished by presence of secondary granules; cytoplasm begins to turn light yellow-orange; round nucleus with early chromatin condensation; ± nucleolus
Metamyelocyte	Resembles myelocyte, but with indented (kidney bean–shaped) nucleus with increased chromatin condensation
Band neutrophil	Deeply indented (horseshoe-shaped) but not segmented nucleus; mature cytoplasm
Segmented neutrophil	Nucleus segmented into distinct lobes

Neutrophil, eosinophil, and basophil maturation follows parallel pathways; they can be differentiated at the myelocyte stage, when secondary (specific) granules appear.

Megakaryocyte and Platelet (Thrombocyte) Production

Platelets are derived from bone marrow **megakaryocytes**, which are large cells with multilobated nuclei and abundant finely granular light gray-blue cytoplasm. Megakaryocytes become polyploid, with a deoxyribonucleic acid (DNA) content up to 32 to 64n, by a process of **endomitosis** (chromosome replication without cell division). Megakaryocytes have cytoplasmic projections extending through the walls of sinuses into the lumen; fragments of cytoplasm break off into the sinus as platelets.

Monocyte Maturation

Monocytes are derived from the CFU-GEMM. Monocytes circulate through the blood and then enter the tissues to become either phagocytes (macrophages) or professional antigen presenting cells (Langerhans' cells and dendritic reticulum cells).

Lymphocyte Maturation

Lymphocyte maturation begins in the bone marrow; B cells complete initial development in the marrow and then circulate to peripheral lymphoid tissues (lymph node, spleen, and mucosal surfaces) to await antigen exposure and final maturation into plasma cells. T-cell maturation also begins in the bone marrow; T-cell precursors then travel to the thymus (initially the cortex of the thymus, progressing down into the medulla of the thymus), where they complete maturation before being released into the blood to travel to tissues. Differentiation into T helper and T suppressor subsets occurs in the thymus.

HEMATOPOIETIC GROWTH FACTORS

Hematopoietic growth factors are proteins or glycoproteins that regulate the production and differentiation of hematopoietic precursors. They act on specific cell surface receptors on hematopoietic precursor cells and may either stimulate or inhibit cell proliferation and differentiation. A large number of growth factors have been identified, including various **interleukins** (produced by lymphocytes), **colony-stimulating factors** (**CSFs**), and others. The majority are produced within the marrow and act locally. Erythropoietin and thrombopoietin are produced outside the marrow and reach the marrow through the blood. Growth factors may affect multiple cell lines and act at multiple stages; a few are relatively lineage specific (for example, the effects of erythropoietin are primarily limited to erythroid precursors). There are complex interactions between different growth factors in the differentiation of different cell types.

Growth factors may have effects on mature cells, as well as on the proliferation and maturation of hematopoietic precursors. For example, granulocyte colony-stimulating factor (G-CSF) can activate mature neutrophils, and granulocyte-macrophage colony-stimulating factor (GM-CSF) can activate both monocytes and granulocytes. Several growth factors are available for therapeutic use and are widely used in cancer treatment and bone marrow transplantation.

Examples of important growth factors:

- **Stem Cell Factor** (Steel factor, **c-*kit* ligand**): Stem cell factor is critical at the level of pluripotent stem cells. It also has effects on the later maturation stages of several cell lineages.
- **Granulocyte Colony-Stimulating Factor** (**G-CSF**, filgrastim, Neupogen): Stimulates granulocyte differentiation and maturation and stimulates the action of mature neutrophils. Available commercially, G-CSF is widely used in bone marrow transplantation, neutropenia induced by chemotherapy, and other conditions to increase the granulocyte count.
- **Granulocyte-Macrophage Colony-Stimulating Factor** (**GM-CSF**, Leukine): GM-CSF stimulates differentiation and maturation of granulocytes and monocytes, and also the function of mature cells. Commercially available, GM-CSF has clinical uses similar to those of G-CSF.
- **Erythropoietin** (**EPO**; Epogen or Procrit): EPO is produced predominantly in the kidney (a small amount is produced in the liver) in response to renal hypoxia. It is required for erythrocyte production and appears relatively specific for erythroid cells. Recombinant human erythropoietin is widely used for the anemia of chronic renal failure and for some cases of anemia of chronic disease, including acquired immunodeficiency syndrome (AIDS).
- **Thrombopoietin** (**TPO**, Mk-CSF, megakaryocyte growth and differentiation factor): TPO is critical in megakaryocyte growth and differentiation and is produced predominantly in the liver. It has been cloned and synthesized, but appropriate clinical indications are still being sought.

3

Metabolism and Function of Erythrocytes and the Metabolism of Iron

Erythrocytes, or red blood cells, are simple cells that perform an essential function: the exchange of respiratory gasses. These cells are faced with a number of challenges. They lack nuclei, ribosomes, and other cellular organelles and have no protein synthesis or repair capability. They carry oxygen (O_2), a toxic substance, but cannot use it in the process of energy generation like other cells of the body. They must maintain a high internal concentration of potassium and low internal concentration of sodium, against the concentration gradient for both ions, which requires energy. They must be flexible to squeeze through small capillaries and must also withstand the shear stresses of blood flow at high arterial pressures.

ERYTHROCYTE METABOLISM

Erythrocytes generate energy from glucose via the **Embden-Meyerhof pathway** (anaerobic glycolysis), which turns glucose into lactate and generates adenosine triphosphate (ATP) for energy (Figure 3–1). Approximately 10% of glucose is shunted into the **hexose monophosphate shunt**, which generates reducing potential for the cell in the form of NADPH, the reduced form of nicotinamide adenine dinucleotide phosphate (NADP). The first enzyme in the pathway is glucose-6-phosphate dehydrogenase. An additional accessory pathway off the Embden-Meyerhof pathway is the **Rapoport-Luebering shunt**, which generates **2,3-diphosphoglycerate (2,3-DPG)**, which is the primary physiologic regulator of the oxygen affinity of hemoglobin. Another product of the Embden-Meyerhof pathway is reducing equivalents in the form of NADH, the reduced form of nicotinamide adenine dinucleotide (NAD).

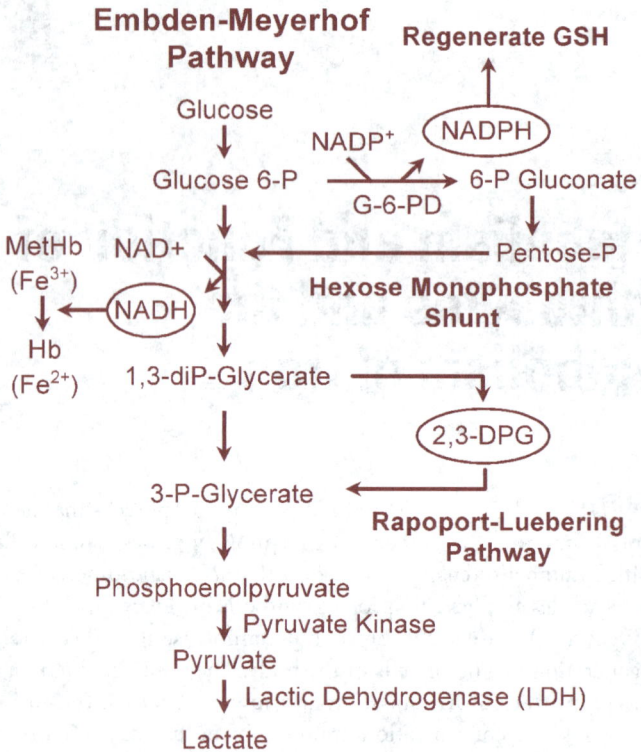

Figure 3–1 Erythrocyte metabolism.

In the normal functional state, the iron atoms in hemoglobin are in the ferrous (Fe^{2+}) state. The iron atom can be oxidized to the ferric (Fe^{3+}) state with the production of **methemoglobin** and **superoxide** (O_2^-). Methemoglobin, in which iron atoms are in the ferric (Fe^{3+}) state, is useless as an oxygen carrier. Unless it is reduced back to hemoglobin (Fe^{2+}), methemoglobin may be oxidized to form **hemichromes** and then aggregates of denatured hemoglobin called **Heinz bodies**. Hemichromes and Heinz bodies can attach to and damage the cell membrane and, if present in sufficient quantity, can cause lysis of the erythrocyte. Methemoglobin is reduced back to hemoglobin by the **methemoglobin reductase** enzyme system, which requires NADH, generated as part of glycolysis.

Superoxide (O_2^-) is a potent oxidizing agent and will damage the erythrocyte unless it is neutralized. Superoxide is converted to hydrogen peroxide (H_2O_2) by the enzyme **superoxide dismutase;** hydrogen peroxide is itself an oxidizing agent and must be neutralized by reduced **glutathione** (GSH). Oxidized glutathione (GSSG) is reduced by the enzyme **glutathione reductase**, which requires NADPH generated by the hexose monophosphate shunt.

If methemoglobin is not reduced to hemoglobin, or GSSG reduced back to glutathione, the result is premature destruction of the erythrocyte (**hemolysis**).

HEME SYNTHESIS AND HEMOGLOBIN

Hemoglobin consists of two components: a protein chain (**globin**) and a **heme** molecule. Heme consists of a protoporphyrin ring into which a ferrous iron atom has been inserted. The initial reaction in the heme synthesis pathway is the combination of glycine and succinyl coenzyme A (CoA) to form δ-aminolevulinic acid (ALA), which is catalyzed by the enzyme aminolevulinic acid synthetase (**ALA synthetase**). Pyridoxal 5'-phosphate (derived from pyridoxine, or vitamin B$_6$), is an essential cofactor in the reaction. The final step in the pathway is insertion of the ferrous iron atom into protoporphyrin IX, catalyzed by the enzyme ferrochelatase (Figure 3–2). Defects in various enzymes in the heme synthesis pathway cause the **porphyrias** (such as porphyria cutanea tarda); other defects in the heme synthesis pathway result in the **sideroblastic anemias**.

The hemoglobin molecule is a tetramer composed of four globin chains, each of which contains a heme ring. The four globins consist of two α-chains and two non-α chains (either β, δ, or γ); in the major adult hemoglobin, Hgb A, the tetramer consists of two α-β dimers. Each globin chain can carry one molecule of oxygen, so a hemoglobin tetramer can carry four oxygen molecules. The four globin chains of hemoglobin can take up different three-dimensional configurations that have different affinities for oxygen. Factors that change the structure of the hemoglobin tetramer favor oxygen loading or unloading. These changes in configuration allow the oxygen affinity of hemoglobin to be regulated as needed and make hemoglobin a much more efficient supplier of oxygen to the tissues.

The affinity of hemoglobin for oxygen can be depicted by the **hemoglobin-oxygen dissociation curve** and is quantified by the **P$_{50}$**, or the partial pressure of oxygen at which hemoglobin is 50% saturated with oxygen. The hemoglobin-oxygen dissociation curve has a sigmoid shape. There is little change in oxygen saturation at the high oxygen tensions present in the alveoli of the lung, but there is a rapid drop in affinity at lower concentrations. This drop in affinity allows the hemoglobin to unload oxygen effi-

Glycine + Succinyl CoA

ALA Synthetase
Pyridoxal 5'-P

δ-aminolevulinic acid (ALA)

Porphobilinogen

Negative
Feedback
Inhibition

Protoporphyrin IX
Fe^{2+}

Ferrochelatase

Heme

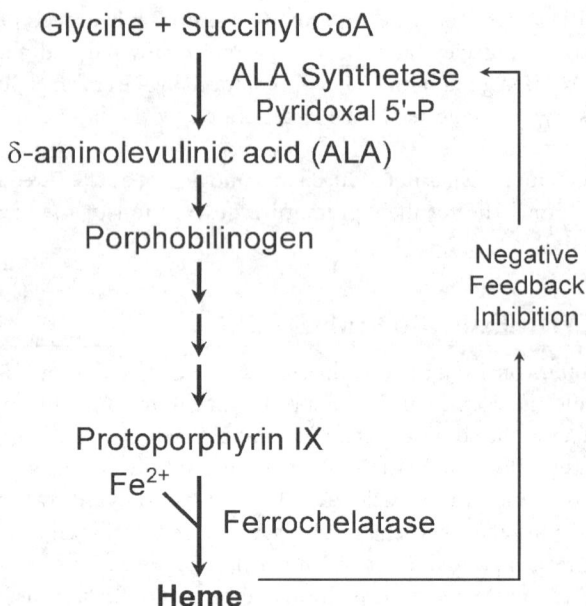

Figure 3–2 Heme synthesis pathway.

ciently at the lower oxygen tension present in tissues. A rightward shift in the hemoglobin-oxygen dissociation curve results in decreased oxygen affinity and increased oxygen delivery to tissues; a leftward shift has the opposite effect. The P_{50} increases as oxygen affinity decreases; thus, a higher P_{50} results in lower oxygen affinity and increased oxygen supply to tissues.

The affinity of hemoglobin for oxygen is regulated by several factors, the most important of which are **2,3-DPG**, **pH**, and **temperature**. The primary regulator of oxygen affinity is the intracellular concentration of 2,3-DPG, which is generated by the Rapoport-Luebering shunt. An increase in the concentration of deoxyhemoglobin leads to an increase in the concentration of 2,3-DPG; this decreases the affinity of hemoglobin for oxygen and increases oxygen delivery to tissues. Acidosis decreases the oxygen affinity of hemoglobin (the **Bohr effect**), as does an increase in temperature. Acidosis and increased temperature are associated with conditions in which the oxygen requirement is likely to be increased, such as exercise, and thus an increase in oxygen supply is physiologically beneficial.

THE ERYTHROCYTE LIFE CYCLE: EXTRAVASCULAR AND INTRAVASCULAR HEMOLYSIS

Heme Breakdown

Erythrocytes are born in the bone marrow. After losing their nucleus, they still contain ribonucleic acid (RNA) and continue to synthesize hemoglobin for 4 days (reticulocytes). Normally, three of these days are spent in the marrow and the fourth in the circulation. After ~120 days, the majority of erythrocytes (90%) are phagocytized and destroyed by the spleen (**extravascular hemolysis**). The hemoglobin is broken down into the heme ring and the globin proteins. The iron is removed from the heme ring and either returns to the bone marrow to be inserted into new erythrocytes or enters the iron storage pool. The tetrapyrrole ring of the heme molecule is opened, with release of one molecule of carbon monoxide and production of biliverdin. The biliverdin is transformed to bilirubin, which circulates to the liver bound to albumin (**unconjugated** or ***indirect*** bilirubin). In hepatocytes, bilirubin is conjugated to glucuronic acid and is excreted into the bile. The majority of bilirubin is excreted in the stool, but a small amount is absorbed in the ileum and returns to the liver via the portal vein; this is the source of **conjugated** (***direct***) **bilirubin** in plasma.

A minority of erythrocytes, normally ~10%, are destroyed in the circulation (**intravascular hemolysis**). The released hemoglobin can meet several different fates:

- The majority of hemoglobin complexes with a plasma protein called **haptoglobin**. The hemoglobin-haptoglobin complex is removed from circulation by hepatocytes. In pathologic intravascular hemolysis, the concentration of haptoglobin in the circulation drops and may become insufficient to tie up all of the released hemoglobin.
- Excess heme can complex with another plasma protein called **hemopexin**. The heme-hemopexin complexes are then cleared from the circulation by the liver.
- Free heme, which exceeds the capacity of the hemopexin system, may bind to albumin, forming **methemalbumin**. This may circulate for several days until the liver can synthesize additional hemopexin.
- In pathologic intravascular hemolysis, excess free hemoglobin may be filtered through the glomeruli of the kidneys into the urine. Some is phagocytized by renal tubular epithelial cells, but if the amount spilled into the urine exceeds the phagocytic capacity of the tubular cells, the excess appears in the urine, causing it to appear pink or red. The renal

tubular cells are eventually shed and may be visualized in the urine with an iron stain such as Prussian blue (**urine hemosiderin**).

IRON ABSORPTION, TRANSPORT, AND STORAGE

Iron is a two-edged sword; it is both necessary for life and potentially life threatening. Iron is required for hemoglobin and is also present in myoglobin, cytochrome oxidase, and several other enzymes.

- Deficiency of iron results in anemia, a weakened immune system, and impaired physical and intellectual performance.
- An excess of iron (**hemochromatosis**) can result in cirrhosis of the liver, hepatocellular carcinoma, cardiac failure and arrhythmias, diabetes mellitus, hypopituitarism, and arthritis.
- **The body iron store is primarily regulated by limiting absorption**. Iron excretion is relatively fixed, and the body has no means of ridding itself of excess iron.

Iron Absorption

The majority of iron absorption occurs in the proximal small intestine, predominantly the duodenum. Iron has to complete two sequential steps in order to be absorbed: (1) absorption into the mucosal cells lining the gastrointestinal (GI) tract and (2) movement across the mucosal cells into the plasma on the other side.

There are two proposed mechanisms that regulate the size of the body iron stores. One mechanism has been termed the **store regulator**, the second has been called the **erythroid regulator**. The store regulator primarily controls absorption of nonheme iron from the GI tract; absorption is inversely proportional to iron stores. The erythroid regulator is driven by erythropoiesis; increased erythropoiesis increases iron absorption. The erythroid regulator can override the store regulator, so someone with chronically increased erythropoiesis (such as a patient with a chronic hemolytic anemia) will continue to absorb iron at a high rate despite increased body iron stores. Transfer across the mucosal cells into the plasma appears to be the primary limiting factor in iron absorption.

Dietary Iron

The average diet in the United States provides approximately 10 to 20 mg of iron per day (approximately 6 to 7 mg per thousand calories). Normally, about 1 or 2 mg of this is absorbed. Iron absorption can be increased approximately fivefold in states of iron deficiency and can be decreased to approximately 0.5 mg per day in conditions of iron excess. Dietary iron is considered to be of two types: **heme iron** and **nonheme iron**. Heme iron is easily and efficiently absorbed into the mucosal cells, and absorption is not affected by other components of the diet. Nonheme iron is absorbed much less efficiently and can be inhibited by many dietary factors.

Heme iron comes from meat. It represents about 10 to 15% of dietary iron in the United States—less in underdeveloped countries, where meat is a smaller part of the diet. The heme ring is absorbed intact into the mucosal lining of cells. After the heme has entered the cytoplasm of the mucosal cell, the iron is split off and enters a common pool with nonheme iron. Heme iron completes the first absorption step easily and efficiently; however, it has the same difficulty completing the second step that nonheme iron does.

The majority of dietary iron is in the nonheme form. This comes from vegetables, grains, and cereals. The majority of nonheme iron is in the ferric (Fe^{3+}) state, which must be converted to the ferrous (Fe^{2+}) state in order to be absorbed. Conversion of ferric to ferrous iron requires gastric acid and is facilitated by ascorbic acid. Absorption is decreased by iron chelators, such as phytates in grains, tannates in tea and coffee, phosphates, calcium, and zinc. Some vegetable proteins also inhibit iron absorption. Egg proteins and cow's milk also inhibit iron absorption, whereas human breast milk increases it. Ascorbic acid facilitates the conversion of ferric to ferrous iron and thus increases absorption; lack of gastric acid (achlorhydria) inhibits absorption because ferric iron cannot be converted to ferrous iron.

Iron Requirement

Iron is lost through cells lining the GI tract and through the superficial squamous cells of the skin as they are shed; a small amount of iron is also lost in sweat. This **obligatory iron loss** averages approximately 1 mg per day in adult men and postmenopausal women and approximately 2 mg per day in menstruating women. Times of increased iron need include the first 18 months of life (particularly in premature infants), the adolescent growth spurt, and pregnancy. A woman loses approximately 750 mg during the average term pregnancy; approximately 225 mg of this is taken by the fetus, mostly during the last trimester.

Iron Transport

Iron is transported in the plasma bound to **transferrin**. Transferrin is a plasma protein synthesized by the liver, which has high affinity for ferric (Fe^{3+}) iron. Each molecule of transferrin can carry up to two iron atoms.

There are specific cell surface receptors for the iron-transferrin complex on almost all cells; the highest concentration is on developing erythroblasts. After iron-transferrin complexes bind to the transferrin receptor, clusters of transferrin receptors with their attached transferrin-iron complexes are phagocytized into the cell. The iron is released from the transferrin, the transferrin receptor returns to the cell surface, and the transferrin protein is released into the circulation so it can transport more iron.

Iron Storage

The major sites of iron stores are macrophages in the bone marrow and reticuloendothelial cells in the liver (Kupffer's cells). There are two storage forms of iron: **ferritin**, which stores iron for immediate use or short-term storage, and **hemosiderin**. Hemosiderin serves as the long-term storage form; iron stored as hemosiderin is not immediately available for use.

Body Iron Content

The average adult man contains a total of about 4 g (4,000 mg) of iron. Approximately half of this is in red cell precursors and erythrocytes (the **erythron**); another quarter is in other tissues; a small amount (3–6 mg) is circulating in the plasma bound to transferrin; and the remainder (approximately 1 g) makes up the body iron storage pool. The average woman, being slightly smaller, has slightly less iron in red cells, other tissues, and plasma; her iron stores are also much smaller. During her childbearing years, the average woman has only 250 to 300 mg of iron stored in ferritin and hemosiderin, and many have almost no iron stores at all.

The Iron Cycle

In the average man, approximately 25 mL of red blood cells, containing about 25 mg of iron, are phagocytized by macrophages of the reticuloendothelial system every day. About 20 mg of this iron is rapidly recycled back into hemoglobin for newly formed erythrocytes. A few milligrams are transferred to tissue cells, and most of the remainder is transferred to body iron stores. Approximately 1 mg is lost from the GI tract, skin, and sweat, and an equal amount is absorbed from the diet. A woman in her childbearing years has to absorb an additional 1 mg daily, on average, to make up for her menstrual blood loss.

Iron Indices

Four values are used to describe body iron status: serum iron, serum transferrin or iron binding capacity, transferrin saturation, and serum ferritin. The transferrin saturation is the serum iron as a percent of the total iron binding capacity. **In the absence of inflammation or illness, the ferritin level is directly proportional to body iron stores and is the most useful single measurement.** A newer test, the serum transferrin receptor level, has become available and may prove useful in the diagnosis of anemia.

4

Introduction to Anemia

A*nemia is defined* clinically as a blood hemoglobin or hematocrit value that is below the appropriate reference range for that patient. The reference range is derived from the hemoglobin or hematocrit values of a group of persons who are presumed to be without hematologic disease (in other words, normal). It is defined as the range of values containing 95% of the population (two standard deviations above and below the median value). The reference range needs to be adjusted for the age and sex of the patient since the hemoglobin and hematocrit vary with age and sex (in adults). It should also be adjusted for other factors, such as altitude (the normal range for Denver, Colorado, would be different from that for Death Valley, California). However, for general purposes, anemia can be defined as **hemoglobin values less than 14 g/dL (140 g/L) in adult men and less than 12 g/dL (120 g/L) in adult women**. Normal hemoglobin values for children vary with age; values begin to reach the adult range after puberty. The lower limit of the normal hemoglobin in the geriatric population is somewhat controversial. Some studies have found that the normal hemoglobin range in the older population is the same as that in younger adults, whereas other studies have found a slightly lower normal limit. It is probably best to use the same normal range as for younger adults in order not to miss correctable (and potentially serious) causes of anemia in older patients, while recognizing that no cause will be found for some cases of mildly decreased hemoglobin in older individuals.

Problems with the Definition of Anemia

This definition of anemia is satisfactory for most purposes but does have some limitations:

- Of the normal population, 2.5% will have hemoglobin values below the defined reference range and will therefore be considered anemic. (Another 2.5% of the normal range will have hemoglobin values above the upper limit of the reference range and will be considered polycythemic.)
- There is overlap between the normal and abnormal populations.
- Anemia, thus defined, ignores physiologic factors; for example, a person with a hemoglobin variant that has a low oxygen affinity will have a low blood hemoglobin because the variant hemoglobin allows him or her to maintain a normal tissue oxygen supply at a lower hemoglobin level, and, therefore, the kidneys produce less erythropoietin. Thus, although the person appears anemic based on the complete blood count (CBC), he or she is physiologically normal.
- The hemoglobin value does not change with acute blood loss; this is not really a problem since the bleeding is usually clinically apparent.
- The blood hemoglobin does not always reflect the true red cell mass. A patient with expanded plasma volume may have a low hemoglobin, although his or her red cell mass may be perfectly normal.
- A final problem, perhaps the most serious, is that the variation in hemoglobin levels in the normal population greatly exceeds the amount of hemoglobin variation over time in a single individual. For example, a hemoglobin level of 14.0 g/dL would be considered normal for an adult man but would be a significant drop for a man whose hemoglobin is usually 16 g/dL (like me!).

However, despite these limitations, the blood hemoglobin and hematocrit assays are clinically useful, are quickly and reliably measured by modern hematology analyzers, and can be easily obtained.

It should always be kept in mind that anemia is not a *diagnosis*; it is a *laboratory abnormality that requires explanation*. Therefore, anemia alone is not a satisfactory explanation; "iron deficiency anemia due to occult blood loss from colon carcinoma" is. After you identify the *presence* of anemia, your job is not finished until you have also identified the *cause* of the anemia.

The following discussion will be limited to conditions in which anemia is the sole or primary hematologic abnormality. Anemia is seen in association with other abnormalities in a wide variety of hematologic conditions, but these will be discussed in other sections.

CLASSIFICATION OF ANEMIA

Anemia can be approached from two perspectives: **morphologic** and **pathophysiologic** (also called **functional** or **kinetic**).

Morphologic Approach

The morphologic approach to anemia begins with review of the CBC, particularly the mean corpuscular volume (MCV), and the peripheral blood smear. The initial distinction is based on the red cell size: anemias are classified as microcytic, normocytic, or macrocytic (Table 4–1). The presence of abnormally shaped erythrocytes (poikilocytes) may suggest a specific disease or cause (see Table 1–6). A problem with the morphologic approach is that the morphologic changes in early anemia may be subtle and easy to miss. A second problem is that one morphologic abnormality may have several possible causes.

Pathophysiologic (Functional or Kinetic) Approach

The pathophysiologic approach[1] is based primarily on the reticulocyte count. Anemias are classified into three broad categories: **hypoproliferative**

Table 4–1
Classification of Anemia Based on Erythrocyte Size

Microcytic	Normocytic	Macrocytic
Iron deficiency	Anemia of chronic disease (most cases)	Megaloblastic anemia: folate or cobalamin deficiency
Thalassemia	Iron deficiency (early)	Hemolytic anemia (reticulocytosis)
Sideroblastic anemia	Anemia of renal disease	Liver disease
Anemia of chronic disease (severe cases)	Combined nutritional deficiency: iron plus folate or cobalamin	Hypothyroidism
	Marrow failure	Myelodysplasia
	Hypothyroidism	

anemias, **maturation defects**, and **hemorrhagic/hemolytic (hyperproliferative) anemias** (Table 4–2):

- In **hypoproliferative anemias**, the marrow fails to appropriately respond to the anemia, but the cells that are produced are usually normal. The reticulocyte count or reticulocyte production index is low; erythrocyte morphology is unremarkable.

Table 4–2
Pathophysiologic Classification of Anemia

Hypoproliferative	Maturation Defects: Cytoplasm	Maturation Defects: Nuclear	Hyperproliferative (Hemorrhagic/ Hemolytic)
Iron deficiency	Severe iron deficiency	Megaloblastic anemia: • Cobalamin (vitamin B_{12}) deficiency • Folic acid deficiency	Acute blood loss
Anemia of chronic disease (anemia of chronic inflammation)	Thalassemia	Intrinsic marrow disease: • Myelodysplasia	Acute hemolysis: • Intravascular • Extravascular
Decreased erythropoietin: • Chronic renal disease • Endocrine disorders	Sideroblastic anemia		Chronic hemolysis: • Environmental disorders • Membrane defects • Metabolic defects • Hemoglobinopathies • Paroxysmal nocturnal hemoglobinuria (PNH)
Marrow damage: • Stem cell damage • Structural damage • Autoimmune (Table 4–3)			

Table 4–3
Marrow Damage Anemias

Stem Cell Damage	Structural Damage	Autoimmune or Unknown
• Chemotherapy	• Radiation	• Infections: hepatitis, Epstein-Barr virus, HIV
• Drugs: antibiotics, antidepressants	• Metastatic malignancies	• Rheumatic disorders: systemic lupus erythematosus (SLE)
• Chemicals: solvents, heavy metals	• Myelofibrosis	• Aplastic anemia/ pure red cell aplasia
• Infections: bacterial or viral	• Granulomatous diseases: tuberculosis, fungal infections	• Graft-versus-host disease
• Aplastic anemia	• Storage diseases: Gaucher's disease	• Congenital: Blackfan-Diamond

Adapted from Hillman RS, Finch CA. Red cell manual. 7th ed. Philadelphia: FA Davis; 1996.

- In **maturation defect** anemias, the bone marrow is attempting to respond to the anemia, but the cells produced are unable to enter the circulation and most die within the bone marrow (ineffective erythropoiesis). The reticulocyte count is low, and, in contrast to the hypoproliferative anemias, erythrocyte morphology is abnormal. The maturation defect anemias are subclassified into **cytoplasmic maturation defects**, which are generally associated with microcytic erythrocytes, and **nuclear maturation defects**, which are associated with macrocytic erythrocytes.
- In **hemorrhagic/hemolytic (hyperproliferative) anemias,** there is increased destruction or loss of erythrocytes. The bone marrow is attempting to respond to the anemia and is producing mature erythrocytes but is unable to fully compensate for the increased red cell loss. The reticulocyte production index is high (>3) and the MCV is frequently high since reticulocytes are larger than normal mature erythrocytes.

RETICULOCYTE COUNT, CORRECTED RETICULOCYTE COUNT, AND THE RETICULOCYTE PRODUCTION INDEX (RPI)

Reticulocyte Count: The **reticulocyte count** is the proportion (percent) of young erythrocytes containing ribonucleic acid (RNA), which can be visually identified as reticulin using a special stain such as new methylene blue. Under normal conditions, approximately 1% of red blood cells (RBCs) are turned over each day; an erythrocyte contains RNA for approximately one day after leaving the marrow, so the normal reticulocyte count is approximately 1%. The reticulocyte count increases if RBC production by the marrow increases, so an increased reticulocyte count is the primary indicator of increased RBC production. However, in order to be useful in an anemic patient, the reticulocyte count must be corrected to take into account both the anemia and the possibility of premature release of reticulocytes from the marrow under the stimulus of increased erythropoietin.

Corrected Reticulocyte Count

Since the reticulocyte count represents a ratio (number of reticulocytes divided by the total number of erythrocytes), a decrease in the total RBC count may result in an increase in the reticulocyte count even if reticulocyte production by the marrow is not increased. In order to correct for this, the reticulocyte count is multiplied by the patient's hematocrit divided by a normal hematocrit (45%):

Corrected reticulocyte count = reticulocyte count × (patient hematocrit ÷ 45)

Reticulocyte Production Index (RPI): Under severe erythropoietin stimulus, reticulocytes may be released from the bone marrow prematurely and must finish their maturation in the peripheral blood (**shift reticulocytes**). Since these prematurely released cells exist as reticulocytes for more than 1 day, they are, in effect, "counted" more than once in the reticulocyte count (remember: the normal reticulocyte count presumes that the cells exist as reticulocytes for only 1 day, rather than 2 or more days). In order to correct for these shift reticulocytes, the corrected reticulocyte count has to be divided by a correction factor, giving the RPI. The correction factor varies depending on the severity of the anemia (Table 4–4):

Table 4–4
Reticulocyte Production Index Correction Factors

Hematocrit	Correction Factor
40	1.0
35	1.5
25	2.0
15	2.5

$$RPI = \text{corrected reticulocyte count} \div \text{correction factor}$$

The RPI can be used to indicate whether the marrow is successfully responding to the anemia:

RPI > 3: Good marrow response (hyperproliferative)
RPI < 2: Inadequate response (hypoproliferative)
RPI > 2 but < 3: Appropriate for mild anemia (hemoglobin >10–11 g/dL) but borderline for more severe anemia

A healthy marrow with adequate nutrition (iron, vitamin B_{12}, and folate) should be able to increase RBC production four- to fivefold (RPI = 4 to 5). Under prolonged stress (for example, a chronic hemolytic anemia such as sickle cell anemia), the marrow can increase RBC production seven- to eightfold.

⇨ It may take a few days for the bone marrow to begin to respond to erythrocyte destruction or loss. Therefore, the RPI may be low during the first few days after blood loss or during the first few days of hemolysis.

Example: A patient is found to have a hematocrit of 15% and reticulocyte count of 10%. Is this an appropriate reticulocyte response for this degree of anemia?

First, calculate the corrected reticulocyte count:

Corrected reticulocyte count = 10 $\times$ (15 $\div$ 45) = 3.3%
3.3% is increased, but is it increased enough for the degree of anemia?

Second, calculate the RPI:

RPI = 3.3 $\div$ 2.5 = 1.3
An RPI of 1.3 is too low for this severe degree of anemia and indicates that the marrow is not appropriately responding to the anemia. This would be consistent with a hypoproliferative anemia.

⇨ I always calculate the corrected reticulocyte count but don't bother to calculate the RPI unless it appears that the RPI will be borderline.

An alternative to calculating the RPI is to determine the **absolute reticulocyte count**, which can be done by many modern hematology analyzers. A value >100 $\times$ 10^9 cells/L indicates that the marrow is responding to the anemia with increased erythrocyte production.

SYMPTOMS AND SIGNS OF ANEMIA

Common symptoms of anemia include **decreased work capacity**, **fatigue**, **weakness**, **dizziness**, **palpitations**, and **dyspnea on exertion**. The severity of symptoms may vary widely depending on the degree of anemia, the time period over which anemia developed, the age of the patient, and other medical conditions that are present. If the anemia developed gradually (months or years), compensatory mechanisms such as an expanded plasma volume and increased 2, 3-diphosphoglycerate (2,3-DPG) have time to take effect. Consequently, the patient may not experience any symptoms with a hemoglobin level down to 8 g/dL, or even lower. If the anemia developed more rapidly, the patient may note symptoms with a hemoglobin level as high as 10 g/dL. Children may tolerate remarkably low hemoglobin levels with few symptoms, whereas older patients with cardiovascular or pulmonary disease tolerate even mild anemia poorly. Angina pectoris may be the initial symptom of anemia in patients with coronary atherosclerosis.

Physical signs of anemia include **pallor**, **tachycardia**, **increased cardiac impulse** on palpation, **systolic "flow" murmur** heard at the apex and along the left sternal border, and a **widened pulse pressure** (increased systolic blood pressure with a decreased diastolic blood pressure). Pallor is best noted in the conjunctiva, mucous membranes, palmar creases, and nail beds, especially in people with darkly pigmented skin.

GENERAL APPROACH TO A PATIENT WITH ANEMIA

Clinical History

Key questions to include in the medical history are listed in Table 4–5.

Physical Examination

Specific items in the physical examination worthy of particular attention in the anemic patient are listed in Table 4–6.

Laboratory Tests

Important laboratory tests include a CBC with erythrocyte indices, white cell count and leukocyte differential, and platelet count. Examination of a well-made peripheral blood smear is critical and may be diagnostic. Important chemistries include serum creatinine, calcium, liver profile including total and direct bilirubin, lactic dehydrogenase, total protein, and albumin. A reticulocyte count (corrected for anemia) and RPI should be performed.

After the initial laboratory studies have been performed, a selection of additional tests should be performed based on the clinical situation and the results of initial studies. These additional tests could include iron indices (serum ferritin or serum iron/transferrin/saturation), folic acid and cobal-

Table 4–5
Clinical History: Important Questions

Question	Significance
Onset of symptoms: insidious or abrupt	Nutritional deficiency likely to be insidious in onset; hemolysis more likely to be abrupt
Duration of symptoms	Nutritional deficiency is likely to be of longer duration; hemolysis is more likely to be of recent onset
Previous CBC? When and what circumstances?	A previous normal CBC helps exclude an inherited disorder
Previous diagnosis of anemia? When and what circumstances?	Possible recurrence of previous disease
Iron, folate, or B_{12} treatment? When and what circumstances?	Possible recurrence of previous disease
Family history of anemia	Possible inherited hemoglobinopathy, thalassemia, membrane defect, or enzyme deficiency
Change in bowel habits? Black or tarry stools? Hematochezia?	Iron loss due to peptic ulcer disease, colon carcinoma, or other GI tract malignancy; malabsorption in folate or B_{12} deficiency
Diet: meats, dairy products, fresh fruits and vegetables	Does the patient have adequate intake of iron (meat), folic acid (fresh fruits and vegetables), and B_{12} (meat, dairy products)?
Medications	Interference with folate metabolism (sulfa drugs, trimethoprim, antiepileptic medications); oxidant drugs causing hemolysis in enzyme deficiency; blood loss from gastritis or peptic ulcer due to nonsteroidal anti-inflammatory drugs
Past medical history	Anemia of chronic disease due to inflammatory diseases or malignancy; decreased erythropoietin production in renal disease
Alcohol consumption	Alcohol interferes with folate metabolism; liver disease
Menstrual history (women)	Iron loss in menorrhagia
Reproductive history (women)	Iron loss in pregnancy
Occupational history and hobbies	Exposure to chemicals that are toxic to bone marrow (organic solvents, hydrocarbons)
Jaundice or dark urine	Hyperbilirubinemia could indicate hemolysis or ineffective erythropoiesis
Weight loss	Common with malignancies; also occurs in megaloblastic anemia

Continued

Table 4–5
Clinical History: Important Questions—Continued

Question	Significance
Fevers, night sweats	Common in malignancies; could indicate chronic infection
Abdominal discomfort or fullness	Splenomegaly occurs with lymphoma, chronic liver disease, myeloproliferative disorders
Sores in mouth or sore tongue	Common in megaloblastic anemia; may also occur in iron deficiency
Paresthesias, clumsiness, weakness	Neurologic disease due to B_{12} deficiency

amin (vitamin B_{12}) levels, hemoglobin electrophoresis, and direct antiglobulin (Coombs') test, among others. The most efficient and cost-effective approach is to establish a differential diagnosis of the most likely causes, perform selected tests to confirm or exclude the most probable causes, choose additional tests, if necessary, based on the results of the first round of tests, and so on, until you have a diagnosis. The common practice of

Table 4–6
Physical Examination of Anemic Patients

System	Significance
General appearance	Jaundice due to hemolysis or megaloblastic anemia; cachexia; tremor or myxedema due to thyroid disease; "spider" angiomata in liver disease; "spoon nails" in iron deficiency
Eye examination	Scleral icterus due to hemolysis; retinal hemorrhages in iron deficiency and other anemias
Head and neck	Glossitis or angular stomatitis in iron deficiency or megaloblastic anemias
Cardiac	Murmurs due to bacterial vegetations in endocarditis; flow murmur in anemia
Abdomen	Splenomegaly in chronic hemolytic anemias; hepatosplenomegaly in lymphoma or myeloproliferative disorder; mass due to intra-abdominal malignancy
Lymphatic system	Lymphadenopathy in lymphoma
Nervous system	Peripheral neuropathy, cerebellar or cortical dysfunction due to cobalamin deficiency

ordering a "shotgun" battery of tests to cover every possible cause (ferritin, iron/transferrin/iron saturation, folate and B_{12} levels, hemoglobin electrophoresis, and reticulocyte level) is often a considerable waste of money and indicates a lack of thought on the part of the ordering physician.

A general approach to the laboratory diagnosis of the anemic patient will be given, based largely on erythrocyte size (MCV). Naturally, the approach for each individual case will be modified by the history, physical examination, and other clinical and laboratory information for that specific patient.

Evaluation of a Microcytic Anemia (MCV < 80 fL)

The key initial steps in the evaluation of a microcytic anemia are **iron indices** and **examination of a blood smear**. The most common cause of microcytic anemia is iron deficiency. If the iron indices confirm the presence of an iron deficiency, the next step is to discover the cause (blood loss, insufficient dietary iron) and begin replacement therapy. If the iron studies do not suggest iron deficiency, the next step is to order a hemoglobin electrophoresis to diagnose β-thalassemia (increased hemoglobin A_2) or a hemoglobinopathy. α-Thalassemia is usually diagnosed largely by exclusion—a microcytic anemia in the absence of iron deficiency or increased hemoglobin A_2 is most likely α-thalassemia. Consider the ethnic origin and family history of the patient. A blood smear could be done to check for target cells and basophilic stippling. Complete blood counts and blood smears from relatives might be helpful in this circumstance. Consider the possibility of a chronic inflammatory process that might be causing anemia of chronic disease. If none of these appear to be responsible for the anemia, a bone marrow examination with an iron stain to look for ringed sideroblasts might be required.

Evaluation of a Macrocytic Anemia (MCV > 100 fL)

The most important initial step in the evaluation of an anemia with an increased MCV is to differentiate **megaloblastic anemia** from **macrocytic, non-megaloblastic anemia**. Examine a blood smear for hypersegmented neutrophils and oval macrocytes, which would suggest a megaloblastic anemia. The MCV can also prove helpful; the MCV in megaloblastic anemia is often ≥120 fL, whereas in non-megaloblastic anemias, it is usually ≤115 fL. The first laboratory studies should be **serum cobalamin, serum folate,** and **red cell folate** levels. If one of these is abnormal, the cause must be determined and therapy started (see the section on megaloblastic anemias in Chapter 5). If these are all normal, a reticulocyte count and RPI should be done to check for a hemorrhagic or hemolytic process. A careful examination of the blood smear may also be helpful; for example, the presence of polychromasia would indicate reticulocytosis, and the presence of target cells would suggest liver disease. If reticulocytosis is confirmed, the underlying hemolytic or hemorrhagic process should be determined. Tests that might be helpful in this circumstance include a direct antiglobulin (Coombs') test, a hemoglobin electrophoresis, and a screen for glucose-6-phosphate dehydrogenase (G6PD) deficiency.

Evaluation of a Normocytic Anemia (MCV 80–100 fL)

The first step in the evaluation of a normocytic anemia is to assess the clinical history. Does the patient have some process that would cause an anemia of chronic disease? Does the patient have renal insufficiency, thyroid disease, or another endocrine disease? Check iron studies and folate/vitamin B_{12} levels to look for early iron deficiency or combined nutritional deficiency. If the reticulocyte count is increased, follow with hemoglobin electrophoresis to look for a hemoglobinopathy, a screen for G6PD deficiency, and, possibly, a direct antiglobulin test. If the reticulocyte count is low, consider anemia of chronic disease, chronic renal insufficiency, thyroid disease, or marrow damage. If the cause is not apparent, a bone marrow aspirate and biopsy should be done.

Anemia with Increased Reticulocyte Production Index

Anemia in the presence of increased reticulocyte production suggests blood loss (hemorrhage) or increased erythrocyte destruction (hemolysis). Anemia due to acute or recent hemorrhage will usually be apparent on clinical history and physical examination. Hemolytic anemias will usually fall into one of the following general groups:

- Obvious exposure to infectious, chemical, or physical agents
- Positive direct antiglobulin (Coombs') test (immune hemolytic anemia)
- Spherocytic anemia, but with a negative antiglobulin test (most likely hereditary spherocytosis)
- Hemolytic anemia with specific morphologic abnormalities on blood smear (sickle cells, elliptocytes, schistocytes)
- Miscellaneous conditions including hemoglobinopathies, thalassemias, enzyme defects, metabolic abnormalities, and paroxysmal nocturnal hemoglobinuria

The diagnostic approach is to initially confirm or exclude hemorrhage and then attempt to place the patient into one of the above categories of hemolytic anemia. Review the clinical history for evidence of blood loss.

Does the patient have a family history of anemia or ethnic background that may be predisposed to an inherited hemolytic anemia (sickle cell anemia in African Americans; thalassemias in people from Africa, the Mediterranean basin, and the Far East). Some medications may cause oxidative stress in someone with an inherited enzyme deficiency. A morphologic abnormality in the blood smear may suggest a specific cause (sickled cells, spherocytes, "bite" or "blister" cells). If there is no obvious explanation, a direct antiglobulin (direct Coombs') test and antibody screen (indirect Coombs') test should be performed. Consider a sickle solubility test or hemoglobin electrophoresis if there is a possibility of an inherited hemoglobinopathy.

Reference

1.   Hillman RS, Finch CA. Red cell manual. 7th ed. Philadelphia: FA Davis; 1996.

5

Iron Deficiency Anemia, Anemia of Chronic Disease, Sideroblastic Anemias, and Megaloblastic Anemias

Iron deficiency anemia and **anemia of chronic disease** (sometimes called **anemia of inflammation**) are discussed in this section because both are characterized by decreased serum iron, both can be microcytic, and differentiating between them can occasionally be difficult. The **sideroblastic anemias** are typically microcytic and hypochromic and thus enter into the differential diagnosis of iron deficiency. **Megaloblastic anemias** are due to deficiencies in cobalamin (vitamin B_{12}) or folic acid. In contrast to iron deficiency anemia and anemia of chronic disease, the megaloblastic anemias are characterized by an increase in erythrocyte size (macrocytosis).

IRON DEFICIENCY

⇨ Iron deficiency is the most common cause of anemia in the United States, and one of the most common conditions seen in general medical practice.

One study of the prevalence of iron deficiency in the United States found that a low serum iron was present in about 14% of adult women and 5% of adult men, and anemia was present in approximately 4 to 6% of women and 3% of men.[1] A study of high socioeconomic status girls found that 24% had an absence of storage iron and 42% had suboptimal iron stores.[2] It has been estimated that 10 to 30% of the world's population is iron deficient.

Note that **iron deficiency** is not synonymous with **iron deficiency anemia**. Many people have suboptimal or absent storage iron and are therefore iron deficient, but are not anemic. However, even in the absence of anemia, iron deficiency may have deleterious consequences, such as impaired growth and psychomotor development in children and impaired work capacity and mental function in adults. Anemia is a late manifestation of iron deficiency; marrow iron stores will be totally consumed before the hemoglobin begins to decrease. A decrease in the mean corpuscular volume (MCV) occurs even later. The blood hemoglobin drops before the MCV decreases, although microcytic erythrocytes may be present on the blood smear before the MCV falls below the normal range.

⇨ The absence of microcytosis does **not** exclude anemia due to iron deficiency!

Causes of Iron Deficiency

Iron absorption and the iron cycle were discussed in Chapter 3. Iron deficiency is due to insufficient iron intake, malabsorption of iron despite adequate intake, or iron loss in excess of iron absorption (Table 5–1). Inadequate dietary iron may be the cause of iron deficiency during times of greatest iron need, including infancy and early childhood, the adolescent growth spurt, and pregnancy. Inadequate dietary iron may lead to deficient storage iron in menstruating women, particularly those with heavy menstrual bleeding. Multiparous women are at high risk for iron deficiency: each pregnancy results in the loss of ~500 to 700 mg of iron, and an additional 450 mg is needed to expand the blood volume. On average, 2.5 mg of iron must be absorbed daily over the course of the pregnancy. Iron deficiency due to inadequate diet is particularly common in economically deprived areas in the United States and in developing countries worldwide.

- The most common cause of iron deficiency in adult men, and the second most common cause in adult women, is gastrointestinal (GI) bleeding. In adult men and postmenopausal women, iron deficiency should be presumed to be due to occult GI bleeding until proven otherwise. Failure to identify the cause of iron deficiency may allow an early treatable GI carcinoma to progress to a metastatic incurable one.
- The average blood loss per menstrual period is 35 mL, with a range of about 20 to 80 mL. A woman's impression of whether her menstrual periods are normal or heavy is very unreliable. Indications of excessive menstrual flow include inability to control bleeding with tampons alone; use of more than 12 pads per period, or more than 4 per day; passage of clots, especially if more than 2 cm in diameter; and duration of period exceeding 7 days.

Table 5–1
Causes of Iron Deficiency

Decreased Iron Intake
  Inadequate dietary iron

Decreased Iron Absorption
  Achlorhydria
  Gastric resection
  Celiac disease (gluten-sensitive enteropathy)
  Pica

Increased Iron Loss
  Gastrointestinal blood loss:
  • Neoplasms
  • Erosive gastritis due to nonsteroidal anti-inflammatory drugs
  • Peptic ulcer disease
  • Erosive esophagitis
  • Inflammatory bowel disease (Crohn's disease, ulcerative colitis)
  • Diverticular disease
  • Hemorrhoids
  • Meckel's diverticulum
  • Infections: hookworm, schistosomiasis
  Excessive menstrual blood flow
  Frequent blood donation
  Hemoglobinuria: paroxysmal nocturnal hemoglobinuria, malfunctioning artificial
      heart valve
  Hereditary hemorrhagic telangiectasia (Rendu-Osler-Weber syndrome)
  Hemodialysis
  Idiopathic pulmonary hemosiderosis
  Runner's anemia

Increased Iron Requirements
  Infancy
  Pregnancy
  Lactation

Adapted from Lee GR. Iron deficiency and iron deficiency anemia. In: Lee RG, Foerster J, Lukens J, et al, editors. Wintrobe's clinical hematology. 10th ed. Baltimore: Williams & Wilkins; 1999. p. 979–1010.

• Iron deficiency is common in infancy, especially in premature or low birth weight infants and in infants of multiple gestation.

Malabsorption of iron does occur but is uncommon. Loss of gastric acid production (achlorhydria) results in impaired absorption of ferric (Fe^{3+}) iron, but heme iron and ferrous iron are absorbed adequately. Iron deficiency and anemia are commonly seen after gastric surgery, including partial or total gastrectomy or vagotomy with gastroenterostomy. This is particularly common if the duodenum is surgically bypassed since the majority of iron absorption normally occurs in the duodenum. Iron deficiency can also be seen with malabsorption syndromes such as tropical sprue and celiac sprue (gluten-sensitive enteropathy).

Clinical Features

In general, the symptoms of iron deficiency anemia are those of anemia of any cause: fatigue, dyspnea on exertion, and dizziness. There are a few signs and symptoms that are relatively unique to iron deficiency anemia, including "spoon" fingernails, glossitis (atrophy of the papillae of the tongue, with burning or soreness), ulcerations or fissures at the corners of the mouth (angular stomatitis), and dysphagia due to esophageal webs or strictures. The combination of dysphagia, angular stomatitis, and hypochromic anemia has been called the **Plummer-Vinson** or **Paterson-Kelly** syndrome. These extreme signs of iron deficiency are now uncommon.

Pica is the habitual consumption of unusual substances. It can be both a manifestation and a cause of iron deficiency. Specific examples of pica include *geophagia* (consumption of earth or clay), *pagophagia* (ice), and *amylophagia* (laundry starch). Food pica is the compulsive eating of one kind of food, often crunchy foods such as celery, potato chips, carrots, or raw potatoes. In most cases, pica is a symptom of iron deficiency and disappears when the iron deficiency is relieved. However, pica can also be a cultural phenomenon and, in these instances, can induce iron deficiency. Laundry starch and clay can impair iron absorption. Laundry starch is also extremely poor in iron, so if starch constitutes a significant proportion of caloric intake, the diet is likely to be deficient in iron.

Laboratories

The anemia of iron deficiency is classically microcytic (decreased MCV) and hypochromic (increased central pallor in red blood cells [RBCs]) (Figure 5–1). However, in early iron deficiency, the MCV will be normal. Occasional microcytic and hypochromic RBCs may be present on the blood smear, if carefully looked for.

- In iron deficiency, bone marrow iron stores will be completely depleted before the hemoglobin begins to drop. The hemoglobin begins to fall before the MCV begins to decrease. The reverse occurs in megaloblastic anemia: the MCV begins to increase before the hemoglobin begins to fall.
- The MCV may be normal in combined nutritional deficiency (deficiency of iron plus either cobalamin or folic acid). However, on the blood smear you should see hypersegmented neutrophils and possibly a dimorphic smear with both microcytes and macrocytes.

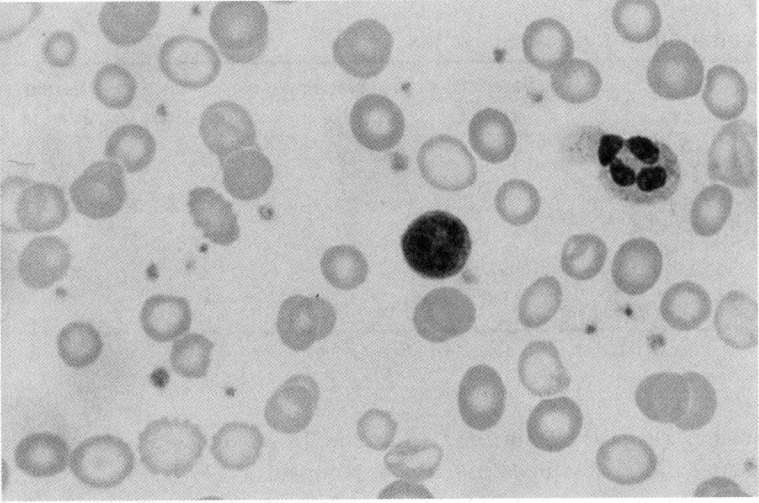

Figure 5–1 Iron deficiency. Note the decreased size of erythrocytes (compared with normal size that approximates a lymphocyte nucleus) and the widened central pallor.

Iron Indices

The critical laboratory values in the evaluation of iron status are serum iron concentration, serum transferrin or total iron-binding capacity (TIBC), iron saturation, and serum ferritin level. The serum iron decreases in iron deficiency and the anemia of chronic disease. The transferrin (TIBC) tends to increase in iron deficiency and decrease in anemia of chronic disease. Iron saturation decreases in both iron deficiency and the anemia of chronic disease but tends to decrease more in iron deficiency (usually <10% in iron deficiency and >10% in anemia of chronic disease). Serum ferritin is decreased in iron deficiency but is usually normal or increased in anemia of chronic disease (Table 5–2).

The single most efficient test to assess body iron stores is the serum ferritin. In the absence of a complicating factor, the serum ferritin level is directly proportional to body iron stores. However, ferritin acts as an acute phase reactant (increases with inflammation), so the serum ferritin can be difficult to interpret in the presence of acute or chronic inflammation. A low serum ferritin (less than 15 ng/mL or 15 μg/L) is strong evidence for iron deficiency, with or without inflammation. A serum ferritin that is increased or high in the normal range (greater than ~150–200 ng/mL or 150–200 μg/L) is strong evidence against iron deficiency, whether or not there is inflammation. A serum ferritin between these two levels, in the presence of an inflammatory condition, requires additional laboratory tests

Table 5–2
Iron Indices in Disease States

Disease	Serum Iron	Transferrin (TIBC)	Saturation	Serum Ferritin
Iron deficiency	↓	↑	↓↓	↓
Anemia of chronic disease	↓	↓	↓	↑
Combined	↓	↓	↓	↓ or normal
sideroblastic anemia	↑	Normal or ↑	↑	↑

↓ = decreased;; ↓↓ = severely decreased; ↑ = increased.

such as serum iron/TIBC/iron saturation. In rare cases, a bone marrow examination and stain for iron may be required.

Differential Diagnosis of Iron Deficiency

The primary differential diagnosis of iron deficiency primarily includes the other forms of microcytic anemia: thalassemia, anemia of chronic disease (severe cases), sideroblastic anemias, and some hemoglobinopathies. Lead poisoning is also a consideration in children living in older homes that might have lead paint.

Diagnostic Evaluation

Since iron deficiency is by far the most common cause of microcytic anemia in the United States, the initial focus of evaluation should be to confirm or exclude iron deficiency. The history should emphasize possible reasons for such a deficiency, such as excessive menstrual blood loss in premenopausal women or GI blood loss. On physical examination, look for glossitis, angular stomatitis, and spoon fingernails. Examination of the stool for occult blood should be performed.

Laboratory Evaluation

The first step in laboratory evaluation should include serum ferritin or serum iron, TIBC, and iron saturation. If the iron studies indicate iron deficiency, the next step is to determine the cause. If the iron studies are not consistent with iron deficiency in a patient with a microcytic anemia, the next step is hemoglobin electrophoresis to diagnose β-thalassemia or a hemoglobinopathy. A serum lead level should be done in children when iron deficiency is excluded. A bone marrow examination should seldom be necessary to diagnose iron deficiency, but if the iron studies are indeterminate, a bone marrow examination should be performed and stained for iron. Marrow deficient in iron usually shows mild erythroid hyperplasia; late erythroid precursors appear ragged, poorly hemoglobinized (grayish), and small. Storage iron must be completely absent; the presence of *any* stainable iron in the bone marrow *excludes* the diagnosis of iron deficiency.

⇨ Note for pathologists and others who look at bone marrows: Decalcification of a bone marrow biopsy also removes iron, so the absence of stainable iron on a Prussian blue (iron) stain on a decalcified biopsy does not conclusively prove that iron is absent. To be sure that iron is completely absent, an iron stain must be done on an aspirate smear or aspirate clot section that has not been decalcified.

⇨ An elevated *zinc erythrocyte protoporphyrin* level (**ZEP**, also called *free erythrocyte protoporphyrin*) has been recommended as a screening test for iron deficiency since it is very sensitive and can be easily and inexpensively measured. However, it is also elevated in anemia of chronic disease, lead poisoning, and other conditions. It is therefore useful in screening *populations* for iron deficiency (since iron deficiency is the most common cause of elevated ZEP in the general population) but is less useful in diagnosis of the individual patient.

Treatment of Iron Deficiency

Any primary cause of iron deficiency (excessive menstrual blood loss, gastrointestinal neoplasm) should be treated appropriately. The most effective and inexpensive way to replace iron stores is iron supplements given orally. In general, oral supplementation is the treatment of choice unless there is a significant GI condition that precludes absorption of iron. Parenteral iron administration can be done but is much more expensive than oral therapy and has potential side effects.

Oral Iron Replacement

Ferrous (Fe^{2+}) iron salts are the least expensive way to give iron orally. Various preparations are available (Table 5–3). The aim is to give approximately **200 mg of elemental iron daily** for adults. Side effects of oral iron therapy include heartburn, nausea, abdominal cramps, and diarrhea or constipation. The patient should be warned that the stool will become black. The incidence of side effects is decreased when the iron is taken with food, but this decreases iron absorption. Tolerance to oral therapy is improved by

Table 5–3
Oral Iron Preparations

Preparation	Size	Iron Content	Adult Daily Dose
Ferrous sulfate:			
• Tablets	300 mg	60 mg	3 tablets
• Syrup and elixirs	40 mg/mL	8 mg/mL	25 mL
• Pediatric drops	125 mg/mL	25 mg/mL	—
Ferrous gluconate	300 mg	37 mg	5 tablets
Ferrous fumarate	200 mg	67 mg	3 tablets
	300 mg	100 mg	2 tablets

Adapted from Lee GR. Iron deficiency and iron deficiency anemia. In: Lee GR, Foerster J, Lukens J, et al, editors. Wintrobe's clinical hematology. 10th ed. Baltimore: Williams & Wilkins; 1999. p. 979–1010.

starting at a low dose (ie, one tablet of ferrous sulfate daily); after a week or two, the dose can be increased to two and then three tablets per day. If the patient cannot tolerate iron on an empty stomach, it can be taken with a few crackers or milk. If iron therapy is started at a low dose, gradually increased, and properly encouraged, most patients can tolerate oral iron therapy.

- **It is important to monitor the response to therapy.** The reticulocyte count should increase within 5 to 10 days and the hemoglobin should increase by about 2 g/dL within 3 to 4 weeks. Failure to respond appropriately suggests that the diagnosis of iron deficiency was incorrect, that there is some complicating factor (such as cobalamin or folate deficiency, anemia of chronic disease, GI disease that prevents adequate iron absorption, or continuing blood loss), or that there is failure to comply with the therapy.
- It is important to continue iron therapy for 3 to 6 months after the hemoglobin returns to normal to replenish body iron stores.

Parenteral Iron Therapy

Indications for parenteral therapy include inability to tolerate oral therapy, continuing blood loss faster than can be compensated for with oral therapy, or a GI disease such as ulcerative colitis that prevents iron absorption or that would be aggravated by oral therapy. Parenteral therapy is significantly more expensive than oral therapy and may have serious side effects. The most common preparation is iron dextran complex (Imferon), which contains 50 mg of iron per milliliter of solution. It can be administered intramuscularly or intravenously.

- Intramuscular injections should be given in the upper outer quadrant of the buttock. The skin should be laterally displaced prior to injection (z-track technique) to prevent staining of the skin. The maximum recommended daily dose is 2 mL (100 mg of iron). At the beginning of therapy, a test dose of 0.5 mL should be given first and if there are no side effects after at least 1 hour, the full dose can be given. Absorption from the injection site takes several days to a few weeks, and approximately one-quarter of administered iron seems to be unavailable. Side effects of intramuscular injection include pain at the injection site and discoloration of the skin. Hypersensitivity reactions can also occur.
- Intravenous therapy avoids the discomfort of repeated intramuscular injections but has a higher incidence of systemic side effects including rare anaphylactoid reactions. A test dose of 0.5 mL should be given initially, and if there is no reaction after 1 hour, 2 mL of undiluted iron dextran complex can be given at a rate of 1 mL per minute. Pain in the injected vein, flushing, and a metallic taste in the mouth can occur with rapid intravenous injection. These usually disappear if the rate of injection is slowed.

Systemic reactions can occur with both intramuscular and intravenous administration and can include both immediate and delayed reactions. Immediate reactions include hypotension, headache, malaise, nausea, hives, and anaphylactoid reactions. Delayed reactions include fever, muscle and joint pain, and lymphadenopathy. Most systemic reactions are mild and transient, but the anaphylactoid reactions can be life-threatening; these are fortunately uncommon.

Several formulas for calculating the total iron dose for parenteral therapy have been proposed. One example is as follows:

$$\text{Dose (mg iron)} = [15 - \text{patient's hemoglobin (g/dL)}] \times \text{body weight (kg)} \times 3$$

Iron Supplementation

Prophylactic iron supplementation has been suggested for groups at special risk for iron deficiency, such as infants (particularly those born prematurely), pregnant women, adolescents, women with menorrhagia, and regular blood donors. Full-term infants can get an adequate iron supply (approximately 1 mg/kg per day) by eating iron-fortified cereals. Infants born prematurely have a higher requirement, approximately 2 mg/kg per day. One tablet of ferrous sulfate (300 mg) should be adequate for most adults. Patients with chronic severe blood loss, such as those with hereditary hemorrhagic telangiectasia (Rendu-Osler-Weber syndrome), may require continuous full-dose iron therapy (300 mg of ferrous sulfate three times daily).

Acute Iron Intoxication[3]

Accidental iron overdose usually occurs in children who mistake the iron tablets for candy. It is estimated that more than 25,000 cases occur yearly in the United States. Ingestion of >60 mg of iron per kilogram body weight may be associated with severe symptoms. The initial symptoms of iron poisoning (within the first 6 hours) include nausea, vomiting, hematemesis, diarrhea, and melena, due to irritation of the GI mucosa, with ulceration and hemorrhage. Perforation of the GI tract with peritonitis may occur. Dyspnea, lethargy, coma, and shock may follow; metabolic acidosis is common. Hepatic failure may occur 2 to 5 days after ingestion. Intestinal obstruction may occur as a late complication, due to scarring and strictures.

Treatment of acute ingestion includes gastric lavage; however, iron tablets may clump, making lavage ineffective. Abdominal radiography may show iron tablets; however, the radiograph will be negative if the iron has already been absorbed. Repeat radiographs can be used to determine the effectiveness of lavage. Blood should be drawn for serum iron at ~3 to 5 hours and ~6 to 8 hours after ingestion. Levels of <350 μg/dL generally indicate minimal toxicity, levels of 350 to 500 μg/dL are associated with moderate toxicity, and levels >500 μg/dL may be lethal. Deferoxamine, an iron chelator, may be given intravenously at a rate of 15 mg/kg body weight per hour for severe poisoning. Standard supportive measures for hypotension, shock, and acidosis should also be employed.

ANEMIA OF CHRONIC DISEASE

Anemia of chronic disease (also called **anemia of chronic inflammation**) is a common condition characterized by **anemia**, **decreased serum iron**, and **adequate storage iron in the bone marrow**. Another name that more precisely describes the condition is *hypoferremic anemia with reticuloendothelial siderosis.* (Fortunately, this hasn't had widespread use!) Anemia of chronic disease can be confused with iron deficiency anemia because both present with low serum iron and both can be microcytic. The distinction between anemia of chronic disease and iron deficiency anemia is usually fairly simple, but the two can coexist (for example, a patient with active rheumatoid arthritis could have blood loss from erosive gastritis due to high doses of nonsteroidal anti-inflammatory drugs). Deciding whether a patient with a known chronic inflammatory condition also has coexistent iron deficiency can be difficult.

- Anemia of chronic disease is the second most common cause of anemia after iron deficiency and probably the most common cause of anemia in hospitalized patients.

Causes of Anemia of Chronic Disease

Any disease condition that is associated with inflammation, and that lasts more than 1 or 2 months, can cause anemia of chronic disease (Table 5–4). In some cases, the inflammation is obvious (chronic infections or rheumatic disorders, for example); in other cases, the inflammation is less obvious (malignancies). Chronic illnesses that are not associated with inflammation (for example, hypertension or diabetes mellitus) are not usually associated with the anemia of chronic disease.

Table 5–4
Causes of Anemia of Chronic Disease

Chronic Infections
    Pulmonary infections: abscesses, bronchiectasis, tuberculosis, pneumonitis
    Infective endocarditis
    Pelvic inflammatory disease
    Osteomyelitis
    Chronic urinary tract infections
    Chronic fungal infections
    Human immunodeficiency virus (HIV) infection

Rheumatic (Autoimmune) Diseases
    Rheumatoid arthritis
    Rheumatic fever
    Systemic lupus erythematosus (SLE)
    Vasculitis: temporal arteritis, polymyalgia rheumatica, others
    Others

Malignancies
    Carcinomas
    Hodgkin's disease
    Non-Hodgkin's lymphoma
    Others

Miscellaneous
    Burns
    Severe trauma
    Alcoholic liver disease
    Others

Adapted from Means RT. The anemia of chronic disorders. In: Lee RG, Foerster J, Lukens J, et al, editors. Wintrobe's clinical hematology. 10th ed. Baltimore: Williams & Wilkins; 1999. p. 1011–21.

Pathophysiology

Five basic processes are believed to be involved in anemia of chronic disease:

- **Inflammatory cytokines:** Inflammatory cytokines appear to play a central role in the anemia of chronic disease, particularly interleukin 1 (IL-1), tumor necrosis factor (TNF), and the interferons (α-INF, β-INF, and γ-INF). All of these suppress erythropoiesis by the marrow and may also decrease erythropoietin production by the kidney.
- **Decreased erythrocyte survival:** There is usually a modest decrease in RBC survival. Part of this may be due to the deposition of immune complexes on erythrocytes, leading to phagocytosis by macrophages of the reticuloendothelial system.
- **Decreased erythropoietin production:** Erythropoietin production by the kidneys is impaired. Erythropoietin levels are usually increased but less than anticipated for the degree of anemia.
- **Decreased marrow response:** The marrow fails to respond appropriately to the anemia. This may be due in part to decreased erythropoietin levels, but the marrow response to erythropoietin also appears to be blunted.
- **Blockage in iron transfer:** Patients with anemia of chronic disease usually have adequate or increased iron stores, unless the primary illness also causes blood loss or there is some other condition causing iron deficiency. However, the serum iron is decreased, and transfer of iron to developing erythrocytes is blocked.

Laboratory Diagnosis

The anemia due to chronic disease is usually mild or moderate: blood hemoglobin levels ≥8 to 10 g/dL. However, the anemia may be more severe in chronic illnesses with marked inflammation. The anemia is usually normocytic and normochromic but can be microcytic in severe cases. In such cases, the MCV is usually only mildly decreased (≥70 fL). The reticulocyte count is low. Laboratory measures of inflammation such as the erythrocyte sedimentation rate are usually increased. The serum iron is low, the serum transferrin (iron-binding capacity) is decreased, and the iron saturation is decreased, although usually not as low as in iron deficiency anemia. The serum ferritin is usually increased, unless there is coexistent iron deficiency.

Treatment

The *primary treatment* is to *treat the underlying condition*. Most patients are asymptomatic from the anemia, and no specific treatment for the anemia is required. Iron supplementation is unnecessary and will not be beneficial unless there is coexistent iron deficiency. In occasional severe cases, in which the primary illness cannot be effectively treated, recombinant erythropoietin (Procrit or Epogen) may be helpful. Rarely, patients with severe anemia may require transfusion, particularly if there is an urgent need for surgery or some other procedure.

SIDEROBLASTIC ANEMIAS

The **sideroblastic anemias** are a heterogeneous group of illnesses characterized by **abnormalities in the synthesis of the heme molecule**: either defective protoporphyrin synthesis or impaired incorporation of iron into the protoporphyrin ring. The result of the defect in heme synthesis is the accumulation of iron in the mitochondria of developing erythroblasts. Sideroblastic anemia may be inherited or acquired, and acquired cases may be reversible or irreversible (Table 5–5). The key feature of sideroblastic anemia is the presence of **ringed sideroblasts** in a bone marrow aspirate stained for iron (Figure 5–2). The "rings" in ringed sideroblasts represent mitochondria loaded with iron, which cluster around the nucleus and resemble rings on an iron stain. By definition, a ringed sideroblast must have five or more granules, which must encircle one-third or more of the diameter of the nucleus. At least 15% of nucleated erythrocyte precursors must have rings for the anemia to be classified as sideroblastic.

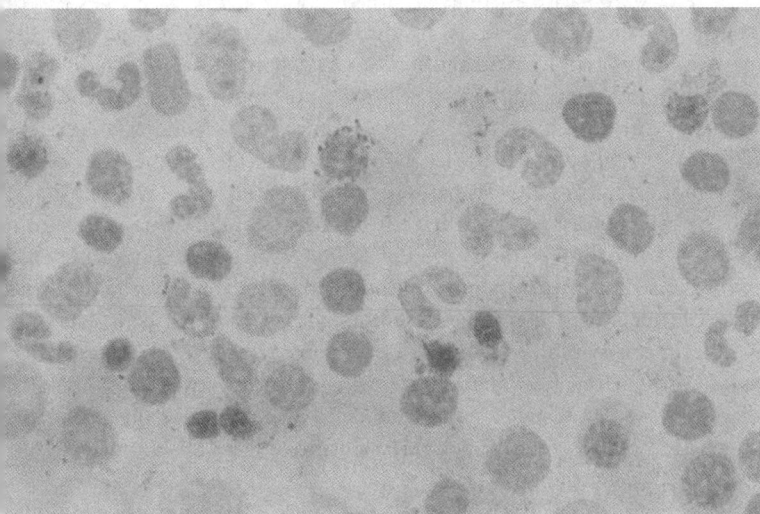

Figure 5–2 Sideroblastic anemia. Bone marrow aspirate with iron stain. Note the iron granules forming a ring around the nucleus.

Table 5–5
Causes of Sideroblastic Anemia

Congenital
    X-linked (majority)
    Autosomal: dominant or recessive
    Sporadic

Acquired
    Idiopathic
    Associated with myelodysplasia

Reversible
    Alcoholism
    Drugs: isoniazid, chloramphenicol
    Copper deficiency
    Zinc excess

⇨ A *sideroblast* is a nucleated RBC precursor that has cytoplasmic iron granules on Prussian blue stain; a *siderocyte* is an anucleate RBC with iron granules. Nucleated RBC precursors are also called *erythroblasts* (to be distinguished from ***pro****erythroblasts*, which are the earliest recognizable RBC precursors).

Inherited Sideroblastic Anemia

Inherited sideroblastic anemias are uncommon. The majority of cases of inherited sideroblastic anemia are due to mutations in the gene for the enzyme **aminolevulinic acid synthetase** (**ALA synthetase**), which catalyzes the first and rate-limiting reaction in protoporphyrin synthesis. The gene for ALA synthetase is on the X chromosome, and thus inheritance is X-linked. A smaller number of cases are due to mutations in other enzymes in the protoporphyrin synthesis pathway; inheritance of these is variable.

The severity of anemia in inherited sideroblastic anemia varies from mild to severe. Some patients present in infancy, whereas other cases may not be diagnosed until well into adulthood. Erythrocytes are usually microcytic. Clusters of small granules resembling stacked cannonballs that stain as iron on Prussian blue stain may be seen in erythrocytes (*Pappenheimer bodies*). The serum iron and transferrin saturation are usually increased. Diagnosis of sideroblastic anemia is made by demonstrating the pathologic ringed sideroblasts on a bone marrow aspirate. The inheritance is confirmed by family studies.

Pyridoxine (**vitamin B$_6$**) at a dose of 50 to 200 mg per day should be tried. About one-third of cases linked to mutations in the ALA synthetase gene improve with this therapy. Patients who respond should be kept on pyridoxine lifelong, at the minimum effective dose. Pyridoxine may be discontinued if there is no response within 3 months. Transfusion may be necessary for severe cases that fail to respond to pyridoxine. Iron overload can be a significant problem; this can be due to both increased iron absorption (driven by ineffective erythropoiesis) and transfusions. Chelation therapy with deferoxamine may be necessary to avoid complications of iron overload (hepatic cirrhosis, cardiomyopathy, diabetes mellitus). Patients should be cautioned to avoid iron supplements and excessive ascorbic acid (vitamin C), which increases both iron absorption and the tissue toxicity of iron.

Acquired Sideroblastic Anemia

Acquired sideroblastic anemia is more common than the inherited type. Acquired cases are divided into **reversible** (*secondary*) and **irreversible** (*idiopathic*) forms. Most reversible cases are due to toxic chemicals or drugs, such as alcohol, isoniazid (INH), or chloramphenicol. Sideroblastic anemia associated with alcohol usually occurs in alcoholics with multiple nutritional deficiencies, as seen in "skid rows" and inner-city hospitals; it is rare in the well-nourished, middle-class alcoholic. Sideroblastic anemia occurs in a minority of patients given INH (people who are slow acetylators of the drug) and can be prevented by giving pyridoxine (25–50 mg/day). Sideroblastic anemia is also a predictable dose-related toxicity of chloramphenicol and will occur in virtually all patients given a sufficiently high dose of the drug (>2 g/day) for prolonged periods. This is distinct from the rare idiosyncratic aplastic anemia for which chloramphenicol is notorious.

Copper is an essential factor for some of the enzymes in the protoporphyrin pathway, and, therefore, copper deficiency can also be associated with sideroblastic anemia. Copper deficiency may occur in patients given total parenteral nutrition lacking copper supplementation. High zinc intake inhibits the absorption of copper from the GI tract, and thus excessive zinc consumption can induce copper deficiency. With the increasing popularity of unregulated zinc supplements, sideroblastic anemia related to excess zinc consumption may become more frequent. Diagnosis of suspected zinc-induced sideroblastic anemia can be confirmed by finding an elevated serum zinc level and a decrease in serum copper and ceruloplasmin levels.

Treatment of acquired reversible sideroblastic anemia consists of finding the cause and eliminating it. Patients consuming excessive alcohol should be advised to stop. Patients with sideroblastic anemia due to INH can be given supplemental pyridoxine, and alternative antibiotics can be substituted for chloramphenicol. Patients taking excessive zinc should discontinue it.

Irreversible variants of acquired sideroblastic anemia are due to genetic mutations in hematopoietic stem cells or early hematopoietic precursors. These are clonal proliferations, and they fall into the general category of the myelodysplastic syndromes. There are usually morphologic abnormalities (dysplastic changes) in erythrocyte precursors (*dyserythropoiesis*), sometimes accompanied by dysplastic changes in the other cell lineages. Cases with dysplasia limited to the erythroid series have sometimes been designated *idiopathic acquired sideroblastic anemia* (**IASA**). Cases with dysplastic changes in the other series are classified as *refractory anemia with ringed sideroblasts* (**RARS**). The distinction between IASA and RARS is subjective at best; some authorities do not use the category of IASA and classify all cases as RARS. Treatment for IASA and RARS is the same; patients with dysplastic changes in multiple lineages may have shorter survival and a higher rate of transformation to acute leukemia.

The anemia in IASA and RARS is usually macrocytic (MCV ~100–110 fL) rather than microcytic, as in the inherited varieties. Erythrocytes may appear dimorphic on blood smear. The white cell count and platelet count are usually normal, except in those cases with multilineage dysplastic changes.

Patients with IASA or RARS should be given a trial of pyridoxine, 100 to 200 mg per day for approximately 3 months. Only a minority of patients respond, and response tends to be partial. Patients who do respond should be kept on pyridoxine lifelong, at the minimum effective dose. Other patients should be given blood transfusions as necessary. Patients should be advised to avoid iron supplements, and iron chelation therapy may become necessary. Median survival of patients with IASA is relatively long (4–6 years). A minority of patients transform to acute leukemia (~3–12%). Patients with cytogenetic abnormalities may have shorter survival and a higher rate of transformation to acute leukemia than patients without chromosomal abnormalities.

⇨ *Pyridoxine deficiency* is sometimes listed as a cause of sideroblastic anemia. In reality, true pyridoxine deficiency is extremely uncommon. Some patients have *pyridoxine-responsive* sideroblastic anemia, but the dose of pyridoxine required is far in excess of the normal daily requirement.

ANEMIA OF LEAD POISONING

Lead interferes with protoporphyrin synthesis at several levels and also appears to block iron delivery to the site of incorporation into the protoporphyrin ring. A characteristic feature in lead poisoning is prominent *basophilic stippling in erythrocytes*. Anemia is a relatively late complication of lead poisoning; abdominal pain, constipation, encephalopathy (lethargy, malaise, drowsiness), and peripheral neuropathy are more common. However, anemia due to lead poisoning can be a problem in inner cities, where old buildings still contain lead paint. The diagnosis of lead poisoning is made by demonstrating elevated blood lead levels (>25 μg/dL).

THE MEGALOBLASTIC ANEMIAS: COBALAMIN (VITAMIN B_{12}) AND FOLATE DEFICIENCIES

The **megaloblastic anemias** result from **interference in DNA synthesis**. Although the term megaloblastic **anemia** implies that the primary manifestation is on developing erythroblasts, the same process affects granulocyte precursors, megakaryocytes, the lining of the GI tract, and other replicating cells throughout the body. The most common causes of megaloblastic anemia in clinical practice are deficiencies of cobalamin (vitamin B_{12}) and folic acid. A similar process also occurs in patients on chemotherapy drugs that interfere with DNA synthesis, some nucleoside analogues used to treat HIV infection, and sometimes with medications that interfere with folate metabolism (antifolate drugs such as methotrexate, sulfa antibiotics, trimethoprim). Cobalamin deficiency can also be associated with neurologic abnormalities.

It is important to differentiate between *megaloblastic* anemias and *macrocytic* anemias. Both are associated with an increase in red cell size (increased MCV), but whereas nearly all cases of megaloblastic anemia are macrocytic, many cases of macrocytic anemia are not megaloblastic. Com-

Table 5–6
Macrocytic Anemias: Megaloblastic versus Non-Megaloblastic

Megaloblastic	Non-Megaloblastic
Folate deficiency	Liver disease
Cobalamin deficiency	Myelodysplasia
Antifolate drugs	Reticulocytosis
Cancer chemotherapy	Hypothyroidism
	Alcoholism
	Chronic obstructive pulmonary disease (COPD)

mon causes of *macrocytic* anemia include liver disease, reticulocytosis, and alcoholism (Table 5–6). The MCV is usually only mildly elevated in most macrocytic anemias (~100–110 fL) but can be dramatically increased in the megaloblastic anemias (≥130 fL).

- **Megaloblastic anemia** is caused by interference with DNA synthesis, usually due to a deficiency of cobalamin or folic acid.
- **Pernicious anemia** is megaloblastic anemia due to autoimmune chronic gastritis with destruction of the gastric parietal cells. Pernicious anemia is not synonymous with megaloblastic anemia; it is a subset of megaloblastic anemias.
- **Vitamin B$_{12}$**, strictly speaking, is *cyanocobalamin*; **cobalamin** is the generic term for members of the cobalamin family. Cyanocobalamin is an artifact of manufacturing, not a natural form, but it is used therapeutically. The terms vitamin B$_{12}$ and cobalamin are used interchangeably.

Folic Acid

Folic acid (folate) is actually *pteroylglutamic acid*. Folic acid is required for the transfer of one-carbon fragments such as methyl groups in numerous chemical reactions. Folic acid is synthesized by higher plants and microorganisms; it is abundant in vegetables, fruit, cereals, and dairy products. Folic acid is heat labile, and much is destroyed by cooking. Therefore, the **primary dietary source** for folic acid is **fresh uncooked fruits and vegetables**. It is primarily absorbed in the jejunum. The daily requirement is ~50 μg. The body has stores of approximately 5 to 10 mg, primarily in the liver. An enterohepatic circulation is required for redistribution of hepatic folate stores to the rest of the body. Folate stores can be exhausted in a few weeks to a few months—much faster if the enterohepatic circulation is disrupted.

   Pregnancy is worth special mention here. It is believed that folate deficiency during pregnancy predisposes the fetus to neural tube defects and that folate supplementation will reduce the risk of such defects. **Every woman who is pregnant, or who is considering becoming pregnant, should take folic acid.**

Causes of Folate Deficiency

Most cases of folate deficiency are due to inadequate diet (Table 5–7). Malabsorption is less common. Chronic alcoholics are at particular risk for folate deficiency because they are less likely to eat fresh fruits and vegetables and because alcohol interferes with folate metabolism.

Table 5–7
Causes of Folate Deficiency

Inadequate Diet (most common)
Alcoholism
Lack of fresh fruits and vegetables

Malabsorption (less common)
Gluten-sensitive enteropathy (celiac sprue)
Tropical sprue
Extensive small bowel resection
Inflammatory bowel disease (regional enteritis)

Rare Causes
Hemodialysis
Antiepileptic drugs
Antifolate drugs
Increased requirements: chronic hemolytic anemia, psoriasis, pregnancy
Oral contraceptives (uncommon)
Exposure to nitrous oxide (N_2O)

Cobalamin

The primary dietary sources of cobalamin are meat, eggs, milk, and cheese. The daily requirement is ~0.1 µg/day. The average American diet contains ~5 to 15 µg/day, and body stores (primarily in the liver) contain 2 to 4 mg (2,000–4,000 µg). Thus, body stores can supply daily needs for many years. **Most cases of cobalamin deficiency are due to malabsorption** (Table 5–8),

Table 5–8
Causes of Cobalamin Deficiency

Malabsorption (most common)
Pernicious anemia: loss of IF production and gastric acid
Gastrectomy: loss of IF production and gastric acid
Inflammatory bowel disease: loss of absorption in terminal ileum
Resection of terminal ileum: loss of absorption by specific IF-B_{12} receptors
Pancreatic insufficiency: inability to digest R-binders off of B_{12}
Blind loop syndrome: bacterial overgrowth; bacteria compete for B_{12}
Congenital deficiency of intrinsic factor (rare)
Fish tapeworm (*Diphyllobothrium latum*): competition for B_{12}

Dietary Deficiency (extremely rare in US)
Strict vegans
Infants breast-fed by vegetarian mothers

Congenital Deficiency of Transcobalamin (rare)

IF = intrinsic factor.

with pernicious anemia being the most common cause. *Insufficient dietary intake of cobalamin is extremely uncommon in the United States*; only strict vegans who consume no eggs, fish, cheese, or other dairy products are at risk of insufficient dietary intake.

Absorption of cobalamin from the GI tract is a multistep process, with several places for possible problems. Absorption requires **intrinsic factor** (**IF**), which binds to B_{12}. There are specific receptors for the IF-B_{12} complex in the terminal ileum. B_{12} bound to IF is efficiently absorbed, but very little unbound B_{12} can be absorbed. Intrinsic factor is produced by gastric parietal cells, which also produce gastric acid. Dietary B_{12} is bound to proteins and must first be released by gastric acid and proteases.

The **steps in cobalamin absorption** are as follows:

1. B_{12} is digested off of food protein by pepsin and gastric acid. The released B_{12} is then bound to B_{12}-binding proteins (R proteins) produced by the salivary glands, which blocks binding of IF.
2. The B_{12} is released from the R proteins by pancreatic enzymes, allowing IF to bind to the B_{12}.
3. The B_{12}-IF complex is absorbed in the terminal ileum.

Cobalamin circulates in the blood bound to proteins called **transcobalamins**. The physiologically important transcobalamin is designated **transcobalamin II** (**TCII**); there are receptors on cell surfaces for the TCII-B_{12} complex. There is an enterohepatic circulation of cobalamin, similar to that of folate.

Causes of Cobalamin Deficiency

The most common cause of cobalamin deficiency is pernicious anemia (see Table 5–8). Pernicious anemia is an autoimmune chronic gastritis, resulting in destruction of the parietal cells and loss of IF production. It occurs in all ethnic groups, although the highest incidence appears to be in persons of Scandinavian, English, Scottish, and Irish descent. In Caucasians, the average age of onset is about 60 years, although it can be seen at all ages, including children. The average age of onset is younger in African Americans; in this population, there is a high incidence in relatively young women. There is a familial predisposition to pernicious anemia. There is also a strong association between pernicious anemia and other autoimmune disorders, including thyroid disease (Graves' disease, Hashimoto's thyroiditis), Addison's disease, vitiligo, and hypoparathyroidism. Patients with pernicious anemia may have serum antibodies against gastric parietal cells (*anti–parietal cell antibodies*) or antibodies against intrinsic factor (*anti-IF antibodies*). Patients with pernicious anemia have an increased risk of gastric carcinoma compared to the general population; the increase in risk is significant, but the overall risk for the individual patient is low.

Pathophysiology of Megaloblastic Anemia

The metabolic pathways of cobalamin and folic acid are complex; however, only a few key reactions are needed to understand megaloblastic anemia (Figure 5–3). The primary defect is an inability to produce **deoxythymidine monophosphate (dTMP)** from deoxyuridine monophosphate, which is catalyzed by the enzyme **thymidylate synthetase**. 5,10-Methylene-tetrahydrofolate (methylene-FH_4) is required for the reaction. Cobalamin is involved in the regeneration of methylene-FH_4, so cobalamin deficiency, in effect, results in folate deficiency. Deoxythymidine monophosphate is converted to deoxythymidine triphosphate (dTTP), which is required for DNA synthesis. In the absence of adequate dTTP, deoxyuridine triphosphate (dUTP) is inserted into DNA, resulting in abnormal DNA synthesis including DNA strand breaks. Since RNA synthesis is unimpaired, cytoplasmic maturation is relatively normal; the cell continues to synthesize hemoglobin while waiting for DNA synthesis and cell division to be completed, resulting in increased cell size. There is marked ineffective erythropoiesis; the marrow is markedly hypercellular, but most cells die before leaving the marrow. This results in massive intramedullary hemolysis.

Key Reactions (1)

- 5,10-methylene tetrahydrofolate required for dUMP conversion to dTMP by **thymidylate synthetase**
- dTMP required for DNA synthesis
- Cobalamin required for regeneration of methylene-FH_4
  - Without cobalamin, folate trapped as methyl-FH_4

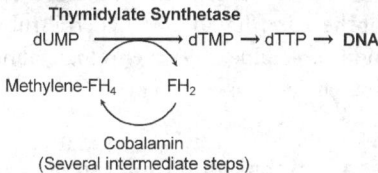

$$\text{dUMP} \xrightarrow{\text{Thymidylate Synthetase}} \text{dTMP} \rightarrow \text{dTTP} \rightarrow \textbf{DNA}$$

Methylene-FH_4 FH_2

Cobalamin
(Several intermediate steps)

Key Reactions (2)

- Conversion of **homocysteine** to **methionine** by **methionine synthetase**
- Requires methyl-FH_4 and cobalamin

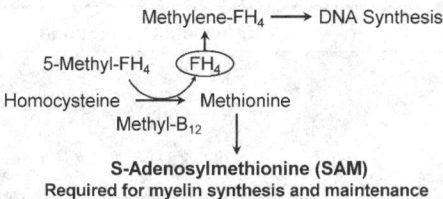

Methylene-FH_4 ⟶ DNA Synthesis

5-Methyl-FH_4 FH_4

Homocysteine ⟶ Methionine

Methyl-B_{12}

S-Adenosylmethionine (SAM)
Required for myelin synthesis and maintenance

Figure 5–3 Key metabolic reactions in megaloblastic anemias. dUMP = deoxyuridine monophosphate; dTMP = deoxythymidine monophosphate; dTTP = deoxythymidine triphosphate.

A second key reaction is the conversion of homocysteine to methionine, which requires 5-methyl-FH$_4$ and methyl-cobalamin. Methyl-FH$_4$ is converted to tetrahydrofolate (FH$_4$), which is subsequently converted to methylene-FH$_4$ for DNA synthesis. Methionine is a precursor of S-adenosylmethionine (SAM), which is required for myelin synthesis and maintenance. Deficiency of SAM is probably important in the neurologic complications of cobalamin deficiency.

Symptoms

Megaloblastic anemia presents with an insidious onset of weakness, fatigue, abdominal pain, nausea, diarrhea, or constipation. Patients may complain of soreness of the tongue or mouth or pain on swallowing. Weight loss is common (Table 5–9). Since the onset of anemia is gradual, allowing time for physiologic compensation, patients often tolerate astounding degrees of anemia without symptoms. Various neuropyschiatric abnormalities may be present in cobalamin deficiency, including altered mental status or obtundation, dementia, hallucinations, and paranoid ideation. Currently, many patients are asymptomatic, and the anemia is detected because of abnormalities on routine blood counts.

Physical Examination

Physical examination characteristically shows pallor and a peculiar "lemon yellow" coloration of the skin (due to mild hyperbilirubinemia). A "beefy" red tongue is common (see Table 5–9). Neurologic abnormalities may be present in cobalamin deficiency (see below).

Neurologic Disease in Cobalamin Deficiency

Cobalamin deficiency may be complicated by neurologic disease, a feature that separates cobalamin from folate deficiencies. The degree of neurologic

Table 5–9
Symptoms and Signs of Megaloblastic Anemia

Symptoms	Physical Examination
Weakness, fatigue	Pallor, "lemon yellow" skin
Painful tongue and mouth	Dry, smooth, "velvety" skin
Weight loss	Smooth, red, "beefy" tongue
Loss of appetite, nausea, vomiting	Silver coloration or premature graying of hair
Loose, semisolid stools	

disorder does not correlate with the degree of anemia, and patients may have severe neurologic disease without significant hematologic abnormalities. The primary neuropathologic change in cobalamin deficiency is demyelination of the dorsal and lateral columns of the spinal cord and the cerebral cortex. Both sensory and motor systems are affected, leading to the terms *subacute combined degeneration* and *combined system disease*. The earliest and most common symptom is paresthesias in the distal extremities. The earliest changes seen on physical examination are decreased vibration and position sensation in the extremities. These symptoms progress to weakness, clumsiness, and an unsteady gait. In severe disease, the patient may have severe weakness and spasticity. In more advanced cases, the patients may have hyperreflexia, clonus, and positive Romberg and Babinski signs. Early cerebral signs include depression and impairment of memory. More severe cortical changes include delusions, hallucinations, and paranoid and schizophrenic states (*megaloblastic madness*); however, these are uncommon.

Laboratory Evaluation

A summary of laboratory abnormalities associated with megaloblastic anemia is presented in Table 5–10. The CBC shows anemia, which can be quite striking. The MCV is increased (often ≥120 fL). The white cell count and platelet count are typically decreased, but usually to a lesser degree than the

Table 5–10
Laboratory Abnormalities in Megaloblastic Anemia

Decreased hemoglobin

Increased MCV (often ≥120 fL)

Oval macrocytes

Leukopenia

Hypersegmented neutrophils:
- >5 nuclear lobes in any cell
- ≥5% of neutrophils have 5 nuclear lobes

Thrombocytopenia

Increased lactic dehydrogenase (LD)

Increased bilirubin

Decreased haptoglobin

Bone marrow:
- Megaloblasts (enlarged erythrocyte precursors with immature nuclear chromatin)
- Giant bands and metamyelocytes

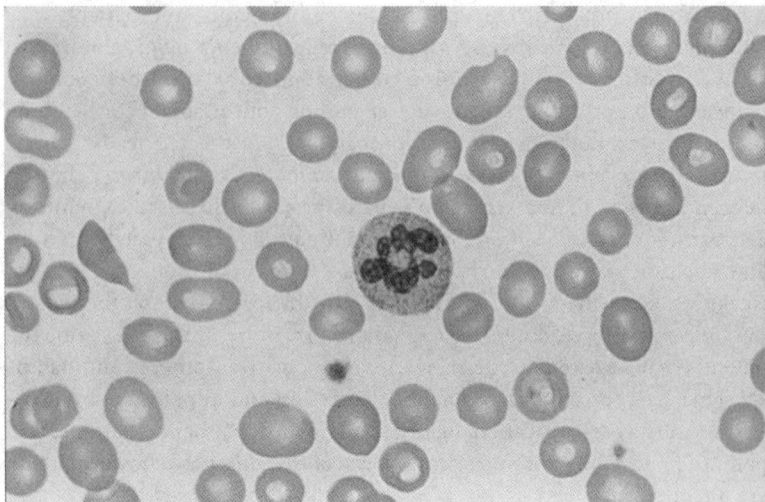

Figure 5–4 Megaloblastic anemia blood smear. Note the hypersegmented neutrophil and the large oval erythrocytes.

hemoglobin. On blood smear (Figure 5–4), erythrocytes show both macrocytosis and ovalocytosis; the presence of *oval macrocytes* is very suggestive of megaloblastic anemia. In severe cases, there may be teardrop and fragmented RBCs, Howell-Jolly bodies, and nucleated RBCs. The characteristic finding in granulocytes is *hypersegmented neutrophils*. Hypersegmented neutrophils are defined by the **Rule of Fives**: either more than five distinct nuclear lobes in any cell or ≥5% of neutrophils have five distinct nuclear lobes.

- **Hypersegmented neutrophils** are one of the earliest blood findings of megaloblastic anemia and may precede both anemia and macrocytosis. They are also one of the last morphologic changes to disappear after therapy is started (several days to 2 weeks). The presence of hypersegmented neutrophils in a patient with a macrocytic anemia is a strong indication that the process is megaloblastic anemia.
- It is important to note that a patient can have cobalamin deficiency without having either macrocytosis or anemia. In fact, it has been suggested that patients with the worst neurologic disease tend to have the mildest hematologic disease and vice versa. **The absence of anemia (or macrocytosis) does not exclude neurologic disease due to cobalamin deficiency!**

The marked intramedullary hemolysis results in an increase in serum **lactic dehydrogenase** (**LD** or **LDH**) and **bilirubin** and a decrease in serum haptoglobin. The LD is often several thousand international units.

Bone Marrow

The bone marrow is hypercellular, with an increase in erythroid precursors. The characteristic cell is a *megaloblast*, which is a large erythroid precursor with an immature-appearing ("open") nucleus (Figure 5–5). The nucleus of a megaloblast has been likened to the cut surface of salami. Another characteristic feature is *giant metamyelocytes* and *band neutrophils*.

Laboratory Diagnosis

Serum cobalamin, serum folate, and erythrocyte folate levels will establish the cause of a megaloblastic anemia in most cases (Table 5–11).

- The serum folate level is labile and may easily fluctuate with meals. Therefore, if a patient with folate deficiency is admitted to the hospital and the blood sample is drawn after a couple of good meals, then the serum folate level may be normal. The erythrocyte folate level, on the other hand, is likely to remain depressed for several days.

Two additional tests that may be useful are serum levels of **methylmalonic acid** (MMA) and **homocysteine**. An increase in MMA is very sensitive for cobalamin deficiency and may be clearly increased when the serum cobalamin is borderline and before the hemoglobin begins to decrease. Both the MMA and homocysteine levels are increased in cobal-

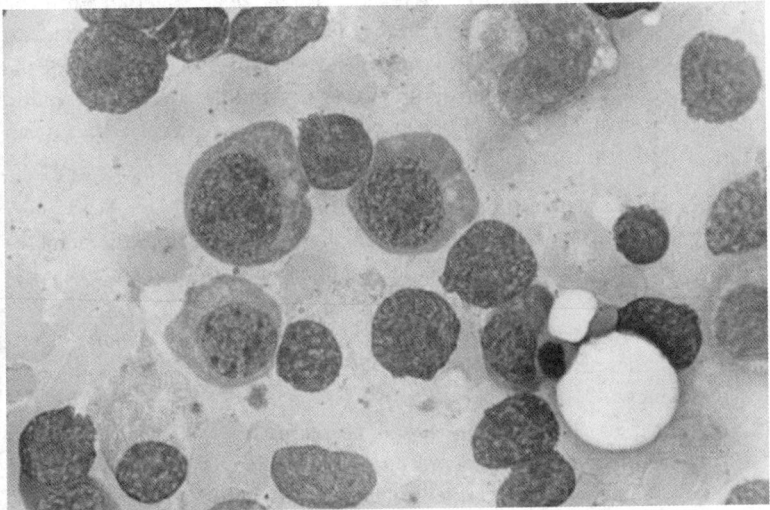

Figure 5–5 Megaloblastic anemia bone marrow aspirate. Note the large erythroid precursors with open nuclear chromatin.

Table 5–11

Laboratory Diagnosis of Megaloblastic Anemias

Test	Cobalamin Deficiency	Folate Deficiency
Serum cobalamin	Decreased	Usually normal
Serum folate	Normal to increased	Decreased
Erythrocyte folate	Decreased	Decreased
Serum methylmalonic acid	Increased	Normal
Serum homocysteine	Increased	Increased (moderately)

amin deficiency. In folate deficiency, homocysteine is characteristically increased, whereas the MMA is usually normal.

Schilling Test

The standard method to diagnose pernicious anemia, once cobalamin deficiency is confirmed, is the **Schilling test**. Radiolabeled cobalamin is given orally, a large dose of unlabeled B_{12} is given intramuscularly, and urine is collected for 24 hours. The amount of radioactivity in the urine indicates how much B_{12} was absorbed orally. Typically, recovery of <6% in the urine indicates malabsorption of B_{12}. If the initial value is abnormal, a second stage is performed in which intrinsic factor is given together with the labeled B_{12}. An increase in the amount of B_{12} absorbed during the second stage of the Schilling test indicates pernicious anemia. (The purpose of the intramuscular "cold" B_{12} is to saturate the B_{12}-binding sites in the serum, and thereby flush all of the orally absorbed B_{12} into the urine, where it can be measured. It took me a long time to figure that out.)

- The Schilling test can be done even if the patient has been on B_{12} therapy for months or years. Cobalamin therapy will correct the hematologic complications of pernicious anemia but will not correct the gastric atrophy or the lack of IF production.
- The Schilling test is done to investigate the cause of *cobalamin* deficiency; there is no reason to do a Schilling test in a patient with *folate* deficiency.
- Some experts believe that there is no reason to do a Schilling test in cobalamin deficiency; they presume that pernicious anemia is the most likely diagnosis, and treatment of cobalamin deficiency of any cause is the same.

Assay of serum *anti–parietal cell* or *anti-IF antibodies* can also be useful in diagnosis of pernicious anemia:

- **Anti–parietal cell antibodies** are very *sensitive* for pernicious anemia (~90%) but are not very *specific*. They are found in about 8% of normal older individuals and 50 to 60% of patients with atrophic gastritis not associated with pernicious anemia.
- **Anti-IF antibodies** are very *specific* for pernicious anemia but not very *sensitive* (~50–60%).

Treatment of Megaloblastic Anemia

It is critical to determine whether the deficiency is due to folic acid or cobalamin; giving the wrong treatment is ineffective and potentially dangerous.

Oral folate supplementation is the treatment of choice for most cases of folate deficiency. One 0.4 or 1.0 mg (400- or 1,000-μg) tablet daily should be adequate. Parenteral therapy may be required for rare cases of folate malabsorption.

Treatment of pernicious anemia and other causes of cobalamin malabsorption requires parenteral therapy. Available preparations include cyanocobalamin and hydroxocobalamin. A typical treatment regimen would be 1,000 μg (1 mg) of cyanocobalamin weekly for 5 weeks, followed by 1,000 μg monthly for life. **It is critical that once cobalamin deficiency is documented, therapy must be continued for life.** Discontinuing therapy may result in the devastating neurologic complications of cobalamin deficiency.

The response to therapy is usually dramatic, with rapid symptomatic improvement. Reticulocytosis should appear after about 2 to 3 days, with a maximum response at 5 to 8 days. The hemoglobin should begin to rise after about 1 week, with normalization of the hemoglobin by 4 to 8 weeks. The granulocyte count usually reaches a normal level within 1 week; hypersegmentation of neutrophils usually disappears within 2 weeks. The platelet count usually returns to normal within 1 week. The bone marrow shows dramatic improvement, with disappearance of megaloblasts within 1 to 2 days. The serum LD and bilirubin drop rapidly.

- It is important to monitor the response to therapy; failure to respond appropriately indicates either an incorrect diagnosis or some complicating factor such as coexistent iron deficiency.
- Treatment with high doses of folic acid can partially reverse the hematologic manifestations of cobalamin deficiency but will not help the neurologic disease. In fact, treatment of cobalamin deficiency with folic acid may *accelerate* the progression of neurologic disease.

Cobalamin therapy halts the progression of neurologic disease due to cobalamin deficiency, and most patients demonstrate improvement. The degree to which the neurologic disease is reversible is variable and difficult to predict. Neurologic symptoms of recent onset (within a few months) are likely to be completely reversible. Abnormalities that have been present for 6 months or more are likely to result in permanent residual deficits. It usually takes 6 months or longer to achieve maximum benefit; however, some patients continue to show neurologic improvement up to 1 year.

References

1. National Center for Health Statistics. Hematological and nutritional biochemistry reference data for persons 6 months to 74 years of age: United States, 1976–1980. In: Fulwood R, Johnson CL, Bryner JD, et al. Vital and Health Statistics Series II, No. 232. Washington (DC): US Government Printing Office; 1982. DHHS Publ. No.: (PHS) 83-1682.
2. Scott DE, Pritchard JA. Iron deficiency in healthy young college women. JAMA 1967;199:147–500.
3. Gruber JE. Acute iron and lead poisoning. In: Rosen P, Barkin R, eds. Emergency medicine: concepts and clinical practice. 4th ed. St. Louis: Mosby, 1998. p. 1367–73.

6

The Inherited Hemolytic Anemias: Hemoglobinopathies, Thalassemias, Enzyme Deficiencies, and Membrane Defects

Hemolytic anemias are characterized by premature destruction of erythrocytes (*hemolysis*). Clinically, they are recognized by an increase in the reticulocyte count and reticulocyte production index. Other indications of a hemolytic anemia include increased serum bilirubin and lactic dehydrogenase (LD) and a decrease in the serum haptoglobin.

There are many different types of hemolytic anemia. At the most basic level, hemolytic anemias can be divided into conditions that are **intrinsic** to the erythrocyte and those that are **extrinsic** to the erythrocyte. Virtually all hemolytic anemias that are intrinsic to the erythrocyte are **inherited**, and virtually all hemolytic anemias that are extrinsic to the erythrocyte are **acquired**. The inherited hemolytic anemias will be discussed in this chapter; the acquired hemolytic anemias will be discussed in Chapter 7.

There are four main types of inherited hemolytic anemias:

- **Structural Hemoglobinopathies:** Synthesis of a structurally abnormal hemoglobin protein (globin chain)
- **Thalassemias:** Quantitative abnormality (decreased synthesis) of a globin chain
- **Enzyme Defects:** Absent or decreased function of a metabolic enzyme
- **Membrane Defects:** Abnormalities in the proteins that make up the cytoskeleton of the cell membrane

THE STRUCTURAL HEMOGLOBINOPATHIES

Structural hemoglobinopathies (often simply called *hemoglobinopathies*) are caused by **mutations in the gene for a globin chain**, resulting in the synthesis of a **structurally abnormal hemoglobin**. In most cases, this is due to substitution of a single amino acid. The majority of hemoglobinopathies that are clinically detected are β-chain mutations. Occasional α-chain mutations are found; mutations of the other globin chains (γ, δ) are rare. Since the genes for the hemoglobin chains are on autosomal chromosomes (the α-chain cluster on chromosome 16, the β-chain cluster on chromosome 11), the hemoglobinopathies are inherited in an autosomal fashion. The majority are inherited in an autosomal recessive pattern; homozygotes for the mutation have clinical disease, but heterozygotes are asymptomatic or have mild disease. Some of the hemoglobinopathies can interact; for example, a person heterozygous for *both* hemoglobin S and hemoglobin C has clinical disease, whereas someone who is heterozygous for either one alone is asymptomatic. The hemoglobinopathies can also interact with thalassemias. Someone who is heterozygous for both β-thalassemia and hemoglobin S will have clinical disease, which may be quite severe. Inheriting a gene for α-thalassemia, on the other hand, tends to *decrease* the severity of hemoglobin S.

Hundreds of different hemoglobin mutations have been described; fortunately, most of these are clinically silent. The consequences of a hemoglobinopathy can include hemolytic anemia, increased or decreased oxygen affinity, and a decrease in hemoglobin stability or a tendency for hemoglobin to oxidize to methemoglobin (Table 6–1). Hemoglobin S (sickle cell disease), hemoglobin C, and hemoglobin E will be described in some detail since they are the most common hemoglobinopathies worldwide. Others will be described briefly.

Terminology and Nomenclature

Terminology for the hemoglobinopathies can be confusing. The normal hemoglobins are hemoglobin A ($\alpha_2\beta_2$), hemoglobin A_2 ($\alpha_2\delta_2$), and hemoglobin F (fetal hemoglobin; $\alpha_2\gamma_2$). In the adult, hemoglobin A represents ≥95% of the hemoglobin, A_2 represents ≤3 to 4%, and F represents ≤1 to 2%. Sickle hemoglobin is designated S because erythrocytes with hemoglobin S can transform into a sickle shape. Hemoglobins that tend to oxidize to methemoglobin are designated hemoglobin M. Other hemoglobins are given letter designations based on their migration on routine hemoglobin electrophoresis (alkaline electrophoresis on cellulose acetate). As additional variants were discovered, hemoglobins were designated based on the city,

Table 6–1
Consequences of Hemoglobinopathies

Abnormality	Consequences	Examples
Polymerization or crystallization	Hemolytic anemia	Hemoglobins S and C
Unstable hemoglobin	Intermittent or chronic hemolysis	Hb Hammersmith, Hb Gun Hill, Hb Philly
Increased oxygen affinity	Erythrocytosis	Hemoglobin Yakima
Decreased oxygen affinity	Decreased hemoglobin, cyanosis	Hemoglobin Kansas
Oxidation of iron atom to ferric (Fe^{3+}) state	Methemoglobinemia	Hemoglobin M variants
Decreased RNA synthesis or abnormal RNA	Thalassemic picture	Hemoglobins E and G

Many structural hemoglobinopathies are clinically silent; they may cause altered migration on electrophoresis but no clinical consequences.

place, or hospital in which they were discovered (for example, hemoglobin Kansas, hemoglobin Yakima, and hemoglobin Hammersmith), sometimes in combination with a letter (M-Boston is a methemoglobin variant that was discovered in Boston).

⇨ Hemoglobins are also given scientific names based on the specific amino acid sequence abnormality and the part of the protein where the abnormality is located. For example, the scientific name for hemoglobin S is β6 (A3) Glu→Val—in other words, substitution of valine for glutamic acid in the sixth amino acid of the β chain, which is the third amino acid of the A helix.

An important but sometimes confusing difference is between hemoglobin **genotype** and **phenotype**:

- **Genotype**: The genotypic designation is based upon the specific globin chains that are present. Heterozygous sickle cell would be designated $\alpha_2\beta\beta^S$ (two normal α chains, one normal β chain, one β chain with the sickle mutation). Homozygous sickle cell anemia would be designated $\alpha_2\beta_2{}^S$ (two normal α chains, two β chains with the sickle mutation).

Compound heterozygosity for hemoglobin S and hemoglobin C would be designated $\alpha_2\beta^S\beta^C$.

- **Phenotype:** The phenotypic designation is based on the hemoglobin types that are present. The letter designation for each of the hemoglobins is given, and the hemoglobin in highest concentration should be given first. Therefore, heterozygous sickle cell would be designated hemoglobin AS (since hemoglobin A is usually present in greater concentration than hemoglobin S). Homozygous sickle cell would be designated hemoglobin SS. Double heterozygosity for hemoglobins S and C would be designated hemoglobin SC. A person who is heterozygous for both hemoglobin S and β-thalassemia, where the hemoglobin S concentration is greater than that of hemoglobin A, would be designated hemoglobin SA.

The term phenotype is also used to indicate the clinical features of an abnormal hemoglobin. For example, any hemoglobin characterized by decreased messenger ribonucleic acid (mRNA) synthesis can be described as having a "thalassemic phenotype."

Diagnosis of Hemoglobinopathies

The most common method used to diagnose hemoglobinopathies is hemoglobin electrophoresis, which separates hemoglobins based on differences in size and electrical charge. The initial electrophoresis is usually performed on cellulose acetate at an alkaline pH. Electrophoresis in citrate agar at an acid pH (*acid citrate electrophoresis*) is used to separate hemoglobins that migrate to the same position on alkaline electrophoresis (hemoglobin S from hemoglobin D or G; hemoglobin C from hemoglobin O or E). Other tests include sickle solubility tests, isopropanol test for unstable hemoglobins, and supravital (Heinz body) stains for denatured hemoglobins. Reference hemoglobinopathy laboratories can perform more complex tests, such as isoelectric focusing, electrophoresis of separated globin chains, or globin chain synthesis analysis; however, these tests are not widely available and will not be discussed further.

- If you are going to order hemoglobin electrophoresis, the patient should not have been transfused for at least 90 days before the test is performed because transfused blood may make interpretation of the electrophoresis difficult. Hemoglobin electrophoresis on infants can also be difficult to interpret because of the physiologic elevation in fetal hemoglobin (hemoglobin F).

Sickle Cell Anemia (Hemoglobin S)

Epidemiology

Hemoglobin S (sickle hemoglobin) is the most common hemoglobinopathy worldwide. Hemoglobin S is found most frequently in equatorial Africa and in people of African descent. In parts of Africa, approximately 10 to 40% of the population is heterozygous for hemoglobin S. Approximately 8% of African Americans are heterozygous for hemoglobin S (*sickle trait*), and approximately 1 in 400 to 600 are homozygous (*sickle cell anemia*). There are separate pockets of hemoglobin S in Turkey, along the Mediterranean coast (Sicily, southern Italy, and northern Greece), in Saudi Arabia, and in India. These are areas where falciparum malaria is endemic, suggesting that hemoglobin S arose as a protective mechanism against malaria. Based on genetic analysis, the sickle mutation appears to have arisen independently at least four different times.

Pathophysiology

The abnormality in Hb S is substitution of valine for glutamic acid at the sixth amino acid position ($\beta_6^{\text{Glu}\rightarrow\text{Val}}$). Deoxygenated hemoglobin S tends to polymerize into long rigid structures, which distort the cell into the characteristic sickle shape (Figure 6–1). Anything that causes deoxygenation of hemoglobin predisposes to sickling, including hypoxia, acidosis, and

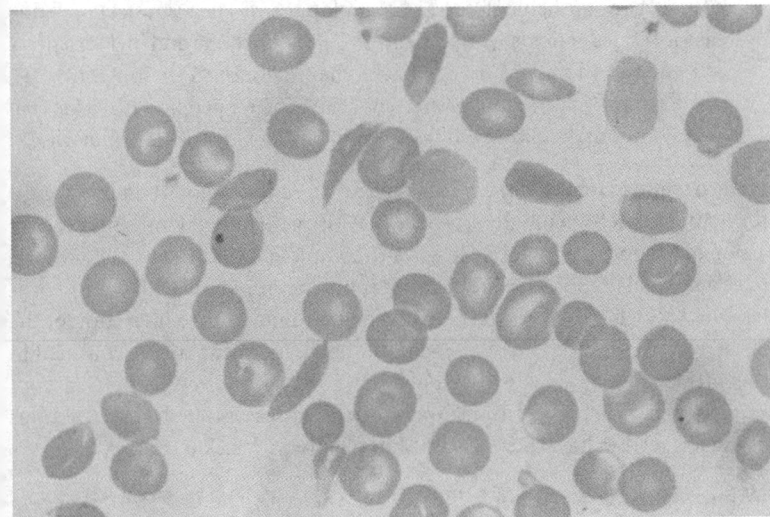

Figure 6–1 Sickle cell anemia. Note the elongated sickled erythrocytes with pointed ends. The erythrocyte center left contains a Howell-Jolly body, indicating asplenism.

increased temperature. The polymerization of hemoglobin S is reversible, and cells that have sickled may return to normal shape with re-oxygenation. However, the repeated cycles of sickling and unsickling damage the cell, and, eventually, the erythrocytes becomes irreversibly sickled. The rigid elongated sickle cells obstruct small blood vessels, resulting in tissue infarction. Sickled erythrocytes are also "sticky" and adhere to endothelial cells, predisposing to thrombosis. Common sites of infarction include the spleen, bone and bone marrow, the medulla of the kidney, mesenteric vessels, and pulmonary vessels.

⇨ There are other hemoglobin mutations that can cause sickling. All sickling hemoglobins have the same $\beta_6^{Glu \rightarrow Val}$ mutation found in typical hemoglobin S, but other sickling hemoglobin variants have additional mutations. Some of these variants have the same migration as common hemoglobin S on alkaline electrophoresis and are thus designated as hemoglobin S variants (for example, S-Travis); however, other sickling hemoglobins can have altered mobility on electrophoresis and are given different alphabet designations corresponding to their migration on alkaline electrophoresis (C-Harlem, C-Georgetown).

Clinical Manifestations and Complications of Sickle Hemoglobin

⇨ Heterozygosity for hemoglobin S (hemoglobin AS) is designated sickle cell **trait**. Sickle cell **anemia** is the preferred term for people who are homozygous for hemoglobin S (hemoglobin SS). The term sickle cell **disease** indicates patients with clinical evidence of sickling and includes sickle cell anemia (hemoglobin SS), sickle/hemoglobin C (hemoglobin SC; $\alpha_2\beta^S\beta^C$), and sickle/β-thalassemia ($\alpha_2\beta^S\beta^{Thal}$). Since people with sickle trait are asymptomatic, sickle cell **trait** is not considered a sickle cell **disease**.

Heterozygous Hemoglobin S (Sickle Trait): People who are heterozygous for hemoglobin S (hemoglobin AS; $\alpha_2\beta\beta^S$) are generally asymptomatic, have a normal blood hemoglobin level and complete blood count (CBC), and have a normal life span. Sickle cell trait is not incompatible with being a professional athlete. Microscopic hematuria is common due to infarction of the renal medulla (the very hypoxic, acidotic, and hyperosmolar environment in the renal medulla can cause even heterozygous cells to sickle). Rare cases of splenic infarcts at high altitudes and sudden death associated with strenuous physical exertion have been reported in people with sickle trait.

Homozygous Hemoglobin S (Sickle Cell Anemia): The severity of illness in sickle cell anemia (hemoglobin SS) is highly variable and can vary even within families. Many children become symptomatic in infancy after 3 to 4 months of age (before that time they are protected by the high levels of hemoglobin F). Other people have very mild disease and may not be diagnosed until adulthood. The reasons for this variability are not clear; the level of hemoglobin F is a factor (an increase in hemoglobin F decreases the severity of sickle cell disease), but other factors also appear to be important.

Sickle Cell Diseases Other Than Sickle Cell Anemia: People who are heterozygous for both hemoglobin S and some other hemoglobinopathy (hemoglobin C, hemoglobin $D_{Los\ Angeles}$ [also called D_{Punjab}], or hemoglobin O_{Arab}), or who are heterozygous for hemoglobin S and β-thalassemia, are often symptomatic and may have many of the same complications as homozygous sickle cell anemia. Patients with sickle/hemoglobin C (hemoglobin SC) tend to have less severe disease than patients with homozygous hemoglobin S; however, they have a particular predisposition to retinopathy, infarcts of the long bones, and complications during pregnancy. They tend to have mild splenomegaly, rather than the splenic infarcts typical of homozygous sickle cell. People with sickle-β$^+$ thalassemia, in which some normal β-globin chain is produced by the thalassemia gene, tend to have relatively mild disease; however, people with sickle-β° thalassemia, in which there is a complete absence of β-globin synthesis by the thalassemia gene, have severe disease that closely resembles homozygous sickle cell anemia. The presence of α-thalassemia tends to decrease the severity of sickle cell disease, possibly by decreasing the concentration of hemoglobin (and thus hemoglobin S) in the cell. Fetal hemoglobin (hemoglobin F) sterically interferes with the polymerization of hemoglobin S; therefore, anything that increases the concentration of fetal hemoglobin in erythrocytes (such as hereditary persistence of fetal hemoglobin [HPFH] and some medications) decreases the severity of sickle cell disease. Sickle cell diseases are summarized in Table 6–2.

Sickle Cell Crises

Three major categories of sickle cell complications have been designated *sickle crises*:

- **Acute vaso-occlusive (painful) crises:** Painful crises are the most common type of crisis and are believed to be caused by occlusion of small blood vessels, with consequent infarction of tissues. Pain can occur in the abdomen, bones, joints, or muscles. Young children often present with pain involving the hands or feet (the *hand-foot syndrome* or *dactylitis*); long bones and the abdomen are more common sites of pain in adults.
- **Sequestration crises:** Sequestration crisis can occur during childhood, usually during the first 3 to 4 years, before the spleen has become

Table 6–2
Sickle Cell Diseases

Severe	Mild or Moderate
Sickle cell anemia (Hb SS)	Sickle-Hb C (Hb SC)
Sickle-β^0 thalassemia*	Sickle-β^+ thalassemia†
Sickle-Hb O$_{Arab}$	Sickle-hereditary persistence of fetal
Sickle-Hb D$_{Punjab/Los Angeles}$	hemoglobin (HPFH)
	Sickle-α thalassemia

*β^0 Thalassemia: complete absence of β-globin synthesis from affected gene.
†β^+ Thalassemia: decreased synthesis of β-globin from affected gene.

infarcted. The spleen suddenly becomes enlarged and engorged with blood; this can sequester a major portion of the total blood volume and can be fatal.

- **Acute aplastic crises:** This occurs as a complication of infections, usually but not always due to **parvovirus B19**. Acute parvovirus B19 infection causes a transient halt in production of erythrocytes, which usually lasts about 5 to 7 days. In normal individuals, in which erythrocytes are being replaced at the rate of about 1% per day, the transient drop in hemoglobin is not significant. Since red cell survival is greatly decreased in patients with sickle cell anemia (10–20 days, compared with 120 days in normal individuals), the hemoglobin drops much more quickly (up to 1 g/dL per day), and without transfusions, the marked exacerbation of anemia can be fatal. Recovery of hematopoiesis usually occurs after about 7 days.

Other Complications of Sickle Cell Disease

- **Infections:** *Infections are the most common cause of death in sickle cell disease.* The risk of death from infection is highest during the first year of life but remains very high during the first 5 years. Overwhelming pneumococcal sepsis is the major risk, due to impaired splenic function and splenic autoinfarction. Starting in infancy, children with sickle cell anemia are usually maintained on penicillin prophylaxis against pneumococcal sepsis. Gram-negative rods are the most common type of infectious agent in adults. Osteomyelitis is common in patients with sickle cell anemia; sickle cell disease has a particular association with osteomyelitis due to *Salmonella*.
- **Cerebrovascular accidents:** Strokes are a major cause of morbidity in sickle cell disease, occurring in 5 to 8% of patients by the age of 14 years. They usually occur in young patients, with a median age below 10

years. Hemiplegia is a common presenting manifestation. Imaging studies indicate that many children have had subclinical undiagnosed strokes. Younger children usually have thrombotic or ischemic strokes; older teens and adults often have hemorrhagic strokes. There is a high risk of stroke recurrence (up to 50–70% within 3 years after the initial event). Chronic transfusion therapy to maintain the hemoglobin S concentration below 30% is recommended for at least 3 to 5 years after the first stroke, to prevent recurrence.

- **Acute chest syndrome (acute lung syndrome):** The acute chest syndrome is the second most common cause of hospitalization (after vaso-occlusive crises) and causes approximately 25% of the deaths from sickle cell disease. Manifestations include *pulmonary infiltrates on chest radiograph, fever, chest pain, hypoxemia, tachypnea, cough,* and *dyspnea.* Infection, fat embolism from infarcted bone marrow, other pulmonary embolism or vascular occlusions, hypoventilation and atelectasis due to rib infarcts or surgery, and pulmonary edema are all possible causes of the acute chest syndrome. Pulmonary fat embolism and other vaso-occlusive events are probably the most common causes; infection may be a precipitating factor in children but is probably not a common cause overall. The acute chest syndrome may occur after surgery or general anesthesia. Patients with recurrent episodes of acute chest syndrome may develop chronic debilitating pulmonary disease.

- **Altered splenic function and splenic infarcts:** Infants and young children with sickle cell anemia often have mild splenomegaly. Later, sickling in the spleen leads to progressive splenic infarction, and by adulthood, the spleen is typically reduced to a small fibrous nodule (*autosplenectomy*). Splenic filtering function appears to be impaired even before the spleen has become infarcted. This predisposes to overwhelming sepsis with *Streptococcus pneumoniae* and other encapsulated bacteria. Autosplenectomy is uncommon in patients with hemoglobin SC and S-β^+ thalassemia; they typically have mild splenomegaly, even as adults.

- **Renal disease:** Infarction of the medulla of the kidney is common, resulting in hematuria (gross or microscopic) and loss of concentrating ability. This can occur in people with sickle trait, as well as those with homozygous disease. Progressive glomerular fibrosis with chronic renal insufficiency or renal failure may also occur in patients with sickle cell disease but is less common.

- **Priapism:** Priapism is a common problem in males with sickle cell anemia, due to infarction of the corpora cavernosa of the penis. Repeated episodes result in impotence.

- **Gallstones:** Bilirubin (pigment) gallstones are common in sickle cell disease, due to increased hemoglobin turnover and bilirubin production; however, serious complications due to gallstones are uncommon.

- **Leg ulcers:** Chronic cutaneous leg ulcers are a common complication of sickle cell disease, usually beginning in late adolescence and early adulthood. They can be a major cause of morbidity and lost time at school and work. Healing of cutaneous ulcers is extremely slow, often requiring years.
- **Aseptic necrosis of the femoral heads:** Aseptic necrosis of the femoral heads is common in patients with sickle cell anemia and sickle/hemoglobin C (hemoglobin SC).
- **Retinopathy:** A proliferative vascular retinopathy resembling diabetic retinopathy occurs occasionally in patients with sickle cell anemia. Interestingly, it is more common in patients with the relatively milder syndromes of hemoglobin SC and S/β+-thalassemia. The retinopathy can cause vitreous hemorrhages, with consequent retinal detachment and blindness. Laser phototherapy decreases the incidence of vitreous hemorrhages and blindness.
- **Complications of pregnancy:** The maternal mortality rate is increased (~1% for each pregnancy) in women with sickle cell anemia. They also have an increased rate of spontaneous fetal loss and low birth weight infants. Pulmonary complications are a common cause of maternal morbidity in pregnancy.

Complications of sickle cell disease are summarized in Table 6–3.

Diagnosis of Sickle Hemoglobin

Patients with sickle trait have a normal CBC and blood smear. The blood hemoglobin in patients with sickle cell anemia is typically 5 to 8 g/dL. The mean corpuscular volume (MCV) is normal. The blood smear shows target cells and the characteristic sickled erythrocytes with sharply pointed ends. Cells with various other shapes ("holly leaf" cells) may also be seen. Howell-Jolly bodies may be present after splenic infarction, and nucleated red blood cells (RBCs) may be present. Smears from patients with hemoglobin SC may have a variety of RBC shapes; rectangular hemoglobin C crystals may be seen within the RBCs. Patients with S/β-thalassemia show prominent target cells and microcytosis, and the MCV is decreased.

Common tests for sickle hemoglobin include sickle solubility tests and hemoglobin electrophoresis. Sickle solubility tests depend on the decreased solubility of deoxygenated hemoglobin S in high-molarity phosphate buffers. The solubility test is usually positive if hemoglobin S comprises more than 10 to 20% of the hemoglobin. It is positive in patients with both sickle trait and sickle cell anemia and therefore cannot be used to distinguish homozygous from heterozygous hemoglobin S. Sickle solubility tests

Table 6–3

Complications of Sickle Cell Disease

Complication	Consequences
Vaso-occlusion	Painful crises: extremities (bones and joints); abdomen; aseptic necrosis of femoral heads
Autosplenectomy	Increased susceptibility to infection, particularly *S. pneumoniae*
Acute chest syndrome	
Cerebrovascular accidents	
Aplastic crises due to parvovirus B19 infection	Acute exacerbation of anemia
Infarction of renal medulla	Inability to concentrate urine; infarction of papillae; hematuria
Vaso-oclusion in and infarction of corpora cavernosa	Priapism and impotence
Chronic hemolysis	Bilirubin gallstones
Leg ulcers	
Proliferative retinopathy	Intraocular hemorrhage; retinal detachment (more common in hemoglobin SC)
Cardiomyopathy	
Restrictive lung disease	

detect all sickling hemoglobin variants (S-Travis, C-Harlem, and others). Sickle solubility tests can be used to confirm hemoglobin S detected on alkaline electrophoresis (ie, distinguish hemoglobin S from other hemoglobins that can migrate in the same position on alkaline electrophoresis but do not sickle, such as hemoglobin D or G).

⇨ Fetal hemoglobin interferes with polymerization of hemoglobin S, and the sickle solubility test can give a false-negative result if hemoglobin F makes up more than ~10 to 20% of hemoglobin in the sample. Therefore, the sickle solubility test is not reliable in infants during the first few months of life.

The other test commonly used to detect hemoglobin S is hemoglobin electrophoresis, usually performed at an alkaline pH on cellulose acetate. Electrophoresis can detect hemoglobin S in infants, who might have a false-negative sickle solubility test. It can also be used to distinguish between sickle trait and sickle cell anemia and can diagnose other sickle cell diseases such as hemoglobin SC. The relative proportions of the major hemoglobins present can be determined by densitometry on the electrophoresis gel. Typically a person with homozygous sickle cell anemia has >80% hemoglobin S, with the remainder being hemoglobin A_2 and hemoglobin F. Hemoglobin A ($\alpha_2\beta_2$) is completely absent (presuming that the patient has not been transfused). A patient with uncomplicated sickle trait always has more hemoglobin A than hemoglobin S (approximately 50–60% A, 35–40% S). If there is more S than A, you should suspect compound heterozygosity for hemoglobin S and β-thalassemia (S/β^{Thal}). A patient with S/β^0-thalassemia (complete absence of β globin synthesis) will resemble hemoglobin SS on electrophoresis (complete absence of hemoglobin A; >80% hemoglobin S) but will have microcytic RBCs on CBC. Distinguishing hemoglobin S from other nonsickling hemoglobins that can migrate at the S position on alkaline electrophoresis (ie, hemoglobins D and G) requires electrophoresis at an acid pH, usually performed on a citrate agar gel. (If the sickle solubility test is negative in a patient with a band in the S position on alkaline electrophoresis, the abnormal hemoglobin is probably either hemoglobin D or hemoglobin G).

Treatment of Sickle Cell Disease

Ideally, patients with sickle cell disease should be referred to a center that has experience treating hemoglobinopathies. General supportive measures, including folic acid supplementation and prophylactic penicillin, are important. Psychological counseling is an important adjunct. It decreases anxiety related to having a chronic and potentially lethal disease, can help patients deal with chronic pain and increase their level of function, and improves compliance with therapy.

Prophylactic penicillin has been shown to reduce mortality from *S. pneumoniae*, and should be started as soon as possible after birth and continued at least through age 5 years. Febrile episodes must be presumed to represent sepsis until proven otherwise and managed accordingly. Children should be vaccinated against *S. pneumoniae*, *Haemophilus influenzae* type b, and *Neisseria meningitidis*.

Treatment of acute painful vaso-occlusive crises is predominantly supportive; the key measures are adequate hydration and pain control. Painful episodes last 4 to 5 days on average, although the duration is highly variable. It is important to exclude other illnesses that may cause or mimic vaso-occlusive crises (osteomyelitis, other infections, stroke, acute appendicitis or other intra-abdominal processes). Many painful crises can be managed on an outpatient basis with oral hydration and analgesia. Severe or intractable crises require hospitalization and parenteral analgesia. Morphine is generlly the preferred parenteral agent for severe pain. Meperidine (Demerol) hould be avoided because seizures may occur due to accumulation of neperidine metabolites. Recently, bolus corticosteroids (methylpred-isolone) have been suggested to be beneficial; long-acting nonsteroidal nti-inflammatory agents may also be helpful. Patient-controlled anesthe-ia is a useful approach.

▷ *Pain in patients with sickle cell anemia should be managed aggressively*. It is a mistake to withhold or under-dose parenteral narcotics for fear of inducing narcotic addiction. Addiction is rare when narcotics are used appropriately.

Red cell transfusions should be considered for acute cerebrovascular ccidents, intractable or recurrent episodes of the acute chest syndrome, or riapism that does not respond to conservative measures. Exchange trans-usion allows the hemoglobin S concentration to be decreased rapidly and s helpful in such instances. Patients who have had a cerebrovascular acci-ent should be considered for chronic transfusions to maintain the hemo-lobin S level below 30% to prevent recurrence. These transfusions should e continued for at least 3 years. Patients with infections should be aggres-ively cultured and treated with antibiotics based on the results of cultures nd antibiotic sensitivity tests.

The acute chest syndrome is treated with supplemental oxygen, empiric ntibiotics pending culture results, adequate analgesia, and transfusions as eeded. Prophylaxis against acute chest syndrome in patients who have had urgery with general anesthesia includes aggressive pulmonary toilet with he use of incentive spirometers, careful fluid management to avoid pul-nonary edema, and adequate analgesia. Preoperative transfusions to attain hematocrit level ≥30% before surgery are frequently given.

An important advance in preventive therapy is the use of **hydroxyurea**. Iydroxyurea has been shown to decrease the number of painful crises, hos-italizations, red cell transfusions, and episodes of the acute chest syndrome n patients with sickle cell anemia. Hydroxyurea increases the percent of etal hemoglobin in the erythrocytes of many patients, which interferes with olymerization of hemoglobin S and therefore decreases sickling. However, ther effects of hydroxyurea (decreasing the granulocyte and reticulocyte ounts) may also be beneficial. The use of a chemotherapy drug for a non-eoplastic condition has raised a concern regarding possible carcinogenic particularly leukemogenic) potential, especially in children; however, the arcinogenic risk of hydroxyurea appears to be low, at least in the short erm. Hydroxyurea has other potential adverse effects, including myelosup-ression, which require close monitoring. Approximately 20 to 25% of atients do not have a significant increase in hemoglobin For a decrease in the number of symptomatic episodes. The decision to use hydroxyurea in patients with sickle cell disease is not a trivial one, particularly in children. Use of hydroxyurea should be restricted to those with special training and/or expertise in treating hemoglobinopathies.

Transfusion therapy in sickle cell disease: The anemia in sickle cell disease is usually well compensated and does not require transfusions. Red cell transfusion to maintain hemoglobin S levels <30% is recommended for patients who have had cerebrovascular accidents and is commonly used in acute cerebrovascular accidents, acute chest syndrome, and priapism that does not respond to conventional therapies. Preoperative transfusion to attain <30% hemoglobin S and a hematocrit level >30% is frequently used prior to major surgery. Transfusion to prevent cerebrovascular accidents has been recommended for children with increased cerebral blood flow velocity on Doppler ultrasonography, who appear to be at increased risk for stroke. Transfusion therapy is associated with significant risks, including iron overload, alloimmunization (antibodies to red cell antigens), hemolytic transfusion reactions, and infections. In many centers, it is standard to type the patient's red cells for antigens that are frequently associated with alloantibodies or hemolytic transfusion reactions, so units compatible with the patient for these antigens can be chosen. Use of leukocyte-depleted red cell units also appears to decrease the risk of alloimmunization. Iron overload requires chelation therapy with deferoxamine (Desferal).

Stem cell therapy (bone marrow transplant): Bone marrow transplant (BMT) or other hematopoietic stem cell therapy has the potential of completely reversing the abnormality in sickle cell disease. Bone marrow transplants have been performed in a number of patients, with generally favorable results. However, BMTs have had short-term mortality rates of up to 10%. Because of the possible mortality associated with BMT, transplant should be reserved for patients at increased risk of serious complications of their disease. In such patients, transplants should be performed as early as possible to prevent permanent injury.

Genetic counseling: Genetic counseling should be offered to couples considering pregnancy if both are hemoglobin S carriers or if one has sickle cell anemia and the other has either sickle trait or one of the syndromes that interact with hemoglobin S. Counseling should include the probabilities of having a child with sickle cell disease or sickle trait and the possibility of prenatal diagnosis. Prenatal diagnosis can be performed by chorionic villus sampling or amniocentesis.

Hemoglobin C

Hemoglobin C is the second most common hemoglobinopathy in the United States and the third most common worldwide. The highest prevalence of hemoglobin C is in the west coast of Africa; approximately 2 to 3% of African Americans are heterozygous for hemoglobin C (hemoglobin C trait), and homozygous hemoglobin C occurs in approximately 1 in 5,000 births in that population. Heterozygosity for both hemoglobin C and hemoglobin S occurs in approximately 1 in 800 African-American births. Like hemoglobin S, hemoglobin C is thought to have arisen as a response to malaria.

Hemoglobin C has a substitution of lysine for glutamic acid at the sixth amino acid of the β globin chain. Like hemoglobin S, hemoglobin C is capable of polymerizing into crystals when deoxygenated.

Heterozygous Hb C (hemoglobin C trait) is clinically silent. The blood hemoglobin level is usually in the normal range; the blood smear shows target cells. People with homozygous hemoglobin C (hemoglobin CC) are usually asymptomatic, with mild microcytic anemia; the blood smear shows small target cells and spherocytes (Figure 6–2).

No treatment is required for hemoglobin C trait or homozygous hemoglobin C.

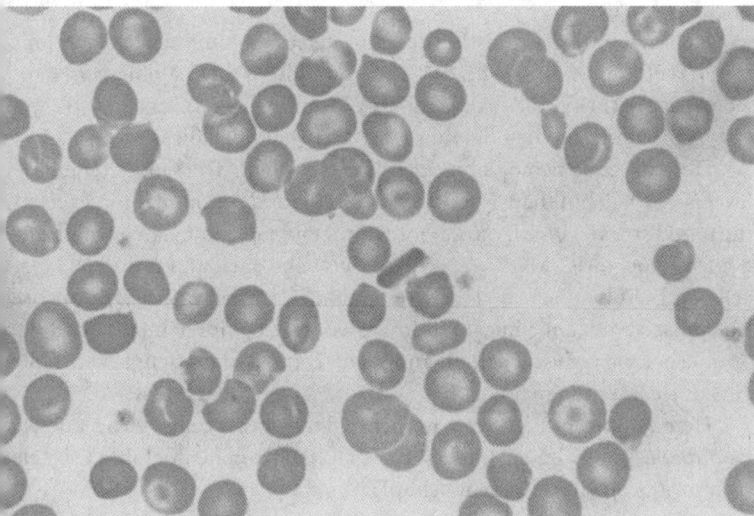

Figure 6–2 Homozygous hemoglobin C. Target cells, spherocytes, and a rectangular hemoglobin C crystal in the center of the photograph.

Compound Heterozygosity for Hemoglobin S and Hemoglobin C

People who are heterozygous for both hemoglobin S and hemoglobin (hemoglobin SC; sickle/hemoglobin C) have a spectrum of complication similar to patients with sickle cell anemia. The severity of illness is variabl but usually milder. Episodic skeletal or abdominal pains are the most com mon manifestation. They often have mild splenomegaly, but splenic infarc tion is unusual. They appear to have a slight increased risk for infection, but overwhelming pneumococcal sepsis is uncommon. Proliferativ retinopathy is a major problem in patients with hemoglobin SC, and ther is a high incidence of the acute chest syndrome during the third trimeste of pregnancy in women with hemoglobin SC. Anemia is mild or absent. Th blood smear shows prominent target cells, occasional hemoglobin C crys tals, and bizarre folded cells, but true sickled erythrocytes are uncommo

Treatment of patients with hemoglobin SC is similar to that of patient with sickle cell anemia. Because of the high incidence of proliferativ retinopathy, patients with hemoglobin SC should be periodically screene with indirect ophthalmoscopy starting in childhood.

Hemoglobin E

Hemoglobin E is the second most common hemoglobinopathy worldwid It is most common in Southeast Asia, particularly Cambodia, Laos, an Thailand. It is seen in the United States in immigrants from that area. Lik hemoglobins S and C, hemoglobin E is thought to have arisen as a conse quence of malaria.

Hemoglobin E has substitution of lysine for glutamic acid at position 2 of the β globin chain ($\beta_{26}^{Glu \to Lys}$). The mutation in the β globin gene cause a decrease in the synthesis of β^E mRNA, resulting in a thalassemia-like phe notype. In addition, hemoglobin E is somewhat unstable.

Heterozygous hemoglobin E is clinically silent. The blood hemoglobi level is normal, but there is mild microcytosis and prominent target cells o the blood smear. Homozygosity for hemoglobin E is associated with promi nent microcytosis (MCV ~55–65 fL), hypochromia, and numerous targe cells on the blood smear. The hemoglobin is normal or mildly decrease The most significant clinical syndrome associated with hemoglobin E is th double heterozygous state for hemoglobin E and β-thalassemia, which pres ents as thalassemia major.

Hemoglobin E migrates with hemoglobin C on cellulose acetate elec trophoresis at alkaline pH; it can be separated from hemoglobin C by elec trophoresis on citrate agar at acid pH.

Other Hemoglobinopathies

- **Hemoglobin D:** Hemoglobin D is actually a heterogeneous group of β globin chain mutations. The most significant variant is $D_{Los\ Angeles}$ (also known as D_{Punjab}). It is significant because heterozygotes for both hemoglobin S and $D_{Los\ Angeles}$ have a sickling illness resembling sickle cell anemia. Hemoglobin D migrates with hemoglobin S on cellulose acetate electrophoresis and with hemoglobin A on citrate agar electrophoresis.

- **Hemoglobin G:** Hemoglobin G is also heterogeneous and includes both α and β globin chain mutations. The most common hemoglobin G variant in the United States is $G_{Philadelphia}$, which is an α chain mutation that occurs in African Americans. Hemoglobin G is not usually associated with significant anemia or other clinical problems; hemoglobin G does *not* interact with hemoglobin S. The electrophoresis pattern of hemoglobin G is similar to that of hemoglobin D.

- **Hemoglobin Lepore:** Hemoglobin Lepore is a fusion protein caused by a crossing over between the genes for the δ globin and the β globin chains. It is synthesized at the low level of the δ chain of hemoglobin A_2 (usually less than about 3%), rather than at the rate of the β globin chain of hemoglobin A, and thus presents with a thalassemic phenotype. Hemoglobin Lepore migrates with S on cellulose acetate electrophoresis but does not sickle.

THE THALASSEMIAS

The thalassemias are characterized by a **quantitative abnormality of globin chain synthesis**. Classic thalassemia is characterized by a complete lack of globin chain synthesis or a decreased amount of a structurally normal globin chain, but some structural hemoglobinopathies also have decreased globin chain synthesis and thus present as thalassemia. The genetic mutation in thalassemia results in the absence of mRNA production from the involved gene, production of a nonfunctional mRNA, or production of an unstable mRNA that is prematurely degraded. The end result is decreased synthesis of the involved globin chain. Thalassemias are, as a group, probably the most common genetic diseases in the world.

The thalassemias are extremely heterogeneous, both in clinical manifestations and molecular (genetic) basis. Hundreds of different mutations have been identified in patients with thalassemia. The majority of thalassemias involve either the α or β globin chains. Cases involving both the δ and β globin chains (δβ thalassemia) or all three β-like chains (γδβ thalassemia) do occur but are rare. There is a high prevalence of thalassemia in areas with endemic malaria, including parts of Africa, the Mediterranean basin, the Middle East, India, Southeast Asia, and southern China (the "thalassemia belt"). Epidemiologic evidence suggests that the thalassemias arose as a defense against malarial infection, but the mechanism of protection is not well understood. Since there is significant overlap between the areas of high prevalence of thalassemia and hemoglobin S and thalassemia and hemoglobin E, people who are heterozygous for thalassemia and either hemoglobin S or hemoglobin E are not uncommon. These hemoglobins can interact with thalassemia, causing clinical symptoms.

The decrease in globin chain synthesis has two consequences:

- **Decreased hemoglobin synthesis**, resulting in anemia and microcytosis
- **Aggregation of the excess free globin chains** produced by the non-thalassemic gene (α chains in the case of β-thalassemia; β chains in the case of α-thalassemia). The aggregates of unpaired globin chains attach to and damage the erythrocyte cell membrane, resulting in hemolysis.

In severe cases, the majority of erythroid precursors are destroyed in the marrow (*ineffective erythropoiesis*). Those that escape into the circulation are prematurely destroyed by macrophages in the spleen and liver.

Complications of Thalassemias

The complications of thalassemia are related to four factors:

- **Chronic anemia:** Chronic anemia causes growth retardation, delayed sexual maturation, cardiac dilatation and congestive heart failure, decreased work capacity, and all of the other complications associated with chronic anemia.
- **Marked expansion of the bone marrow:** The bone marrow becomes greatly expanded due to marked erythroid hyperplasia. Widening of the diploic spaces in the skull gives a characteristic "crewcut" or "hair on end" appearance on radiographs. Hypertrophy of the frontal bones results in frontal bossing. Hypertrophy of the maxillae results in prominent cheeks and dental malocclusions, giving a characteristic "chipmunk" facies. Thinning of the cortex of the vertebrae and long bones results in fractures. Extramedullary hematopoiesis causes enlargement of the spleen and liver. Foci of extramedullary hematopoiesis may occur in soft tissues (*myeloid tumors*), and paravertebral masses may cause spinal cord compression.
- **Iron overload:** There is chronic hyperabsorption of iron by the gastrointestinal tract, driven by the chronic erythropoiesis, and this is exacerbated by RBC transfusions. Iron deposition in the heart causes cardiomyopathy and cardiac arrhythmias. Deposition in the liver causes portal fibrosis and may result in hepatic cirrhosis. Patients with

hepatic cirrhosis are at risk of developing hepatocellular carcinoma (hepatoma).

- **Chronic hemolysis:** Chronic hemolysis causes splenomegaly, hepatomegaly, and bilirubin gallstones. Hypersplenism may develop, increasing transfusion requirements.

The clinical manifestations of the different types of thalassemia (α versus β) are generally similar; however, there are differences in the epidemiology and pathophysiology of α and β thalassemia, and these will be described separately.

α-Thalassemia

Pathophysiology

Most cases of α-thalassemia are due to deletions in the α globin genes. There are two genes for the α globin chain on chromosome 16; the mutation may involve only one or both α genes on each chromosome. The haplotype (single chromosome) is indicated by $\alpha\alpha$/ (normal), -α/ (one gene mutation), or -- (two gene mutation). Since each person has four α genes, there can be a deletion in one, two, three, or all four α genes. The severity of illness depends on the number of α genes with mutations.

- **Single-gene mutation** (-α/$\alpha\alpha$): Clinically silent, without microcytosis or anemia
- **Two-gene mutation** (-α/-α or --$\alpha\alpha$; α-**thalassemia minor** or α-**thalassemia trait**): Mild microcytic anemia; serious complications are uncommon
- **Three-gene mutation** (--/-α; **hemoglobin H disease**): Moderately severe, microcytic anemia. The excess β chains precipitate as β_4 tetramers (hemoglobin H). The clinical picture is variable; patients may or may not have splenomegaly, iron overload, and the skeletal complications seen in severe thalassemia.
- **Four-gene mutation** (--/--; **hydrops fetalis**): Incompatible with life. Most pregnancies spontaneously terminate prematurely. Those infants that survive to delivery have gross anasarca and usually die of congestive heart failure shortly after birth. There is a high incidence of maternal preeclampsia during the pregnancy.

Epidemiology

α-Thalassemia is found around the Mediterranean basin (including Greece and Italy), West Africa, the Middle East (particularly Saudi Arabia), China, and Southeast Asia. The highest frequency is in Southeast Asia and western

Africa. Approximately 3 to 6% of African Americans carry a gene for α-tha-lassemia. The common haplotype in Africa and African Americans is a sin-gle gene mutation (-α/). Mutation of both α genes on the same chromo-some is rare. Therefore, the most common phenotypes in African Americans are single-gene mutation (-α/αα; asymptomatic) or two-gene mutation (-α/-α; mild anemia). Three- or four-gene mutations are uncommon. In Asia however, both one- and two-gene mutations (-α/ and −−/) on the same chromosome are common, and therefore three- (−−/ = α) and four- (−/−) gene mutations (hemoglobin H disease and hydrops fetalis) are distressingly common.

β-Thalassemia

Pathophysiology

There is a single gene for the β globin chain on chromosome 11. Most mutations in β-thalassemia are single-nucleotide substitutions. The muta-tion may result in a complete lack of β chain synthesis (**βº-thalassemia**) or a decrease in β chain synthesis (**β⁺-thalassemia**). The severity of illness depends on how much β chain is synthesized and whether the person is het-erozygous or homozygous for the mutation. The β-thalassemias have been divided into three main clinical syndromes:

- **β-Thalassemia minor** (Figure 6–3): Heterozygosity for β-thalassemia results in a mild clinical syndrome designated β-thalassemia minor. The hemoglobin and the MCV are mildly or moderately decreased (hemoglobin ~9–12 g/dL and MCV ~65–75 fL), and the patient has few symptoms or complications.
- **β-Thalassemia major (Cooley's anemia)** (Figure 6–4): Homozygosity for β-thalassemia results in a severe clinical syndrome characterized by severe anemia and microcytosis (hemoglobin ~3–5 g/dL and MCV <65 fL), total or near total absence of Hb A, marked ineffective erythro-poiesis, marked expansion of the bone marrow with skeletal complica-tions, splenomegaly, and iron overload due to hyperabsorption of iron.
- **β-Thalassemia intermedia:** β-Thalassemia intermedia is *homozygous β-thalassemia that is not transfusion dependent.* It is genetically and clin-ically heterogeneous. The hemoglobin is intermediate between β-tha-lassemia major and minor (~6–9 g/dL), as is the incidence of clinical complications.

(A fourth category, β-*thalassemia minima*, is sometimes added for patients who have a normal CBC but are identified as having β-thalassemia based on screening or family studies.)

Epidemiology

β-Thalassemia is most common around the Mediterranean basin, particularly Greece and Italy. It is also found in northern and western Africa, the Middle East, India, China, and parts of Southeast Asia, although α-thalassemia is more common in these areas. The most common haplotype in Africa is β^+-thalassemia. Mutations producing complete absence of β chain synthesis (β^o) are more common around the Mediterranean basin.

Diagnosis of Thalassemia

A microcytic anemia that is not due to iron deficiency is most likely thalassemia. The first step after identification of a microcytic anemia is to check the serum ferritin or serum iron/transferrin/transferrin saturation. If the results do not indicate iron deficiency, start a workup for thalassemia. Evaluation for thalassemia includes consideration of ethnic background and family history, examination of a well-stained blood smear, and hemoglobin electrophoresis.

The blood smear in mild thalassemia shows microcytosis, hypochromia, and target cells. There may be basophilic stippling (see Figure 6–3). In more severe cases, there is marked microcytosis and anisocytosis, bizarre poikilocytes, polychromasia, and nucleated erythrocytes (see Figure 6–4).

β-Thalassemia is generally diagnosed by the presence of increased hemoglobin A_2 on hemoglobin electrophoresis. Hemoglobin F is often also

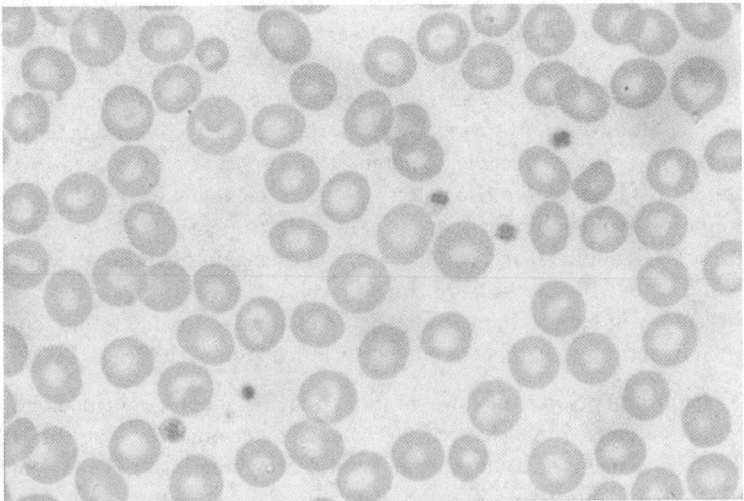

Figure 6–3 Thalassemia minor. Spherocytes and basophilic stippling in one erythrocyte.

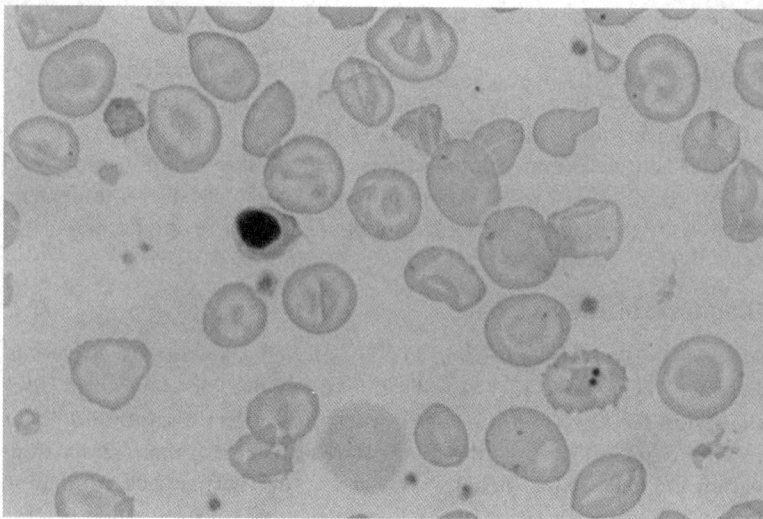

Figure 6–4 β-Thalassemia major (Cooley's anemia). Note the bizarre erythrocyte morphology and the nucleated erythrocyte.

slightly increased. The mean hemoglobin A_2 level in β-thalassemia is about 5% (normal is less than about 3%).

α-Thalassemia trait (two gene mutation) is generally diagnosed by exclusion: a microcytic anemia that is not due to iron deficiency and has a normal hemoglobin A_2 is most likely α-thalassemia. The hemoglobin electrophoresis is normal, except for the first few weeks of life, when γ_4 tetramers (hemoglobin Bart's) is present. A clue to thalassemia is that the erythrocyte count tends to be relatively high for the degree of anemia, in contrast to iron deficiency anemia, for which the erythrocyte count is usually low. Study of family members can also be helpful in confirming the suspicion of α-thalassemia. Hemoglobin H disease can be diagnosed by the presence of hemoglobin H on electrophoresis; hemoglobin H is the fastest migrating hemoglobin on cellulose acetate electrophoresis. The aggregates of excess β globin chains can be visualized by making a smear after incubating a blood sample with brilliant cresyl blue. Under the microscope, erythrocytes will have a characteristic golf ball appearance due to numerous small inclusions that appear evenly distributed around the cell.

➪ **Laboratory Note:** The concentrations of hemoglobin A or hemoglobin S (in patients with sickle cell) are usually determined by densitometry measurements on routine hemoglobin electrophoresis gels. Hemoglobins A_2 or F cannot be accurately determined by densitometry on electrophoresis. Hemoglobin A_2 can be determined by column chromatography, and hemoglobin F can be determined by alkali insolubility. Both can be determined by high-performance liquid chromatography (HPLC).

⇨ **Laboratory Note:** To detect hemoglobin H by electrophoresis, it is important to lyse the erythrocytes with water and use centrifugation to precipitate cell membranes and other debris. If you use an organic solvent such as chloroform to clean up the hemoglobin preparation, the hemoglobin H will be removed and the electrophoresis will be normal.

Prenatal Diagnosis of Thalassemia

Molecular analysis of the globin genes for thalassemia can be done on amniotic cells obtained by amniocentesis or on chorionic villus cells obtained by chorionic villus biopsy.

Treatment of Thalassemia

The cornerstones of thalassemia therapy are *red cell transfusion* and *iron chelation*. Patients with thalassemia minor usually do not require transfusion or other specific therapy. Patients with thalassemia intermedia or hemoglobin H disease may or may not require transfusions to prevent complications of anemia and erythroid hyperplasia. Patients with severe thalassemia are frequently maintained on hypertransfusion regimens— periodic red cell transfusions to maintain the blood hemoglobin >9 to 10 g/dL (some centers try to keep the hemoglobin ≥12 g/dL). This prevents the skeletal complications of thalassemia by shutting off the erythropoietin-driven erythroid hyperplasia, allows normal growth and sexual development, and delays the onset of splenomegaly. A typical transfusion requirement is one to three donor units every 3 to 5 weeks. Complications of transfusion include alloimmunization, iron overload, and transfusion-transmitted infections, particularly viral hepatitis. Alloimmunization can be prevented by phenotyping the patient's red cells for cell surface antigens and selecting units for transfusion that are matched for important antigens.

Iron overload is a serious complication of transfusion therapy (each red cell unit contains 200–250 mg of iron), and chelation therapy is required to prevent the development of secondary hemochromatosis. Deferoxamine is currently the only iron chelation agent licensed for use in the United States. Patients usually start continuous subcutaneous infusions of deferoxamine in the evening and continue overnight. This mobilizes the iron so that it is excreted in the urine. Deferoxamine can cause painful reactions at the site of injection. Other possible side effects include cataracts and hearing loss; therefore, periodic hearing and eye examinations are recommended. If hearing or visual loss is detected, the deferoxamine is discontinued until the sensory abnormality resolves.

Splenomegaly eventually develops in patients with severe thalassemia even with transfusion therapy, and splenectomy will be required. The usual indication for splenectomy is an increase in transfusion requirement. Patients should be immunized against *S. pneumoniae*, *H. influenzae*, and *N. meningitidis* prior to splenectomy.

Bone marrow transplant is potentially curative for thalassemia. Patients with related HLA-matched donors and severe thalassemia should be considered for BMT early, before serious complications occur (particularly before hepatic fibrosis or hepatomegaly develop).

Thalassemia Variants and Related Conditions

Other variants of classic thalassemia include $\delta\beta$-thalassemia and $\gamma\delta\beta$-thalassemia. The level of fetal hemoglobin is markedly increased in $\delta\beta$-thalassemia, and most cases are clinically mild. $\gamma\delta\beta$-Thalassemia presents as a severe neonatal hemolytic anemia, which slowly evolves into relatively mild β-thalassemia.

Some structurally abnormal hemoglobins are synthesized in decreased quantity and thus have the clinical features of thalassemia. Hemoglobin E, hemoglobin $G_{Philadelphia}$, and hemoglobin Lepore were mentioned in the section on structural hemoglobinopathies. **Hemoglobin Constant Spring** is another abnormal hemoglobin that causes a thalassemic phenotype; it is caused by a mutation in the translation termination codon of the α chain, which results in the addition of 31 extra amino acids at the end of the protein. The mutation results in markedly decreased synthesis of the involved protein. Hemoglobin Constant Spring, in combination with other α-thalassemia mutations, is a relatively common cause of α-thalassemia minor and hemoglobin H disease in Southeast Asia and southern China.

Hereditary Persistence of Fetal Hemoglobin

Hereditary persistence of fetal hemoglobin (**HPFH**) is a heterogeneous group of conditions associated with the persistence of a high level of fetal hemoglobin (hemoglobin F) into adulthood. It is relatively common in parts of Africa and the Middle East and is also found in Italy and Greece. Synthesis of hemoglobin A and hemoglobin A_2 is greatly decreased, but the persistence of hemoglobin F results in mild or no anemia. Hereditary Persistence of Fetal Hemoglobin can interact with hemoglobin S and thalassemia, resulting in decreased severity of disease. Some cases are caused by mutation of both the δ and β globin genes; therefore, HPFH is usually discussed in association with the thalassemias.

RED CELL ENZYME DEFECTS

Some defects in erythrocyte metabolic enzymes are associated with hemolytic anemia. By far the most common of these is glucose-6-phosphate dehydrogenase (G6PD) deficiency. Running a distant second is pyruvate kinase deficiency. Deficiencies of other metabolic enzymes are extremely rare.

Glucose-6-Phosphate Dehydrogenase Deficiency

Epidemiology

Glucose-6-phosphate dehydrogenase deficiency is one of the most common genetic diseases in the world, affecting hundreds of millions of people. The gene for G6PD is located on the X chromosome, so G6PD deficiency is inherited as an X-linked trait. As for all X-linked traits, men develop the disease, whereas women are usually asymptomatic carriers. The highest prevalence of G6PD deficiency occurs in parts of Africa, around the Mediterranean basin, and in Southeast Asia, but it is found worldwide. Approximately 12% of African-American men have G6PD deficiency, up to 20% of African-American women are carriers, and perhaps 1% are homozygous or doubly heterozygous for two different G6PD mutations.

Glucose-6-Phosphate Dehydrogenase Deficiency is most common in areas of endemic malaria, and it (like sickle hemoglobin and the thalassemias) probably arose as a defense mechanism against malaria.

Pathophysiology

Glucose-6-Phosphate Dehydrogenase Deficiency is the first enzyme in the hexose monophosphate shunt, which is required to generate the reduced form of nicotinamide adenine dinucleotide phosphate (NADPH) (see Figure 3–1). NADPH is required for the regeneration of glutathione by the enzyme glutathione reductase. In the absence of sufficient glutathione, hemoglobin is oxidized and precipitates in the cell. This damages the cell, resulting in hemolysis. The aggregates of oxidized hemoglobin are plucked out of the cell by the spleen, resulting in characteristic "bite" or "blister" cells. The level of G6PD is highest in reticulocytes and declines with increasing age of the red cell. In normal cells, the half-life of the enzyme is approximately 62 days. The activity level of the enzyme remains sufficient to protect against oxidative stress even in older cells. In patients with G6PD deficiency, the enzyme level declines faster, so older cells are not protected against oxidative stress. In the common African variant, with a half-life of approximately 13 days, enzyme activity remains high enough to prevent increased hemolysis in the baseline condition; however, hemolysis occurs if there is increased oxidative stress, such as oxidative drugs or chemicals. In the common Mediterranean variant, the half-life of the enzyme is measured in hours, and there may be chronic hemolysis even in the absence of increased oxidative stress.

Hundreds of different G6PD variants have been identified. They are classified based on the level of enzyme activity and the severity of hemolysis and anemia:

- **Class I variants:** Severe enzyme deficiency (<10% of normal) and chronic hemolysis
- **Class II variants:** Severe enzyme deficiency, but intermittent instead of chronic hemolysis
- **Class III variants:** Mild to moderate enzyme deficiency (10–60% of normal), with intermittent hemolysis usually precipitated by infection or oxidative drugs or chemicals
- **Class IV variants:** Normal enzyme activity and no anemia or hemolysis
- **Class V variants:** Increased enzyme activity, without anemia or hemolysis

Clinical Manifestations of G6PD Deficiency

The clinical severity of G6PD deficiency is variable. The majority of patients are not anemic and have no hemolysis in the baseline state; a minority of patients have chronic, ongoing hemolysis. It is likely that the majority of people with G6PD deficiency are never diagnosed as such.

The common African variant is a class III deficiency. Under normal conditions, patients have no hemolysis or anemia. Episodes of hemolysis may be precipitated by infection, oxidative drugs or chemicals, surgery, and acidosis. *Infections are probably the most common cause of hemolytic episodes.* Most infection-associated hemolytic episodes are self-limited and mild, although fulminant hemolysis with disseminated intravascular coagulation and acute renal failure can occur. Drugs and chemicals that can cause hemolysis include primaquine and other antimalarial agents, sulfa antibiotics, naphthalene (mothballs) and phenazopyridine (Pyridium) (Table 6–4). Episodes of hemolysis are indicated by sudden onset of jaundice, pallor, dark urine, and abdominal or back pain. The hemoglobin level typically drops about 3 to 4 g/dL. The blood smear may show "bite" and "blister" cells, polychromasia, schistocytes, and microspherocytes (Figure 6–5). Serum bilirubin and lactic dehydrogenase levels are increased; haptoglobin is decreased. A reticulocyte response becomes evident at about 5 days and is maximal at 10 days. Since reticulocytes have protective G6PD levels, hemolysis stops, and the hemoglobin returns to normal after about 2 to 4 weeks even if the oxidative drug is continued.

The common variant in Caucasians (G6PD Mediterranean) is a class II variant. Erythrocytes show severely depressed G6PD activity, but most patients do not have chronic hemolysis. They may experience episodes of

Table 6–4
G6PD Deficiency: Drugs and Chemicals That May Cause Hemolysis

Unsafe for Class I, II, and III Variants		Probably Safe for Class II and III Variants*	
Acetanilid	Primaquine	Acetaminophen	Pyrimethamine
Furazolidone	Sulfa antibiotics	Aspirin	Isoniazid
Nalidixic acid	Thiazolsulfone	Ascorbic acid	Phenacetin
Naphthalene	Toluidine blue	Chloramphenicol	Phenytoin
Nitrofurantoin	Trinitrotoluene	Chloroquine	Quinidine
Phenazopyridine	Doxorubicin	Diphenhydramine	Quinine
Phenylhydrazine		Vitamin K	

*Safe at normal therapeutic doses; may not be safe for Class I deficiency.
Adapted from Glader BE, Lukens JN. Glucose-6-phosphate dehydrogenase deficiency and related disorders of hexose monophosphate shunt and glutathione metabolism. In: Lee RG, Foerster J, Lukens J, editors. Wintrobe's clinical hematology. 10th ed. Baltimore: Williams & Wilkins; 1999. p. 1176–90.

hemolysis similar to those in patients with the African variant, precipitated by the same conditions. However, unlike the African variant, reticulocytes are not protected against oxidative stress, and the patients will have hemolysis until the oxidative drug or other precipitating cause is removed. **Uncooked fava beans** are a notorious cause of hemolysis in patients with G6PD Mediterranean (*favism*). Fava beans will not cause hemolysis in most African Americans or other patients with class III variants. The reaction to fava beans is curiously variable; only a minority of patients with G6PD Mediterranean experience hemolysis with fava beans, and those who do on one occasion may not experience hemolysis on re-exposure.

Severe (class I) G6PD-deficient variants are uncommon. They are usually very unstable and have very low catalytic activity. They may be associated with congenital nonspherocytic hemolytic anemia. Anemia and jaundice are often noted in neonates; exchange transfusion may be required due to hyperbilirubinemia. As patients get older, they have a chronic mild to moderate anemia, with hemoglobin ~8 to 10 g/dL and reticulocyte count ~10 to 15%. Infections, oxidative drugs, or fava beans can cause acute exacerbations of hemolysis. Parvovirus B19 infections can cause episodes of aplastic anemia similar to those seen in patients with sickle cell anemia.

⇨ The G6PD enzyme is also involved in the production of hydrogen peroxide (H_2O_2) and superoxide (O_2^-) for microbial killing action of neutrophils, and it might therefore be expected that patients with G6PD deficiency would also have impaired neutrophil function. In fact, this is

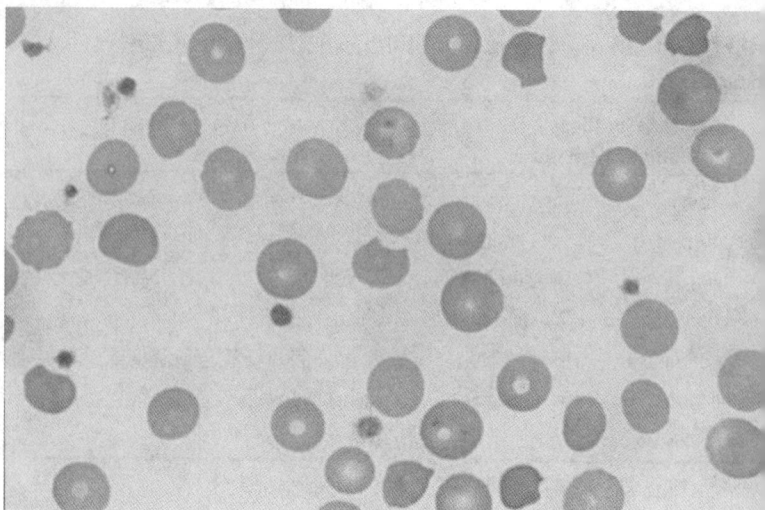

Figure 6–5 Glucose-6-phosphate dehydrogenase deficiency. Note the "bite" cell in the center of the field.

uncommon, although a few patients with class I deficiencies are predisposed to infection due to deficiency in neutrophil killing.

Diagnosis of Glucose-6-Phosphate Dehydrogenase Deficiency

Glucose-6-Phosphate Dehydrogenase deficiency should be an important consideration in any case of acute nonimmune hemolytic anemia. The peripheral smear should be examined for 'bite" or "blister" cells and cells with eccentric "puddles" of hemoglobin; however, the smear is often surprisingly normal. There is an easy fluorescent screening test for NADPH production from glucose-6-phosphate and NADP. If this test is abnormal, a quantitative assay can be performed to confirm the diagnosis and assess the severity of the deficiency.

➫   The G6PD level can be normal in a patient with G6PD deficiency shortly after a hemolytic episode, giving a false-negative result. This occurs if the reticulocyte count is high since reticulocytes have higher G6PD levels than older cells. If you get a normal G6PD level in a patient who you *really* think has G6PD deficiency, repeat the laboratory test in a few weeks.

Treatment of Glucose-6-Phosphate Dehydrogenase Deficiency

The main treatment for G6PD deficiency is to *avoid conditions that predispose to hemolysis.* Patients with G6PD deficiency should not be given medications that cause hemolysis; they should be advised to avoid exposure to naphthalene (mothballs), fava beans, and other hemolytic agents. Infections should be treated promptly. Infants with marked hyperbilirubinemia may require exchange transfusions. Women known to be heterozygous for G6PD deficiency should avoid oxidative drugs while pregnant and nursing to prevent inducing hemolytic episodes in a susceptible fetus or infant.

Pyruvate Kinase Deficiency

Epidemiology

Pyruvate kinase (PK) deficiency is the second most common RBC enzymopathy and the most common enzyme deficiency in the Embden-Meyerhof (glycolytic) pathway (see Figure 3–1). However, it is far less common than G6PD deficiency. It occurs most commonly in people of Northern European and Mediterranean descent. It is inherited in an autosomal recessive manner.

Pathophysiology

Erythrocytes with PK deficiency generate less adenosine triphosphate (ATP) and NADH from glucose. There is decreased Na^+,K^+-ATPase activity, with consequent cellular dehydration. The exact mechanism of hemolysis is unknown, but it is thought that there are abnormalities in membrane function. 2,3-Diphosphoglycerate (DPG) accumulates in RBCs; since increased 2,3-DPG facilitates O_2 unloading, patients tolerate anemia well and are relatively asymptomatic despite decreased blood hemoglobin.

Clinical Manifestations

Neonatal hyperbilirubinemia is common and may require exchange transfusion. Older children and adults have chronic hemolysis, which can vary from mild and compensated to severe and transfusion requiring. Splenomegaly is common. Infections, surgery, and pregnancy may precipitate acute exacerbations of hemolysis. Aplastic crises may occur due to infection with parvovirus B19.

Diagnosis of Pyruvate Kinase Deficiency

A variety of enzyme assays are available. It may be difficult to demonstrate decreased enzyme activity if cells with the most severe deficiency are largely destroyed and cells with higher enzyme levels are relatively preserved. It may be helpful to study relatives, although there is overlap in enzyme levels between heterozygotes and the normal population.

Treatment of Pyruvate Kinase Deficiency

Exchange transfusion may be required for neonatal hyperbilirubinemia. Many older patients tolerate the anemia well and do not require specific therapy. Patients with more severe hemolysis may require transfusion support. Splenectomy can be beneficial in severe cases; it results in striking reticulocytosis (up to 50–60%).

Other Erythrocyte Enzymopathies

Other RBC enzyme deficiencies are extremely rare. Often only a few individuals or families with the deficiency have been described. Some patients with deficiencies of enzymes in the glycolytic pathway have neurologic manifestations, as well as hematologic disease (Table 6–5).

ERYTHROCYTE MEMBRANE DEFECTS

Abnormalities in the red cell membrane can result in hemolytic anemia of variable severity, ranging from mild anemia not requiring treatment to

Table 6–5
Uncommon RBC Enzymopathies

Enzyme	Inheritance	Hematologic Manifestations	Other Manifestations
Glucose phosphoisomerase (GPI)	Autosomal recessive	Neonatal hyperbilirubinemia; hemolytic anemia of variable severity	
Glutathione synthetase	Autosomal recessive	Hemolytic anemia	Metabolic acidosis in some cases
Hexokinase	Autosomal recessive	Hemolytic anemia	
Phosphofructokinase	Autosomal recessive	Hemolytic anemia	Glycogen storage disease
Aldolase	Autosomal recessive	Hemolytic anemia	Glycogen storage disease
Phosphoglycerokinase	X-linked	Hemolytic anemia	Mental retardation; myoglobinuria
Triosephosphate isomerase	Autosomal recessive	Hemolytic anemia	Progressive neurologic abnormalities
Pyrimidine 5' nucleotidase	Autosomal recessive	Hemolytic anemia with prominent basophilic stippling	

chronic transfusion-dependent anemia. These membrane defects mostly result from deficient anchoring of the cell cytoskeleton to the cell membrane or from abnormalities in the cytoskeleton proteins. The most common inherited membrane defects are **hereditary spherocytosis**, **hereditary elliptocytosis**, and **hereditary pyropoikilocytosis** (Table 6–6).

The Red Cell Membrane

The red cell membrane consists of three main components:

- A **phospholipid bilayer**
- Various **integral membrane proteins** and **glycoproteins** embedded in the phospholipid bilayer, some of which extend through the membrane into the cytoplasm (transmembrane proteins). Two of the most important of these cell transmembrane proteins are the **band 3 protein**, an important anion transport protein, and **glycophorin**, which carries red cell antigens. Both of these proteins also serve as anchoring sites for cytoskeleton proteins.
- A **cytoskeleton scaffold**, which gives the red cell its characteristic shape. The cytoskeleton is composed predominantly of **spectrin**.

There are two types of spectrin, designated α and β. One α spectrin spontaneously pairs with one β spectrin to form a heterodimer pair; two α/β heterodimers then join together to form a tetramer. One end of the spectrin tetramer anchors to the phospholipid bilayer at the band 3 molecule, at a structure called the **junctional complex**. The other end of the tetramer anchors to glycophorin. A protein called **ankyrin** is required to bind spectrin to the band 3 protein.

Hereditary Spherocytosis

Epidemiology

Hereditary spherocytosis (HS) is the *most common inherited hemolytic anemia in people of Northern European descent*. Most cases (approximately three-fourths) are inherited in an **autosomal dominant** fashion. The remainder of cases are inherited as autosomal recessive, which are often more severe. A significant number of patients have no family history of the illness and probably represent new mutations. The prevalence of HS in Western countries has been estimated as 1 in approximately 5,000. Hereditary spherocytosis also occurs in Asia and Africa, but its prevalence in these areas is unknown.

Table 6–6
Erythrocyte Membrane Defects

Disorder	Inheritance	Proteins Involved	Hematologic Manifestations	Treatment
Hereditary spherocytosis (HS)	Autosomal dominant (majority)	Ankyrin most common; β spectrin, α spectrin, band 3 protein, others	Spherocytes; increased osmotic fragility; majority have mild to moderate anemia but may have exacerbations; autosomal recessive cases more severe	Folic acid; splenectomy for severe cases
Hereditary elliptocytosis (HE)	Autosomal dominant	α Spectrin most common	Elliptocytes; majority asymptomatic, without anemia; occasional severe anemia in infancy	None in majority of cases
Hereditary pyropoikilo-cytosis (HPP)	Autosomal recessive	α Spectrin most common	Microcytosis, poikilocytosis, RBC fragments; moderate to severe anemia	Splenectomy
Spherocytic elliptocytosis	Autosomal dominant	Unknown	Moderate hemolytic anemia; elliptocytes and spherocytes on smear; increased osmotic fragility	Splenectomy for severe cases
Southeast Asian ovalocytosis	Autosomal dominant	Band 3 protein	No hemolysis or anemia; increased resistance to malarial infection	None

Pathophysiology

The fundamental cause in most cases of HS is *defective vertical attachment* between the phospholipid bilayer and the cytoskeleton scaffold. Hereditary spherocytosis is genetically and clinically heterogeneous; the majority of cases result from mutations in the gene for **ankyrin**. Other cases result from abnormalities in β spectrin, α spectrin, the band 3 protein, or other proteins. Autosomal recessive HS is usually due to mutations in the α spectrin gene.

The result of the defective vertical attachment of the phospholipid bilayer to the cytoskeleton is *loss of phospholipids from the cell membrane*. Consequently, the surface area of the RBC decreases, and the cell gradually assumes the shape of a sphere (the shape with the highest volume to surface area ratio). Spherocytic RBCs are less flexible than normal (biconcave disk) RBCs, and, consequently, they are selectively trapped and destroyed in the spleen. The spleen also plays an important role in the loss of cell membranes by the RBCs (a process known as *splenic conditioning*). An additional metabolic stress on the RBCs in HS is increased permeability to Na^+ and K^+ cations; consequently, the Na^+,K^+-ATPase pump is constantly running at a high rate, and the cells have an increased requirement for glucose. The cells also tend to become dehydrated.

Clinical Manifestations

The clinical manifestations of HS are highly variable, from asymptomatic without anemia to severe chronic hemolysis. Neonatal hyperbilirubinemia is frequent and may require exchange transfusion. The majority of older patients have relatively mild or moderate anemia, and the primary manifestations are hyperbilirubinemia (which may be intermittent) and mild splenomegaly. Bilirubin gallstones are common. Like other patients with chronic hemolytic anemias, patients with HS may have exacerbation of anemia associated with infections, aplastic crises due to parvovirus B19 infection, or megaloblastic anemia associated with folate deficiency.

Patients with autosomal recessive HS may have severe anemia, with hemoglobin as low as 4 to 6 g/dL.

Diagnosis of Hereditary Spherocytosis

The CBC shows a MCV that is normal to slightly low, with an increased mean corpuscular hemoglobin concentration (MCHC). The blood smear shows microspherocytes (Figure 6–6). The reticulocyte count is increased (~5–20%). A direct antiglobulin (Coombs') test should be done to exclude an immune hemolytic anemia.

- *A hemolytic anemia with spherocytes but a negative direct antiglobulin test is most likely HS.*

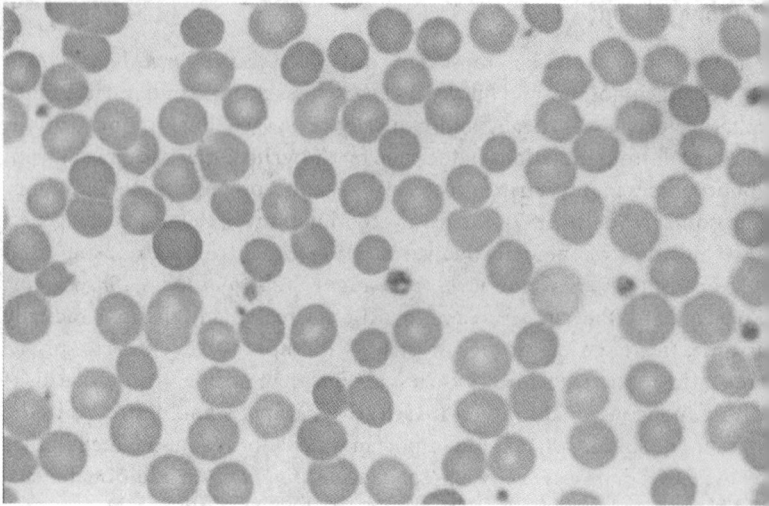

Figure 6–6 Hereditary spherocytosis blood smear. Note the presence of spherocytes.

The classic laboratory test for HS is the **osmotic fragility test**. In this test, erythrocytes are incubated in saline solutions with osmolality ranging from normal to pure water. Percent hemolysis is measured by spectrophotometry. Erythrocytes from patients with HS hemolyze at higher saline concentrations than normal cells. The difference is exaggerated by incubating the cells for 24 hours in the absence of glucose. There may be a component of cells that lyse at nearly normal osmotic pressures, called the "osmotically sensitive tail." This represents cells that have just undergone splenic conditioning and disappears after splenectomy.

- It is important to remember that *increased osmotic fragility is not specific for HS*; any cause of spherocytosis results in increased osmotic fragility.

Treatment of Hereditary Spherocytosis

The standard treatment for HS is splenectomy. Since the spleen is involved in both, causing the membrane loss and removing the spherocytes from the circulation, splenectomy is highly effective. However, because of the risk of overwhelming infection following splenectomy, splenectomy should be performed only on patients having significant complications from anemia, such as growth retardation. It should be delayed until at least 3 to 5 years of age if possible. Patients should receive vaccinations for *S. pneumoniae* and other encapsulated organisms prior to splenectomy and prophylactic penicillin thereafter. Splenectomy does not always correct the anemia in patients with autosomal recessive HS, although there is usually significant improvement. Folic acid supplementation is also recommended.

Hereditary Elliptocytosis

Epidemiology

Most cases of hereditary elliptocytosis (HE) are inherited in an **autosomal dominant** pattern. The estimated prevalence in the United States is about 3 to 5 per 10,000. In the United States, HE is most often seen in African Americans and in people from the Mediterranean basin. A variant called Southeast Asian ovalocytosis is found in Malaysia, New Guinea, Indonesia, and the Philippines. The geographic distribution of HE and its variants suggests a relationship to malaria (malaria *again*!).

Pathophysiology

Hereditary elliptocytosis is due to *defective horizontal stability* in the cytoskeleton. Most cases are caused by mutations in **α spectrin**, resulting in impaired assembly of the α/β spectrin tetramers. A smaller number of cases are caused by mutations in β spectrin or other proteins. Since the α/β spectrin tetramer assembly is defective, the cytoskeleton is less rigid and more easily deformed. Red blood cells are squeezed into an elliptical shape as they pass through capillaries, and eventually RBCs in HE patients become fixed in that shape.

Clinical Manifestations

Most cases of HE in the United States are asymptomatic, with normal RBC survival and no anemia. Many are detected when an individual is tested because a child or other relative is found to have elliptocytosis. Neonatal hyperbilirubinemia is common and may require exchange transfusion. Some infants with HE have severe hemolytic anemia at birth, with marked microcytosis and poikilocytosis, resembling hereditary pyropoikilocytosis (*elliptocytosis with neonatal poikilocytosis*). Such infants usually improve spontaneously and by the age of 1 year have the appearance of mild HE.

Diagnosis of Hereditary Elliptocytosis

Examination of a peripheral blood smear is the key diagnostic test (Figure 6–7). The presence of more than 15% elliptocytes suggests HE. Examining blood smears from parents or siblings may help confirm the presence of an inherited abnormality. Analysis of the cytoskeleton proteins is available but usually not required. The osmotic fragility test is normal in most cases of

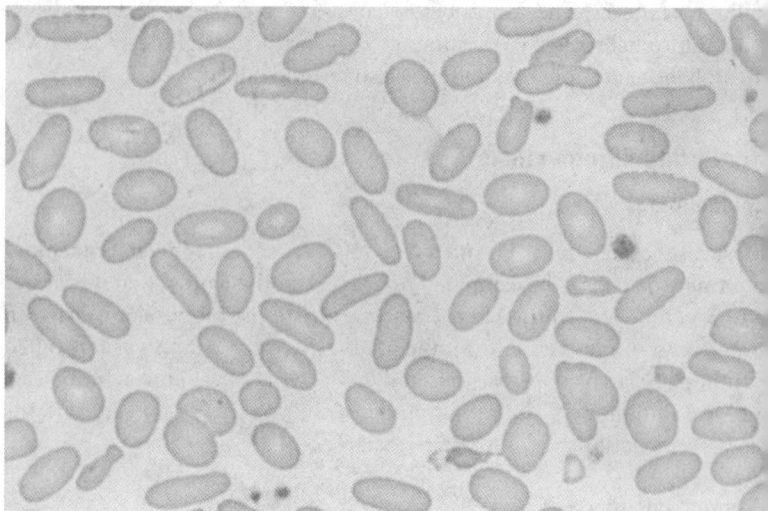

Figure 6–7 Hereditary elliptocytosis blood smear.

HE but may be abnormal in cases with poikilocytosis as well as elliptocytosis.

Treatment of Hereditary Elliptocytosis

The majority of patients with HE do not require any therapy. Splenectomy is not curative but may be beneficial in the rare severe cases that require therapy.

Hereditary Pyropoikilocytosis

Hereditary pyropoikilocytosis (HPP) is a severe chronic hemolytic anemia that begins in infancy and continues lifelong. The blood smear shows marked microcytosis, poikilocytosis, and RBC fragmentation. Hereditary pyropoikilocytosis is inherited in an autosomal recessive fashion; most cases of HPP represent homozygosity for hereditary elliptocytosis or heterozygosity for two different hereditary elliptocytosis mutations. The parents of the patient are often asymptomatic or have minimal anemia. Hereditary pyropoikilocytosis in the United States is most common in African Americans.

Hereditary pyropoikilocytosis involves two abnormalities: defective assembly of α/β spectrin tetramers and an absolute decrease in the amount of spectrin present. One consequence is decreased thermal stability of the spectrin proteins (hence the term "pyro," meaning fire). Spectrin proteins rom patients with HPP denature at approximately 45°C, whereas spectrin rom normal individuals denatures at approximately 49°C.

Review of the blood smear shows the striking changes noted above. Blood smears from one or both parents show elliptocytes.

Transfusions may be required to prevent the complications of chronic hemolysis and erythroid hyperplasia until the child is old enough to undergo splenectomy. Splenectomy is not curative but usually makes transfusions no longer necessary.

Additional Readings

Castro O. Management of sickle cell disease: recent advances and controversies. Br J Haematol 1999;107:2–11.

Serjeant GR. Sickle-cell disease. Lancet 1997;350:725–30.

Steinberg MH. Management of sickle cell disease. N Engl J Med 1999;340:1021–30.

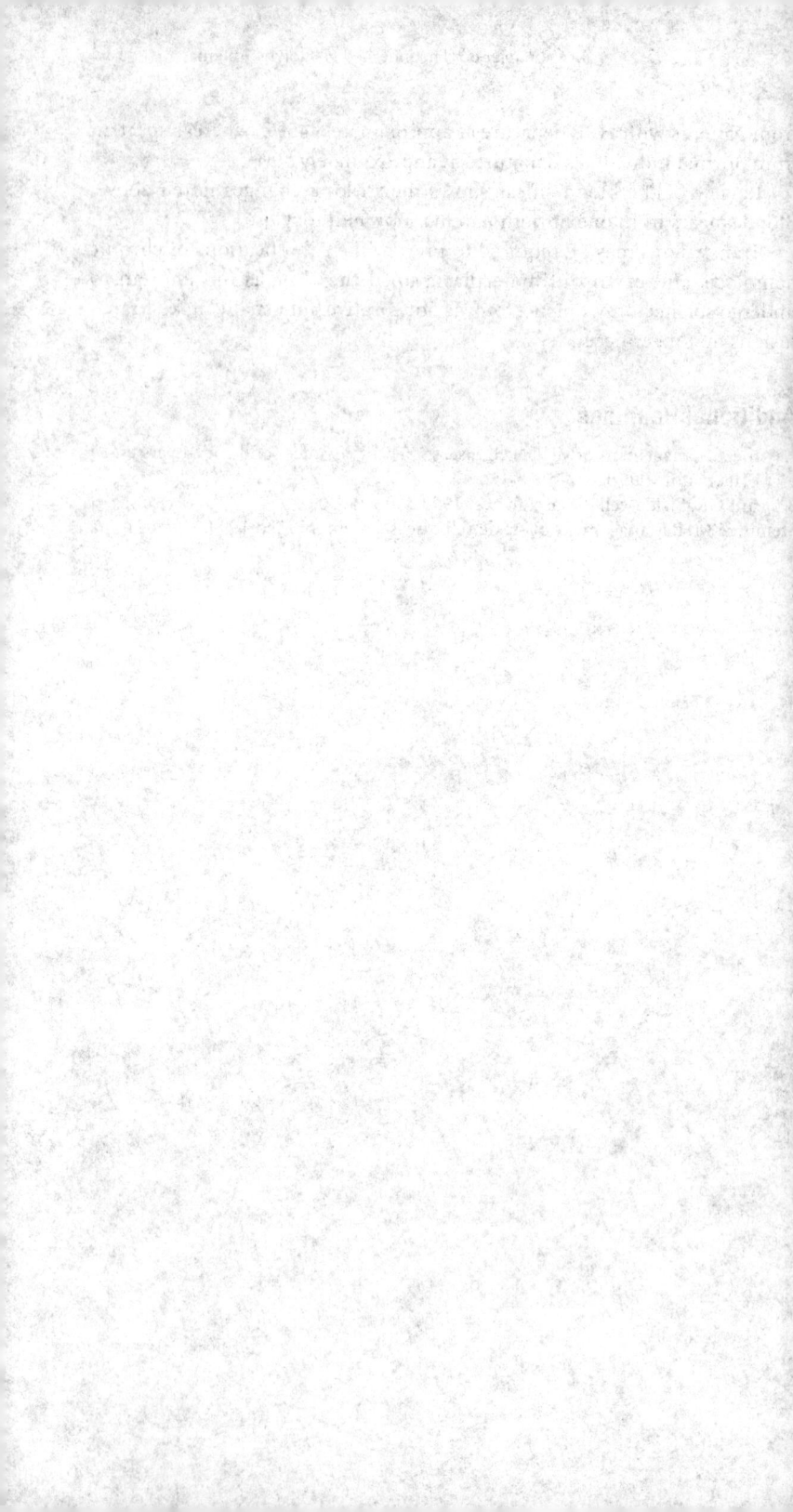

7

Acquired Hemolytic Anemias

Acquired hemolytic anemias are divided into two main types: **immune** and **non-immune**. Unlike the inherited hemolytic anemias, which predominantly involve abnormalities intrinsic to the erythrocyte, the **acquired** hemolytic anemias (with one exception) involve abnormalities that are **extrinsic** to the erythrocyte. The exception to the *acquired = extrinsic* rule is **paroxysmal nocturnal hemoglobinuria** (**PNH**), which is an acquired genetic lesion resulting in increased susceptibility of red blood cells (RBCs) to hemolysis by the complement cascade.

As for the inherited hemolytic anemias, the clues that you are dealing with an acquired hemolytic anemia are an **increased reticulocyte count** (or reticulocyte production index), **increased bilirubin and lactic dehydrogenase**, and **decreased haptoglobin**.

IMMUNE HEMOLYTIC ANEMIAS

The easiest way to approach the immune hemolytic anemias is to divide them according to the mechanism of hemolysis and the type of mediating antibody:

- **Direct complement-mediated (intravascular) hemolysis** versus **phagocytosis by macrophages of the reticuloendothelial system (extravascular hemolysis)** (Table 7–1)
- **Warm-reactive antibodies**, usually immunoglobulin G (IgG), versus **cold-reactive antibodies**, usually IgM (Table 7–2)

Table 7–1
Mechanisms of Immune Hemolysis

Direct Complement Mediated	Phagocytosis by Macrophages of RES
Intravascular	Extravascular
IgM or IgG antibody that fixes complement	Mediated by IgG or complement on cell surface
Complement cascade completed through membrane attack complex (MAC; C5b-9)	Predominantly occurs in spleen and/or liver

RES = reticuloendothelial system.

    Immune hemolytic anemias can be further divided: (1) those with no known precipitating cause (*primary* or *idiopathic*) versus those that are caused by some other disease or condition (*secondary*) and (2) those that are *acute* versus those that are *chronic*. An important additional category of immune-mediated hemolysis is *immune hemolytic anemia due to drugs or medications.*

Table 7–2
IgG versus IgM Antibodies

IgG Antibodies	IgM Antibodies
Usually warm reactive	React at cooler temperatures; initiate complement sequence
May or may not fix complement	Antibodies dissociate from RBC at warmer core temperatures; complement components remain on RBC surface
Hemolysis usually extravascular, predominantly in spleen; liver is usually a minor participant	Hemolysis is usually extravascular, predominantly in liver; spleen is usually a minor participant
Intravascular hemolysis is rare	Intravascular hemolysis may occur
Fcγ receptors on splenic macrophages recognize IgG on RBC surface	Complement receptors on Kupffer's cells recognize inactivated complement on RBC surface (iC3b)
Presence of complement components synergistic with IgG; more avid phagocytosis	High-titer antibody may activate enough complement to complete complement cascade, initiate intravascular hemolysis; Example: antibodies to A or B blood group antigens

Mechanisms of Immune Hemolysis

Direct Complement Mediated (Intravascular)

Direct complement-mediated hemolysis is caused by IgM or IgG antibodies that fix complement. The complement cascade must proceed to the terminal membrane attack complex (MAC; C5b-9); this requires sufficient activation of the complement system to overwhelm the circulating inhibitors of the complement system (C1 inhibitor, C4b binding protein) and the erythrocyte's own defense mechanisms against complement-mediated hemolysis. Important components of the erythrocyte defense system include the *membrane inhibitor of reactive lysis* (**CD59**) and the *decay accelerating factor* (**CD55**). Direct complement-mediated hemolysis is less common than hemolysis due to phagocytosis by macrophages of the reticuloendothelial system.

Phagocytosis by Macrophages of the Reticuloendothelial System (Extravascular)

Macrophages of the reticuloendothelial system have receptors for the Fc component of IgG (Fcγ receptors) and for complement components. The presence of IgG and complement on RBC surfaces results in complete or partial phagocytosis of the erythrocyte. Phagocytosis occurs primarily in the spleen and/or liver by splenic macrophages or Kupffer cells in the liver.

Cold-Reactive Immune Hemolytic Anemia

Cold-reactive immune hemolytic anemia is generally mediated by IgM antibodies that react maximally at approximately 4 to 18°C. They bind to cells at the cooler temperature of the extremities, fix complement, and then dissociate from the cell surface after the RBC returns to the warmer temperatures of the central circulation. The complement components remain on the cell surface after the antibody dissociates. IgM antibodies may cause intravascular hemolysis if the antibody is present in high titer; more often hemolysis is extravascular, predominantly in the liver. IgM antibodies are large and can bridge the distance between two RBCs; thus, IgM antibodies by themselves are able to agglutinate RBCs. (In contrast, IgG antibodies are smaller and alone are not able to agglutinate RBCs.) There are many causes of cold-reactive immune hemolytic anemia (Table 7–3). Most of these fall into the category of **cold agglutinin disease**. Cold agglutinin disease, in turn, is divided into **primary** (**idiopathic**) and **secondary** forms. Cold-reactive immune hemolytic anemia is less common than the warm-reacting type, accounting for approximately 10 to 20% of immunehemolytic anemias.

Table 7–3
Causes of Cold-Reactive Immune Hemolytic Anemia

Cold agglutinin disease:
- Primary (idiopathic)
- Secondary:
    Infections
    Autoimmune disorders
    Lymphoproliferative disorders

Paroxysmal cold hemoglobinuria (PCH)

⇨ Do not confuse *cold agglutinins* with *cryoglobulins*. Cold agglutinins are antibodies that cause agglutination of erythrocytes at cold temperatures. Cryoglobulins are antibodies that aggregate at cold temperatures (no erythrocytes involved).

Primary (Idiopathic) Cold Agglutinin Disease

Primary cold agglutinin disease occurs with no obvious precipitating cause. It usually occurs in older individuals (peak age about 70 years) and is more common in women than men. The course is usually chronic, lasting for months or years. The anemia associated with idiopathic cold agglutinin disease is usually modest; the main symptoms are related to agglutination of erythrocytes on exposure to cold rather than the anemia. Agglutination occurs in the fingers, toes, nose, and ears and causes cyanosis of those areas (*acrocyanosis*). Some patients have a lymphoproliferative disorder such as chronic lymphocytic leukemia (CLL), Waldenström's macroglobulinemia, or non-Hodgkin's lymphoma. Other patients do not have an obvious lymphoproliferative disorder at the onset of the cold agglutinin disease but may develop one later. The antibody is monoclonal, usually IgM with kappa light chain (IgM-κ). Primary cold agglutinin disease thus represents a monoclonal gammopathy.

Secondary Cold Agglutinin Disease

Secondary cold agglutinin disease is most often related to infections, primarily *Mycoplasma pneumoniae* or Epstein-Barr virus (EBV) (infectious mononucleosis). It can occasionally occur with other viral infections (adenovirus, cytomegalovirus, rubella, mumps, HIV), bacterial infections (*Legionella*, *Escherichia coli*, *Listeria*), malaria, syphilis, and others. The patients are usually young and otherwise healthy. The onset is abrupt, usually as the infection is resolving. The patients present with pallor, jaundice, and the other signs of acute hemolytic anemia. Massive acute intravascular hemolysis and acute renal failure may occur but are fortunately rare. Infection-related cases tend to be transient and self-limited, lasting only a few weeks. The antibodies are polyclonal and usually directed against the I/i blood group.

Diagnosis of Cold Agglutinin Disease

Cold agglutinins cause several abnormalities on the routine CBC, including a decreased RBC count, increased mean corpuscular volume (MCV), and increased mean corpuscular hemoglobin concentration (MCHC). Large round clusters of RBCs are seen on the blood smear, which can sometimes be seen as graininess by the naked eye (Figure 7–1). Repeating the CBC and smear after rewarming the sample to 37°C resolves the difficulties, demonstrating the temperature dependence of the reaction. Spherocytes may be present on smear, particularly in cases of acute cold agglutinin disease related to infection. A **direct antiglobulin test** (**DAT** or **Coombs' test**) detects the presence of complement components (but not IgG) on the surface of the patient's RBCs. The titer and thermal amplitude of the antibody should be determined by the blood bank. Attempts can also be made to identify the antibody specificity by testing the antibody against cord blood erythrocytes (which predominantly have the i antigen) and adult erythrocytes (which predominantly have the I antigen). The antibody is often present in very high titer. The thermal amplitude is measured by determining the titer of the antibody at various temperatures, ranging from 4°C to 37°C. Those that retain strong reactivity at higher temperatures are said to have

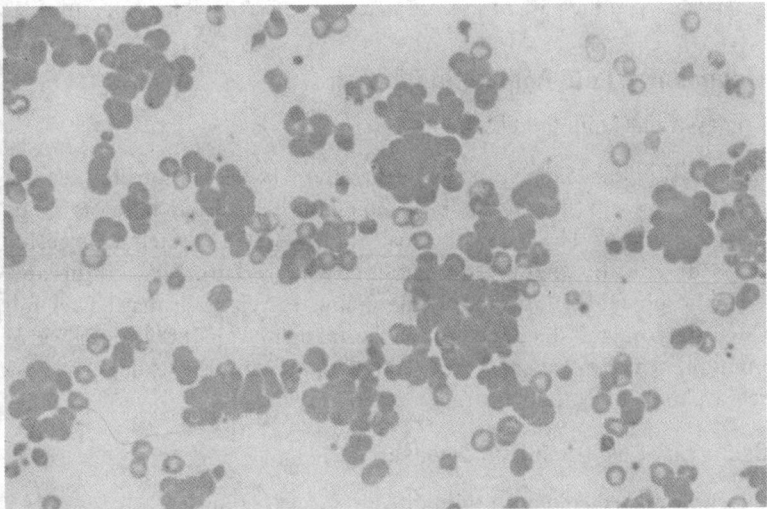

Figure 7–1 Cold agglutinin disease. Note the large round clusters of erythrocytes.

broad thermal amplitude. Clinical severity depends more on thermal amplitude than titer; antibodies that react at higher temperatures are associated with more severe clinical disease.

- The **direct antiglobulin test** (**DAT** or **direct Coombs' test**) tests for antibody or complement on the patient's RBCs. The direct antiglobulin test uses the *patient's cells* and adds a *reagent serum*. It is performed by adding antibodies directed against either human IgG, complement components, or both (the *antiglobulin* or *Coombs' reagent*) to the patient's RBCs and seeing if the cells agglutinate. If there is IgG or complement on the surface of the RBCs, then the added antibodies will cause the cells to agglutinate (positive DAT). If there is no IgG or complement on the RBC surface, the cells will not agglutinate. In cold agglutinin disease, there is complement on the patient's RBCs but no immunoglobulin.

- The **antibody screen** (also called **indirect antiglobulin test** or **indirect Coombs' test**) tests for unexpected anti-erythrocyte antibodies in the patient's serum. The *patient's serum* is added to panels of *reagent red cells*. After the cells and serum have incubated, the cells are washed and an antiglobulin reagent is added. If there are unexpected antibodies in the patient's serum, the reagent cells will agglutinate; otherwise, the reagent cells do not agglutinate. Unexpected antibodies are those that should not be present in a normal person; for example, antibodies against the A or B blood group antigens would be expected in a person who lacks those antigens. Antibodies against other RBC agents would be unexpected. In cold agglutinin disease, there is usually an unexpected antibody in the patient's serum that reacts best at cold temperatures.

Treatment of Cold Agglutinin Disease

Primary Cold Agglutinin Disease

Patients should avoid cold temperatures and take precautions to keep the extremities warm (moving to Florida might be helpful!). In mild cases, this may be sufficient. The anemia is usually mild and does not require transfusions or specific therapy. In patients who require further therapy, cyclophosphamide (Cytoxan) or chlorambucil given orally may be helpful. Corticosteroids and splenectomy (the mainstays of therapy for warm immune hemolytic anemia) are generally *not* helpful. Plasmapheresis to remove the agglutinin may provide temporary benefit.

Secondary Cold Agglutinin Disease

Infection-related cold agglutinin disease is usually transient, lasting only a few weeks. Supportive therapy is usually all that is needed. Blood transfusions should be avoided, if possible, but should be given if necessary. It is often difficult for the blood bank to obtain units that are completely cross-match compatible. It is important for the blood bank to test for red cell antibodies other than the cold agglutinin (alloantibodies). If an alloantibody is detected, units lacking the corresponding antigen should be chosen. It is important to maintain the temperature of the transfused blood at 37°C, using a blood warmer, to prevent the transfused cells from agglutinating as soon as they enter the patient.

Paroxysmal Cold Hemoglobinuria

Paroxysmal cold hemoglobinuria (PCH) is an unusual and now rare syndrome characterized by intravascular hemolysis and consequent hemoglobinuria following exposure to cold. It is caused by a peculiar biphasic IgG antibody that reacts and fixes complement at cold temperatures. After rewarming, the complement cascade goes to completion with formation of the membrane attack complex and intravascular hemolysis due to complement lysis. The antibody has been designated the **Donath-Landsteiner antibody** and is usually directed against the P blood group antigen.

⇨   Warning: Do not confuse *paroxysmal **cold** hemoglobinuria* (**PCH**) with *paroxysmal **nocturnal** hemoglobinuria* (**PNH**).

Paroxysmal cold hemoglobinuria is seen in three clinical forms: (1) an acute form that follows an infection, (2) a chronic form associated with tertiary or congenital syphilis, and (3) a chronic idiopathic form. Syphilis used to be the most common cause, but now most cases occur in children, and are related to viral infection (measles, measles vaccine, mumps, adenovirus, EBV, cytomegalovirus) or *Mycoplasma pneumoniae*. Occasional cases are related to systemic lupus erythematosus (SLE). Paroxysmal cold hemoglobinuria is a relatively common cause of acute hemolytic anemia in children.

Patients experience intermittent episodes of pain in the back, legs, or abdomen; fever; nausea; vomiting; and headache following exposure to cold. The plasma may be red during the acute episode. The urine will be dark red or black, clearing over a few hours. The anemia may be severe. *The DAT is positive for complement but not for IgG.* The diagnosis is confirmed by the **Donath-Landsteiner test**. The patient's serum is incubated in ice water with group O, P+ erythrocytes and fresh normal serum. The mixture is warmed to 37°C, and if the cells hemolyze on rewarming, the test is positive.

Infection-related cases tend to be transient and self-limited. Supportive care and avoidance of cold are usually all that is necessary. Red cell transfusions may be needed for severe anemia. The blood should be transfused through a blood warmer, and the patient should be kept warm. Patients with chronic PCH usually do well enough with avoidance of cold. The rare cases related to syphilis usually resolve after treatment of the syphilis.

Warm-Reactive Immune Hemolytic Anemia

Warm-reactive immune hemolytic anemia is more common than the cold-reactive variant (at least 70% of immune hemolytic anemias). It can be *primary* (idiopathic), *secondary* to a wide variety of different conditions, or *drug-related* (Table 7–4). Most cases (about 80%) are due to some underlying condition, although this may not be apparent at the onset of hemolysis. Hemolytic anemia may be the presenting feature of SLE or other autoimmune disorder.

The idiopathic variety is more common in women and the older population.

Pathophysiology

The antibody is usually a "panagglutinin," meaning that the patient's antibody will react with virtually all cells. In most cases, the antibody appears to be recognizing some antigen in the Rh blood group system, although it is usually impossible to define a specific antigenic reactivity. The antibody is almost always an IgG. Occasionally, an IgA or IgM antibody will be seen along with the IgG or, exceptionally, alone. The antibody often fixes complement to the red cell but usually does not proceed through the complete membrane attack complex.

Red cell destruction is primarily by phagocytosis by splenic macrophages. In many cases, the phagocytosis is partial rather than complete; the RBC

Table 7–4
Causes of Warm-Reactive Immune Hemolytic Anemia

Primary (idiopathic)
Secondary
Infections
Autoimmune disorders: SLE, rheumatoid arthritis
Lymphoproliferative disorders: CLL, non-Hodgkin's lymphomas, myeloma
Hodgkin's lymphoma
Thymoma
Ovarian dermoid cyst or teratoma
Carcinomas
Hypogammaglobulinemia
Acquired immunodeficiency syndrome (AIDS)
Drug related

SLE = systemic lupus erythematosus; CLL = chronic lymphocytic leukemia.

loses a portion of its cell membrane, resulting in a greater loss of surface area than volume. Consequently, the RBC becomes spherocytic. Occasionally, there is sufficient complement activation on the RBC to overwhelm the defense mechanisms against complement, resulting in formation of the membrane attack complex and intravascular hemolysis.

Clinical Manifestations

The severity of illness varies from an asymptomatic increase in red cell turnover completely compensated by increased marrow production to a fulminant illness with prostration, shock, and acute renal failure. The majority of patients experience an insidious onset of fatigue, weakness, and shortness of breath on exertion. Angina may be a presenting feature in older patients with coronary artery disease. Jaundice may be present. Mild splenomegaly and hepatomegaly may be present on examination, as well as mild lymphadenopathy; however, marked hepatosplenomegaly or lymphadenopathy suggests an underlying lymphoproliferative disorder. The course in adults tends to be chronic, lasting months to years, with periodic exacerbations.

The acute fulminant variety is more common in children, usually following a viral infection. These patients may experience back, leg, or abdominal pain; headaches; nausea; or vomiting. They may have dark red or black urine. Although potentially very serious, these episodes are usually transient, are self-limited, and seldom recur.

Diagnosis

The hemoglobin level is variable, from severely decreased to nearly normal. The MCV is typically slightly increased due to reticulocytosis. The peripheral blood smear shows polychromasia and microspherocytes; in severe cases, nucleated RBCs may be present (Figure 7–2). The reticulocyte count and reticulocyte production index are increased (Figure 7–3). The bilirubin and lactic dehydrogenase are variably elevated, and the haptoglobin is decreased.

The most important diagnostic test is the direct antiglobulin test (DAT), which is positive in >95% of cases. In most cases, the DAT is positive for IgG, with or without complement; a smaller number are positive for complement alone (<15%). The antibody screen (indirect antiglobulin test) is positive in about 80% of cases. The blood bank should attempt to identify a specific reactivity for the antibody, but this is usually impossible. It is critical that the blood bank attempt to exclude an alloantibody. If the patient has not been recently transfused, this can be done using an autoadsorption procedure to remove any antibodies against antigens on the patient's own RBCs.

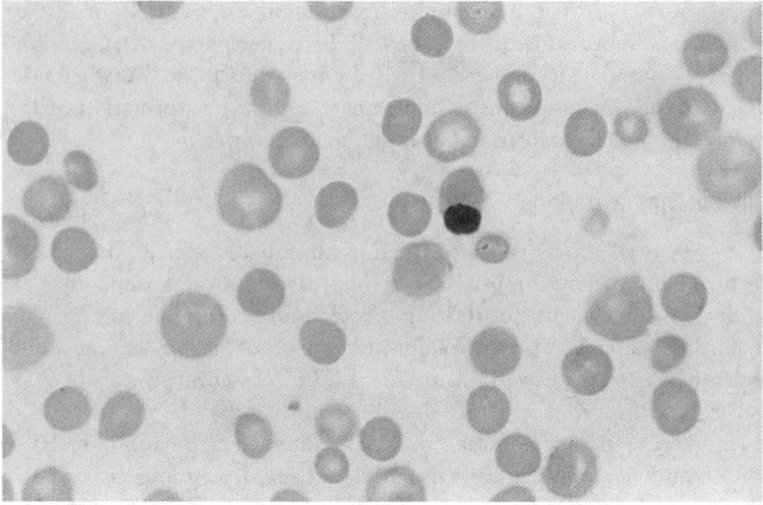

Figure 7–2 Warm-reactive immune hemolytic anemia. Note the small dark spherocytes, polychromasia, and nucleated erythrocyte.

⇨ *A positive DAT does not necessarily mean that the patient has immune hemolytic anemia. A weakly positive DAT can be seen in patients on many medications or due to infections.* In most of these cases, there is no evidence of hemolysis.

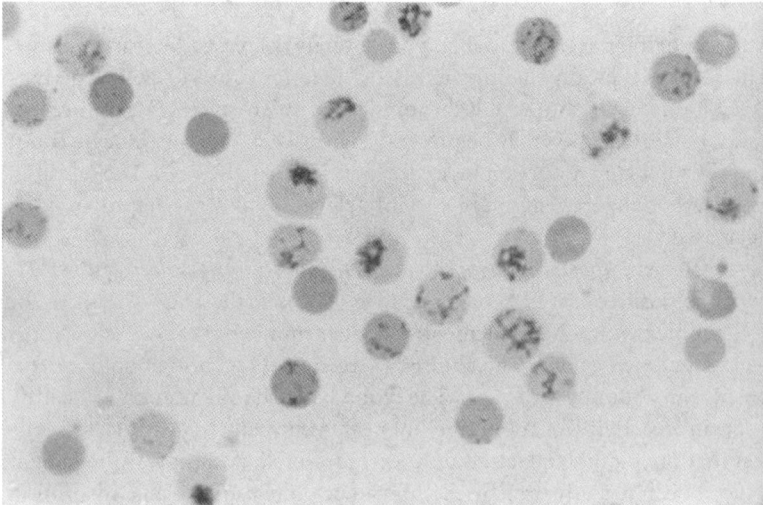

Figure 7–3 Reticulocyte stain. Note the granular aggregates of RNA in the reticulocytes. The reticulocyte count is markedly increased.

Evaluation

Initial evaluation should focus on determining the severity of illness and discovering any possible causes of a secondary hemolytic anemia. Key points to consider:

- **Identify any drugs or medications that the patient has been taking**. All medications that may cause drug-related immune hemolytic anemia should be stopped as much as possible.
- **Determine if the patient has had any transfusions**, particularly within the past 3 months. Recent transfusions raise the possibility of delayed transfusion reactions rather than autoimmune hemolytic anemia. The blood bank should be notified of the circumstances of any recent transfusion. Evaluation is more difficult for the blood bank if the patient has been recently transfused, and their diagnostic evaluation may be altered.
- **History of pregnancies** (including miscarriages or abortions) is critical in women.

Treatment

Any possible primary cause (such as an underlying autoimmune disease or lymphoproliferative disorder) should be treated appropriately.

It is preferable to avoid red cell transfusions, but they should be given if needed. The blood bank will usually not be able to find totally compatible units for transfusion but may be able to select least incompatible units. In general, transfusion does not cause a significant increase in hemolysis, and the transfused red cells survive about as long as the patient's own RBCs.

The mainstay of initial therapy is corticosteroids, such as prednisone (1–2 mg/kg/day in divided doses). Most patients show a response within 3 weeks. Corticosteroids block the macrophage Fc receptors and thus prevent RBC phagocytosis. They can also decrease antibody production by the spleen, but this takes several weeks. Prednisone is usually continued at the original dose until the hemoglobin is ≥10 g/dL; the dose is then slowly tapered down by 5 to 10 mg/week to approximately 10 mg/day. If the hemoglobin remains stable, then the dose is slowly tapered again over 3 to 4 months. About 80% of patients initially respond; however, about two-thirds of responders relapse as the drug is tapered. Some patients can be maintained on no corticosteroids or on a low dose. Patients requiring more than 10 to 20 mg of prednisone per day, or patients having intolerable side effects on prednisone, should be considered for splenectomy.

Splenectomy is the mainstay of therapy for patients who fail to respond to corticosteroids or who require excessive doses to maintain remission. Splenectomy eliminates the primary site of red cell destruction and also removes an important site of antibody production. Approximately 50 to 60% of patients have a good initial response to splenectomy. Patients should be vaccinated against pneumococcus and meningococcus prior to surgery.

Other therapies that are sometimes used include immunosuppressive drugs like cyclophosphamide or azathioprine, intravenous immunoglobulin, plasmapheresis, vincristine or vinblastine, and danazol. Intravenous immunoglobulin and plasmapheresis may be helpful, but the effects are transient.

Drug-Related Immune Hemolytic Anemia

Drugs and medications are common causes of immune hemolytic anemia (~10–20% of cases). The hemolysis is almost always of the warm-reactive type. It is common for patients on a variety of medications to develop a positive DAT; however, *actual hemolysis is rare.*

Three mechanisms of drug-related immune hemolytic anemia have been described. Some medications may cause hemolysis by more than one mechanism, and it may not always be possible to distinguish the mechanism in an individual patient. The three mechanisms are as follows:

- **Drug adsorption (penicillin) type:** In this type, the drug binds tightly to the RBC surface, and an antidrug antibody reacts with the drug that is bound to the red cell. The DAT is positive for IgG, with or without complement. The patient's serum (or antibody eluted from the patient's cells) does not react with untreated red cells but will react with reagent red cells that have been pretreated with the drug. Hemolysis is usually extravascular in the spleen; rarely, there may be intravascular hemolysis if the antibody fixes complement. The hemolysis is usually subacute, not severe. The most common cause of this type of reaction is penicillin. It occurs only with high doses of penicillin (>10 million units/day) in a small minority of patients; a higher proportion of patients develop a positive DAT, without hemolysis. This type of reaction may also be seen with *cephalosporin antibiotics*, *tetracycline*, and *tolbutamide.*

- **Neoantigen (formerly called *immune complex*) type:** In this type, there is a complex of drug and antidrug antibody, which binds to an antigen on the red cell. The antibody can be either IgM or IgG and is often complement fixing. The antibody often has relatively low avidity; it binds to the complex on the cell membrane, fixes complement, and then dissociates from the cell surface. The DAT is therefore positive for complement but usually not for immunoglobulins. The complement cascade often proceeds through formation of the membrane attack complex. **Hemolysis is usually intravascular, often sudden and severe, and may** be associated with acute renal failure. **The reaction may occur with low doses of the medication**. It might be possible to demonstrate the reaction using a combination of the patient's serum, the drug, plus reagent red cells. Medications that can cause this type of reaction include *cephalosporin antibiotics, quinine, quinidine,* and *stibophen.*

- **Autoimmune (α-methyldopa) type:** α-Methyldopa (Aldomet) is capable of inducing an autoimmune reaction. The antibody is directed against a red cell antigen, not against the drug itself. The characteristics are similar to those of idiopathic warm-reactive immune hemolytic anemia. It is common for patients on α-methyldopa to develop a positive DAT (~8–36%), but immune hemolysis is rare (≤1%). The incidence of positive DAT increases with the dose of medication and usually occurs about 3 to 6 months after the medication has been started. The DAT is positive for IgG with or without complement and may be positive even in the absence of the drug. The antibody screen may be positive. This type of drug-related immune hemolysis is now rare since α-methyldopa has largely been replaced by other antihypertensive medications. A similar reaction can be seen with *levodopa* and *procainamide.*

Some drugs may cause nonimmunologic adsorption of proteins to the red cell surface, including immunoglobulins and complement components. This can cause a positive DAT, but does not cause hemolysis. Cephalosporins are the most common medications associated with this type of reaction. *In the absence of hemolysis, a positive DAT alone is* **not** *a reason to discontinue a needed medication!*

Clinical Manifestations

The most common presentation is an insidious onset of fatigue, pallor, and jaundice. Patients with the neoantigen-type reaction are at risk of developing acute fulminant hemolysis with hemoglobinuria and acute renal failure.

Evaluation

It is critical to obtain a complete history of drugs and medications in any case of possible immune hemolytic anemia. The list of medications that may cause hemolysis is long (Table 7–5). For many of these drugs, only a few cases have been described, or a causal relationship has not been conclusively shown. The presence of an immune reaction is confirmed by the presence of a positive DAT. In some cases, it may be possible to demonstrate the reaction using drug-treated red cells or a combination of the patient's serum, drug, and reagent red cells, but most institutions will not test for reactions to unusual or uncommon medications. Therefore, a presumptive diagnosis of

Table 7–5

Drugs Associated with Immune Hemolysis/Autoantibodies

Acetaminophen	Cianidanol	Latamoxef*	Ranitidine
Aminopyrine	Cisplatin	Levodopa	Rifampin
Amphotericin B	Cyclofenil*	Mefenamic acid	Sodium pentothal
Ampicillin	Diclofenac*	Melphalan	Stibophen
Antazoline	Diethylstilbestrol	Mesphenytoin	Streptomycin*
Apazone (azapropazone)*	Diglycoaldehyde	Methadone	Sulfonamides
Buthiazide (butazide)	Dipyrone	Methicillin	Sulfonylurea derivatives
Carbenicillin	Doxepin	Methotrexate	Sulindac
Carbimazole*	Elliptinium acetate	Methyldopa*	Suramin
Carboplatin	Erythromycin	Nafcillin	Suprofen
Catergen*	Fenfluramine*	Nalidixic acid	Teniposide*
Cefotaxime	Fenoprofen	Nomifensine*	Tetracycline
Cefotetan*	Fluorescein	Omeprazole	Thiopental
Cefoxitin*	5-Fluorouracil	p-Aminosalicylic acid	Thioridazine
Ceftazidime	Glafenine*	Penicillin G	Thiazides
Cephaloridine	Hydralazine	Phenacetin*	Tolbutamide
Cephalothin	Hydrochlorothiazide	Podophyllotoxin	Tolmetin*
Chaparral*	Interferon-α	Probenecid	Triamterene
Chlorinated hydrocarbons (insecticides)	Ibuprofen*	Procainamide*	Trimellitic anhydride
Chlorambucil	Insulin	Pyramidon	Zomepirac
Chlorpropamide	Intravenous contrast media	Quinidine	
Chlorpromazine*	Isoniazid	Quinine	

*Medications associated with the autoantibody mechanism as well as the drug-dependent (drug adsorption or neoantigen) type of mechanism.
Adapted from Lee RG, Foerster J, Lukens J, et al, (editors). Wintrobe's clinical hematology. 10th edition. Baltimore: Williams & Wilkins; 1999. p. 1257.

drug-related immune hemolytic anemia is usually made by excluding other causes for immune hemolytic anemia, stopping the drug, and observing to see if the patient improves.

Management

All possible medications should be discontinued and the patient observed. In most cases, the patient will recover without further therapy. Patients with severe hemolysis and anemia may require red cell transfusions. There is usually no difficulty selecting compatible units for transfusion, but the transfused cells may have decreased survival if drug remains in the patient's circulation. Prednisone is of questionable efficacy and is usually not needed.

NON-IMMUNOLOGIC ACQUIRED HEMOLYTIC ANEMIAS

There are a variety of non-immunologic causes of acquired hemolytic anemia (Table 7–6).

Mechanical Hemolytic Anemias

A common cause of mechanical hemolysis is a malfunctioning mechanical heart valve. Erythrocytes are crushed by the valve leaflets as they close, resulting in fragmentation and a chronic intravascular hemolysis. Hemoglobin is filtered by glomeruli and phagocytized by renal tubular epithelial cells. The iron is converted to hemosiderin and eventually lost as the tubular epithelial cells are shed into the urine; this may result in iron deficiency. The diagnosis can be made by noting a heart murmur from the malfunctioning valve, schistocytes on blood smear, and a positive urine hemosiderin test. The treatment is iron supplementation and replacement of the malfunctioning valve if necessary. (This is not a significant problem with properly functioning mechanical heart valves.)

"March hemoglobinuria" can occur during long marches or marathons, resulting from erythrocytes being crushed in the capillaries of the soles of the feet as they pound against the surface. This can be prevented by wearing thicker socks and softer-soled shoes.

The *microangiopathic hemolytic anemias* (sometimes called *thrombotic microangiopathies*) include **thrombotic thrombocytopenic purpura (TTP)**, **hemolytic-uremic syndrome (HUS)**, **preeclampsia/eclampsia**, **malignant hypertension**, and sometimes disseminated intravascular coagulation (DIC). Fibrin strands form within the capillaries, slicing erythrocytes into fragments as they pass through.

Acanthocytosis

Acanthocytes are produced by severe disturbances in lipid metabolism, resulting in abnormalities in the phospholipids of the cell membrane. Causes of acanthocytosis include the following:

Table 7–6
Non-immunologic Causes of Acquired Hemolytic Anemia

Mechanical trauma
  Malfunctioning mechanical heart valve
  "March hemoglobinuria"
  Microangiopathic hemolytic anemias: thrombotic thrombocytopenic purpura (TTP), hemolytic-uremic syndrome (HUS), preeclampsia/eclampsia, malignant hypertension, disseminated intravascular coagulation (DIC)

Acanthocytosis
  Hereditary abetalipoproteinemia
  End-stage liver disease
  Severe starvation, anorexia nervosa

Severe hypophosphatemia
  Intravenous hyperalimentation lacking phosphorous supplementation
  Severe starvation
  Alcoholism
  Prolonged therapy with phosphate-binding antacids

Wilson's disease; copper poisoning

Oxidative drugs or chemicals

Severe burns

Venoms
  Brown recluse spider
  Snakes (cobras)

Infections
  Direct infection of erythrocytes: malaria, babesiasis, bartonellosis, trypanosomiasis
  Clostridium perfringens septicemia
  Other: gram-positive and gram-negative septicemia, leptospirosis, *Borrelia*, others

Paroxysmal nocturnal hemoglobinuria (PNH)

- **Hereditary abetalipoproteinemia:** Hereditary abetalipoproteinemia is a rare genetic defect, most common in Ashkenazi Jews, characterized by an inability to absorb betalipoproteins. As a result, patients are unable to synthesize some of the required membrane phospholipids. Patients frequently have neurologic abnormalities as well.
- **Severe liver disease:** Abnormalities in lipid metabolism also occur in severe liver disease, usually in end-stage cirrhosis. The patients have all the stigmata of terminal liver disease (coagulopathy, gastroesophageal varices, ascites), and just when it seems the situation can't get any worse,

they develop hemolytic anemia with acanthocytes. Survival is short unless the liver disease can be corrected.

- **Severe starvation and anorexia nervosa:** Acanthocytosis may occur with severe starvation or anorexia, again due to disturbances in lipid metabolism. Correction of the malnutrition stops the hemolysis, with disappearance of acanthocytes.

Wilson's Disease: Acute Copper Poisoning

Wilson's disease is due to a mutation in the gene for ceruloplasmin, a copper transport protein. Patients accumulate excessive amounts of copper in their tissues, particularly the liver. Some patients with Wilson's disease develop an abrupt onset of hemolysis due to sudden release of copper from the liver. Excess inorganic copper damages RBC membranes, disrupts cellular metabolism, and accelerates the oxidation of hemoglobin, all of which result in decreased cell survival. Hemolytic episodes tend to occur relatively early in the course of Wilson's disease, often in the patient's twenties, and may be the initial symptomatic manifestation of the disease. Hemolytic episodes are usually transient and self-limited but may be recurrent and severe.

Hemolysis has occasionally been reported in humans and animals exposed to toxic amounts of copper sulfate and after hemodialysis with dialysis solutions contaminated with excessive copper.

Oxidative Drugs and Chemicals

Oxidative drugs and chemicals may cause hemolysis in people with apparently normal erythrocytes, as well as in patients with G6PD and other enzyme deficiencies. Examples of drugs that have been implicated include *sulfonamides, phenazopyridine (Pyridium), nitrofurantoin (Furadantin), phenacetin,* and *cisplatin.* Chemicals that have been implicated in hemolysis include *chlorates, nitrates, naphthalene (mothballs), methylene blue,* and others. Treatment is to stop the drug or exposure and provide support as necessary.

Severe Hypophosphatemia

Severe hypophosphatemia may result in the depletion of intracellular phosphorylated compounds, including adenosine triphosphate and 2,3-diphosphoglycerate. Causes of severe hypophosphatemia include intravenous hyperalimentation lacking phosphorous supplementation, severe starvation, alcoholism, and prolonged therapy with phosphate-binding antacids.

Severe Burns and Thermal Injury

Severe burns and other thermal injury may result in fragmentation of erythrocytes due to denaturation of cell membrane proteins. The blood smear shows schistocytes, spherocytes, and echinocytes.

Infections

A variety of infections can be associated with hemolytic anemia. The most obvious are those with direct infection of the erythrocyte: malaria, babesiasis, bartonellosis, trypanosomiasis (African sleeping sickness), and others. Other infections can cause hemolysis without direct infection of the RBC. A well known but uncommon cause is septicemia with *Clostridium perfringens*; the organism produces a lysolecithinase that damages the RBC membrane. A wide variety of other infections can also be associated with hemolysis including gram-positive and gram-negative septicemia, leptospirosis, *Borrelia*, tuberculosis and toxoplasmosis, among others.

Paroxysmal Nocturnal Hemoglobinuria

Pathophysiology

Paroxysmal nocturnal hemoglobinuria is an acquired genetic disorder that results in increased susceptibility of RBCs to lysis by the complement system. The condition results from an inability to synthesize the **glycosyl phosphatidylinositol** (**GPI**) **anchor**, which anchors a variety of molecules on the surface of erythrocytes and other cells. Among the molecules that use the GPI anchor are the **membrane inhibitor of reactive lysis** (MIRL; **CD59** in the Cluster Designation system for leukocyte antigens), **decay accelerating factor** (DAF; **CD55**), and the **homologous restriction factor** (C8 binding protein), which are all involved in the RBC defense against complement. Lacking these molecules, erythrocytes are unusually sensitive to lysis by complement and are unable to withstand the low level of complement activation that occurs normally. This results in intravascular hemolysis.

Paroxysmal nocturnal hemoglobinuria results from a mutation in the *PIG-A* gene on the X chromosome, which encodes for one portion of the GPI anchor. Analysis of G6PD isoenzymes and other genetic markers has shown that PNH is a clonal disorder. The same defect is found in granulocytes, megakaryocytes, and other blood cells, indicating that the mutation occurs at the level of the hematopoietic stem cell.

- Paroxysmal nocturnal hemoglobinuria frequently arises from, or transforms into, aplastic anemia. This has led to speculation that PNH represents escape from immunologic surveillance. Many cases of aplastic anemia appear to be due to immunologic suppression of hematopoiesis; anything that decreases immunologic recognition could provide a proliferative advantage. Several of the antigens that are missing in PNH are involved in immune recognition, and the absence of these molecules on hematopoietic stem cells would make them less susceptible to recognition by the immune system. Thus, in that circumstance, the PNH clone would have a proliferative advantage over normal cells and would eventually take over the marrow.

Clinical Manifestations

Paroxysmal nocturnal hemoglobinuria occurs at all ages from childhood to old age but is most commonly diagnosed in the fourth and fifth decades. The course is highly variable, from clinically benign to a chronic disabling disorder. The name *paroxysmal nocturnal hemoglobinuria* derived from patients who experienced episodes of dark urine on awakening from sleep; however, this classic presentation occurs in only about one-fourth of patients. The majority of patients have an insidious onset of fatigue, weakness, and jaundice. Many have periodic exacerbations of hemolysis. In most cases, there is no obvious cause for the exacerbations, but some attacks may be precipitated by infections, menstruation, transfusions, surgery, ingestion of iron salts, or vaccinations. The attacks are not precipitated by exposure to cold, distinguishing PNH from paroxysmal *cold* hemoglobinuria. Patients may experience abdominal or back pain, nausea, headaches, malaise, and fever associated with exacerbations of hemolysis. Unexplained pancytopenia may also be a presenting manifestation of PNH. Many patients with myelodysplasia can also be shown to have erythrocytes with increased sensitivity to complement.

Complications

Paroxysmal nocturnal hemoglobinuria is associated with a number of significant complications, including:

- **Thromboemboli:** Thrombotic disease is a common complication in PNH and accounts for approximately half of the deaths. Thrombi predominantly occur in the venous system, including unusual sites such as the cerebral veins, mesenteric veins, portal vein, and hepatic vein (Budd-Chiari syndrome), as well as in the extremities. The reason for the increased risk of thrombosis in PNH is unknown.
- **Infections:** Patients with PNH may be at increased risk of infections due to leukopenia, leukocyte dysfunction, or corticosteroid therapy. Infections can precipitate exacerbations of hemolysis and account for approximately 10% of deaths in patients with PNH.

- **Iron deficiency:** Chronic intravascular hemolysis with hemoglobinuria results in iron deficiency, which further exacerbates the tendency for anemia.
- **Leukopenia, thrombocytopenia, or pancytopenia:** Nearly all patients with PNH develop leukopenia, thrombocytopenia, or pancytopenia.
- **Hemorrhage:** Patients with PNH and severe thrombocytopenia are at increased risk for hemorrhage.
- **Transformation to acute myelogenous leukemia:** Transformation to acute myelogenous leukemia is a rare but well-known complication of PNH.
- **Development of aplastic anemia:** Up to 30% of patients with PNH have a preceding history of aplastic anemia. In addition, an additional 10% of patients may develop aplastic anemia following the diagnosis of PNH.

Diagnosis

The CBC shows anemia, which can vary from mild to severe. The anemia is usually mildly macrocytic but can be microcytic and hypochromic if iron deficiency has developed. Leukopenia and/or thrombocytopenia are also common. Lactic dehydrogenase and bilirubin may be elevated during exacerbations of hemolysis. A test for urine hemosiderin will be positive.

The bone marrow examination in PNH generally shows erythroid hyperplasia; bone marrow cellularity is usually increased but can also be normal or decreased.

The traditional diagnostic tests are the **acidified serum (Ham's) test** and the **sucrose hemolysis test.** Both tests depend on activating the complement system and demonstrating increased sensitivity of the cells to complement-mediated lysis. The sucrose hemolysis test is more sensitive, but the Ham's test is more specific. Demonstration of a decreased expression of GPI-anchored proteins on RBCs or leukocytes by **flow cytometry** has been shown to be more sensitive than either of these tests. Antibodies are available to MIRL (CD59) and DAF (CD55), and these can be used to study erythrocytes or leukocytes by flow cytometry. Other GPI-anchored antigens such as CD14, CD16, and CD24 can also be studied on leukocytes.

Treatment

Standard treatments for PNH include corticosteroids and androgens. Both are helpful in some patients and should be tried. Patients who respond should be maintained on minimally effective doses to avoid side effects. Transfusions may be needed for severe anemia. Iron replacement may be helpful in patients who develop iron deficiency; however, iron replacement can occasionally cause acute exacerbations of hemolysis, so a small test dose is recommended. Thrombotic episodes are treated with anticoagulants or thrombolytic agents.

Hematopoietic stem cell replacement (bone marrow transplantation) has been tried in a few younger patients with histocompatible donors, and has been relatively successful.

Prognosis

The median survival in PNH is approximately 10 to 15 years, and some patients live for 25 years or longer. Rare cases of spontaneous recovery have been reported.

8

Aplastic Anemia, Pure Red Cell Aplasia, and Congenital Dyserythropoietic Anemia

The term aplastic anemia indicates **pancytopenia** in the presence of a **hypocellular (aplastic) bone marrow** (Figure 8–1). Aplastic anemia can be either **inherited** or **acquired**. Causes of acquired aplastic anemia include chemical toxins, drugs and medications, ionizing radiation, and infections (Table 8–1). In at least half of acquired cases, no cause can be determined (*idiopathic aplastic anemia*). Most cases of idiopathic aplastic anemia appear to be caused by immune suppression or destruction of hematopoietic precursor cells.

Pure red cell aplasia (**PRCA**) is defined as **anemia** with an **absence of erythroid precursors in the bone marrow**. In contrast with aplastic anemia, granulocyte precursors and megakaryocytes are preserved in PRCA. Pure red cell aplasia also can be inherited or acquired. There are numerous causes of acquired PRCA, some of which may also cause aplastic anemia.

The **congenital dyserythropoietic anemias** (**CDAs**) are a group of conditions characterized by **anemia** and **abnormal erythroid precursors in the marrow**.

PATHOPHYSIOLOGY OF APLASTIC ANEMIA

Aplastic anemia is caused by a failure of hematopoietic stem cells. Failure may be due to an abnormality of the hematopoietic stem cells themselves or to some factor that suppresses or destroys them.

It is important to distinguish aplastic anemia from other causes of pancytopenia such as myelodysplasia, megaloblastic anemia, and acute leukemia,

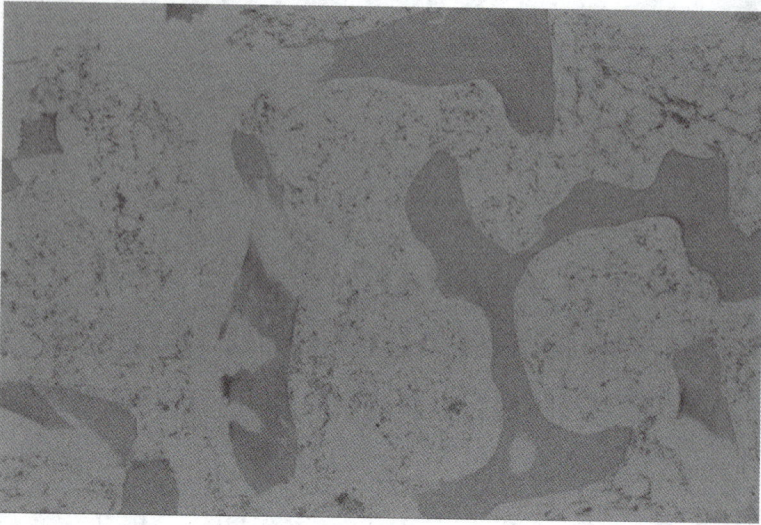

Figure 8–1 Aplastic anemia bone marrow biopsy. Severely hypocellular bone marrow with a predominance of adipocytes and a near total absence of hematopoietic precursors.

among others (Table 8–2). *In aplastic anemia, the cells that are present are normal or have only mild morphologic abnormalities.* The presence of nucleated or abnormally shaped erythrocytes (other than mild macrocytosis),

Table 8–1
Causes of Aplastic Anemia

Familial

Fanconi's anemia

Dyskeratosis congenita

Schwachman-Diamond syndrome (aplastic anemia with pancreatic insufficiency)

Acquired

Chemicals and toxins: benzene, insecticides (DDT, parathion, chlordane), arsenic

Medications: chemotherapy drugs, chloramphenicol, phenylbutazone, anticonvulsants, carbamazepine, Clonazipril, gold compounds, oral hypoglycemic agents

Ionizing radiation

Viral infections: hepatitis, Epstein-Barr virus, HIV, dengue

Miscellaneous: pregnancy, autoimmune disorders (diffuse eosinophilic fasciitis)

Idiopathic

Adapted from Lee RG, Foerster J, Lukens J, et al, editors. Wintrobe's clinical hematology. 10th ed. Baltimore: Williams & Wilkins; 1999. p. 1452–53.

Table 8–2
Causes of Pancytopenia

Aplastic anemia
   Congenital
   Acquired

Bone marrow infiltration
   Metastatic carcinoma
   Aleukemic leukemia
   Lymphoma: non-Hodgkin's, Hodgkin's
   Multiple myeloma
   Myelofibrosis
   Osteopetrosis, metabolic bone diseases
   Granulomas: mycobacterial or fungal infection, sarcoidosis
   Storage diseases: Gaucher's cells

Hypersplenism

Megaloblastic anemia: vitamin B_{12} or folate deficiency

Autoimmune diseases: systemic lupus erythematosus (SLE)

Myelodysplasia

Paroxysmal nocturnal hemoglobinuria

Overwhelming infection

hypersegmented neutrophils or other abnormal leukocytes, immature cells, or megakaryocyte fragments strongly points to a disorder other than aplastic anemia.

INHERITED (CONSTITUTIONAL) VARIANTS OF APLASTIC ANEMIA

Inherited variants of aplastic anemia are rare. The most common (approximately two-thirds of cases) is **Fanconi's anemia**, which is associated with increased chromosomal instability. Less common variants include **Schwachman-Diamond syndrome** (pancreatic insufficiency with pancytopenia) and **dyskeratosis congenita**. It is important to differentiate *congenital* aplastic anemia (ie, present at birth), which can be either inherited or acquired, from *inherited* (also called *constitutional*) aplastic anemia, which may be present at birth or may not become evident until years later.

Fanconi's Anemia

Fanconi's anemia is inherited as an autosomal recessive trait. Abnormalities in at least eight separate genes may be involved. The mechanisms by which defects in these genes cause Fanconi's anemia are unclear.

Clinical Manifestations

The clinical picture of Fanconi's anemia is variable and can include pancytopenia, skeletal abnormalities, neurologic abnormalities, and others (Table 8–3). About 40% of patients have pancytopenia with physical anomalies, ~30% have pancytopenia without physical anomalies, ~25% have physical anomalies without anemia, and rare patients have neither. A characteristic feature of Fanconi's anemia is increased chromosomal fragility. Chromosomes show spontaneous breaks, gaps, rearrangements, reduplications, and exchanges. The frequency of chromosome breaks is increased by ionizing radiation or by culturing the patient's cells in diepoxybutane or mitomycin C.

The hematologic disease usually begins during childhood (median age approximately 7 years) but may not become evident until adulthood. Thrombocytopenia is usually the first manifestation, followed by granulocytopenia and finally anemia. Erythrocytes appear macrocytic; leukocytes and platelets are decreased in number but are morphologically unremarkable. The bone marrow may initially show erythroid hyperplasia but eventually becomes hypocellular.

Patients with Fanconi's anemia are at increased risk for developing malignancies, including myelodysplasia, leukemia (usually acute myelogenous leukemia), and others. The incidence of malignancy begins to rise after patients are about 10 years old and increases progressively with age.

Diagnosis

The main diagnostic test is culturing the patient's lymphocytes in diepoxybutane or mitomycin C and demonstrating increased chromosomal instability.

Table 8–3
Physical Abnormalities in Fanconi's Anemia*

Skin hyperpigmentation: trunk, neck, intertriginous areas

Short stature

Upper limb abnormalities: thumbs, hands, radii, ulnae

Hypogonadism and genital abnormalities (males)

Other skeletal abnormalities: head, face, neck, spine, lower extremities

Anomalies of eyes, eyelids, or epicanthal folds

Renal abnormalities

*Abnormalities seen in ≥25% of cases.

Treatment

The treatment of choice for patients with Fanconi's anemia and pancytopenia is allogeneic bone marrow transplant, preferably from a human leukocyte antigen HLA-identical sibling. This cures the hematologic disease but, unfortunately, does not decrease the risk of malignancy. Androgens may improve the cytopenias if a compatible bone marrow donor is not available.

Other Constitutional Aplastic Anemias

Schwachman-Diamond Syndrome

The Schwachman-Diamond syndrome is an inherited disorder characterized by exocrine pancreatic deficiency, pancytopenia, skeletal changes, and others. Inheritance is autosomal recessive. The cause is unknown, but chromosomal fragility is not increased. Patients with Schwachman-Diamond syndrome also are predisposed to developing myelodysplasia and acute leukemia.

Dyskeratosis Congenita

Dyskeratosis congenita consists of mucocutaneous abnormalities with variable hematologic disorders. The mucocutaneous changes include reticulated pigmentation of skin in the upper body, mucosal leukoplakia, and dystrophic changes in the nails. The inheritance pattern appears to be variable; the majority are X-linked. Chromosomal fragility is not increased. The mucocutaneous changes appear in all patients, usually before the age of 10 years. Aplastic anemia occurs in approximately half of patients, usually in their teens. Patients with dyskeratosis congenita also have an increased risk of malignancy.

ACQUIRED APLASTIC ANEMIA

Acquired aplastic anemia can be due to a variety of causes. Important examples include chemicals, drugs or medications, infections, and pregnancy. However, at least half of cases are idiopathic, in which no underlying cause can be found.

Causes of Acquired Aplastic Anemia

Ionizing Radiation

Bone marrow injury is an inevitable consequence of ionizing radiation, and bone marrow failure is a common cause of death in people exposed to lethal doses of radiation. The dose that is lethal to 50% of people (LD_{50}) is approximately 4.5 Gray (Gy) of total body irradiation. A dose of 10 Gy is lethal to 100%.

Chemicals

Benzene is the chemical that has been most closely tied to aplastic anemia. Benzene and its metabolites bind to DNA, inhibit DNA synthesis, and induce strand breaks. It has been used in the manufacture of a wide variety of products, including leather, shoes, paint, rubber, dyes, drugs, linoleum, batteries, and others. It is also used as a solvent and cleaning solution. Benzene is found in automobile exhaust, some petroleum distillates, and cigarette smoke. Signs of benzene toxicity can occur within a few weeks of exposure or may not occur for many years. Aplastic anemia may develop long after the exposure has stopped. Benzene has also been linked to the development of acute myelogenous leukemia.

Other chemicals that have been linked to aplastic anemia include other hydrocarbons and organic solvents, pesticides, and inorganic arsenic.

Drugs and Medications

Drugs are the second most common cause of aplastic anemia, responsible for approximately 15 to 25% of cases. Drugs can cause aplastic anemia in two ways: an **expected dose-related aplasia** and an **unexpected idiosyncratic reaction**. The first type of reaction will occur in anyone, given a sufficient amount of the medication. The second type of reaction is rare, occurring in only a small proportion of people given the medication, and can occur with small doses.

Cancer chemotherapy drugs are the most common causes of expected dose-related aplastic anemia. Virtually all chemotherapy drugs cause bone marrow suppression as an inevitable result of their cytotoxic effect; however, the effect is transient and reversible.

A wide variety of medications have been associated with aplastic anemia of the idiosyncratic type. The best documented examples are *chloramphenicol* and *phenylbutazone*. Other medications that have been implicated include gold compounds, sulfonamides (trimethoprim-sulfamethoxazole) and other antibiotics, nonsteroidal anti-inflammatory drugs, antithyroid and anticonvulsant medications, and others (Table 8–4). Chloramphenicol can cause both an expected dose-related suppression of erythropoiesis and idiosyncratic aplastic anemia. The mechanism of idiosyncratic reactions to chloramphenicol and other medications is not clear. Hematopoiesis may or may not recover after the medication is stopped.

Table 8–4
Drugs Associated with Aplastic Anemia

Strong Association	Weaker or Rare Association*
Chloramphenicol	Antibiotics: streptomycin, tetracycline, methicillin, ampicillin, mebendazole, flucytosine, mefloquine, dapsone
Phenylbutazone	Nonsteroidal anti-inflammatory drugs: indomethacin, ibuprofen, sulindac, diclofenac, naproxen, piroxicam, fenoprofen, fenbufen, aspirin
Anticonvulsants: hydantoins, carbamazepine, ethosuximide	Antihistamines: cimetidine, ranitidine, chlorpheniramine, tripelenamine
Gold compounds	Sedatives and tranquilizers: chlorpromazine, prochlorperazine, piperacetazine, chlordiazepoxide, meprobamate, methyprylon, remoxipride
Sulfonamides; trimethoprim-sulfamethoxazole	Antiarrhythmics: tocainide, amiodarone
Antithyroid medications: methimazole, methylthiouracil, propylthiouracil	Allopurinol
Oral hypoglycemic agents: tolbutamide, carbutamide, chlorpropamide	Ticlopidine
Carbonic anhydrase inhibitors: acetazolamide, methazolamide, mesalazine	Methyldopa
D-penicillamine	Quinidine
2-Chlorodeoxyadenosine (cladribine)	Lithium Carbimazole Deferoxamine Amphetamines Corticosteroids

*Some of these represent single case reports.
Adapted from Hoffman R, Benz EJ, Shattil SJ, et al, editors. Hematology: basic principles and practice. 3rd ed. New York: Churchill Livingstone; 2000. p. 304.

Viral Infections

Viral infections are a well-documented cause of aplastic anemia. The strongest association is with **hepatitis**. Approximately 5 to 10% of aplastic anemia cases in the United States and Europe appear to be related to hepatitis. The hepatitis virus associated with aplastic anemia has not been identified; aplastic anemia does not appear to be related to any of the known hepatitis viruses (A, B, C, D [delta], E, or G). The signs of aplastic anemia usually appear approximately 1 to 2 months after the onset of hepatitis, occurring most often in young men. Aplastic anemia can also rarely occur with Epstein-Barr virus (EBV), HIV, parvovirus B19, dengue virus, and flavivirus.

Miscellaneous

Aplastic anemia has been reported in *pregnancy*. Completion or termination of the pregnancy is usually followed by hematologic recovery. Aplastic anemia has occasionally been reported in *tuberculosis*. Other causes include *autoimmune diseases* (rheumatoid arthritis, systemic lupus erythematosus, diffuse eosinophilic fasciitis), *thymoma*, *hypogammaglobulinemia*, *immune thyroid diseases*, and *transfusion-related graft-versus-host disease (GVHD)*.

Idiopathic

Despite extensive evaluation, no underlying cause can be found in at least half of the cases (*idiopathic aplastic anemia*). It is now clear that immune-mediated suppression of hematopoiesis is responsible for most cases of idiopathic aplastic anemia. T lymphocytes from patients with idiopathic aplastic anemia have been shown to produce γ-interferon and tumor necrosis factor, which suppress proliferation of hematopoietic progenitor cells. They may cause progenitor cells to undergo the process of *apoptosis* (programmed cell death).

Clinical Manifestations

Aplastic anemia is primarily a disease of younger people, with a peak incidence at 15 to 25 years. Some series show a second peak after about 60 years.

The most common complaints are *fatigue*, *weakness* or *dyspnea on exertion*, and *easy bruising and mucocutaneous bleeding*. Despite granulocytopenia, infections are not a common presenting complaint. The onset of symptoms is usually gradual and insidious but may be abrupt.

Evaluation

History

A complete past medical history and family history (with particular regard to anemia or other hematologic diseases) are required. A complete and detailed medication history is mandatory, including past as well as current medications. It is also important to ask about non-prescription medications, diet supplements, and herbal remedies. A complete occupational history is required, with particular attention to chemical or radiation exposure. It is also important to ask about hobbies, particularly those that might involve solvent or chemical exposure.

Physical Examination

The physical examination in aplastic anemia is generally unremarkable except for pallor and mucocutaneous petechiae or purpura. There may be mild splenomegaly. The presence of lymphadenopathy or marked splenomegaly indicates a disease process other than aplastic anemia.

Laboratory Diagnosis
Complete Blood Count

The complete blood count shows a decrease in at least two cell lines and often all three. The blood smear may reveal mild macrocytosis of red blood cells, but *other morphologic abnormalities, blasts and other immature cells must be absent*. The reticulocyte count is decreased.

Bone Marrow

Both a bone marrow aspirate and biopsy are required. It is important that the biopsy be adequate in size for evaluation (at least 1 cm in length), without extensive aspiration or crush artifact. The marrow must be hypocellular. The aspirate usually has a predominance of lymphocytes and plasma cells; normal hematopoietic precursors of all types are reduced. It is critical to carefully evaluate the aspirate for dysplastic features. There may be dysplastic changes in erythroid precursors (*dyserythropoiesis*), but there should not be any dysplastic changes in granulocyte precursors or megakaryocytes. A careful count of myeloblasts is also required. Marrow cellularity is best assessed on the biopsy. Normal cellularity varies inversely with age but should be ≥30% below age 70 and ≥20% above age 70. Lymphoid aggregates are often present, but fibrosis, granulomas, and metastatic neoplasm must be absent.

➪   Cellularity in the marrow can be variable, and hematopoietic hot spots may be present in aplastic anemia despite an overall decrease in cellularity. Therefore, a single bone marrow biopsy may not be representative of the actual marrow cellularity. It is possible to have both false-positive and false-negative hypocellularity on biopsy due to sampling error.

Differential Diagnosis

Aplastic anemia is a diagnosis of exclusion. The differential diagnosis includes all causes of pancytopenia. Three conditions, in particular, can be difficult to exclude: *hypocellular myelodysplasia, hypocellular acute leukemia,* and *paroxysmal nocturnal hemoglobinuria (PNH).*

- **Hypocellular myelodysplasia** is diagnosed by the presence of dysplastic changes in the granulocytic series and megakaryocytes. Dysplastic changes include abnormal granularity or nuclear-cytoplasmic dyssynchrony in granulocytes, or multinucleate megakaryocytes. A cytogenetic analysis should be done on the marrow; the presence of clonal cytogenetic abnormalities indicates myelodysplasia rather than aplastic anemia.

- **Hypocellular acute leukemia** is diagnosed by a predominance of blasts on the bone marrow aspirate or a predominance of immature cells in the biopsy if an aspirate is not available.

- **Paroxysmal nocturnal hemoglobinuria** can be diagnosed by demonstrating deficient expression of glycosyl phosphatidylinositol (GPI)-linked proteins on the surface of erythrocytes or granulocytes by flow cytometry (see the discussion of PNH in Chapter 7). The distinction between aplastic anemia and PNH is not always clear; patients with aplastic anemia may subsequently develop PNH, and patients with PNH may develop aplastic anemia. Sensitive flow cytometry tests have demonstrated deficient expression of GPI-linked proteins in many patients with aplastic anemia, even without clinical evidence of PNH. Some cases, therefore, appear to represent an overlap between PNH and aplastic anemia.

Treatment

With supportive care alone, the prognosis for severe aplastic anemia is grim, with less than 10% surviving at 1 year. Patients with less severe disease survive longer. The treatment of aplastic anemia can be divided into two phases: *supportive care* and *definitive therapy.*

Supportive Care

Supportive care includes red cell transfusions for symptomatic anemia and platelet transfusions for bleeding due to thrombocytopenia. Prophylactic platelet transfusions should be considered for patients with severe thrombocytopenia (5,000–10,000/μL) even in the absence of bleeding. It is desirable to use single donor platelets as much as possible to avoid alloimmunization and the patient becoming refractory to future platelet transfusions. *Transfusions from relatives or potential bone marrow donors should be avoided to decrease the chance of later marrow transplant rejection.* Antibiotics should also be given for fevers or infection in the presence of neutropenia (absolute neutrophil count ≤500–1,000/μL). Initially, broad-spectrum antibiotics should be used for fever, with specific antibiotics chosen based on results of the cultures.

The patient should have *HLA typing* done immediately after diagnosis, in consideration for possible bone marrow transplantation. It may also assist in selecting platelet transfusions if becoming refractory due to alloimmunization develops.

A decision on definitive therapy needs to be considered early, particularly in patients who are candidates for bone marrow transplantation. Extensive transfusions prior to transplant increases the risk of graft failure.

Definitive Therapy

Options for definitive therapy for aplastic anemia include *bone marrow transplantation* and *immunosuppressive therapy*. Bone marrow transplantation is considered the treatment of choice in young, otherwise healthy patients with severe aplastic anemia who have a related histocompatible donor. Long-term survival rates for patients less than 40 years of age transplanted from HLA-identical siblings are currently approximately 75%. Survival rates for patients less than 40 years of age receiving a transplant from an HLA-matched unrelated donor are approximately 40 to 50%. The major causes of transplant failure include infection or hemorrhage in the immediate post-transplant period, graft failure, and GVHD. The rate of graft failure averages approximately 10%; the risk of graft failure is increased in patients who have been extensively transfused prior to the transplantation. *Graft-versus-host disease* is the major cause of morbidity and mortality after allogeneic bone marrow transplant. Acute GVHD usually begins within the first 6 weeks after transplant. The major organs involved are the skin, the gastrointestinal tract, and the liver. Manifestations include skin rashes, ranging from mild to desquamation; diarrhea, ranging from transient watery diarrhea to bloody diarrhea with ileus; and abnormal liver chemistries to liver failure. Chronic GVHD usually occurs after 100 days from transplantation and can involve the skin, gastrointestinal tract, liver, lungs, and others.

Immunosuppressive therapy includes antithymocyte globulin (ATG) and cyclosporin A. Response rates up to 80% have been shown in different series, with 5-year survival rates for responders of up to 80 to 90%. Unfortunately, responses may be partial (independence from transfusion rather than normalization of blood counts), and patients may relapse or transform to myelodysplasia or PNH. The intense immunosuppression involved also creates a significant risk of infection.

PURE RED CELL APLASIA

Pure red cell aplasia resembles aplastic anemia in many ways: many of the causes and treatment are similar. The primary difference is that there is a selective absence of erythroid precursors in the marrow. Granulocyte precursors and megakaryocytes are normal.

Congenital Hypoplastic Anemia (Diamond-Blackfan Anemia)

Congenital hypoplastic anemia (**CHA**) is heterogeneous in clinical features, pattern of inheritance, and associated anomalies. It probably represents several different conditions, with the common feature of onset during infancy. The estimated incidence is 4 to 7 per million live births. A family history of congenital anemia is present in about 10 to 20% of cases; inheritance appears to be autosomal dominant in most cases. The cause or causes of CHA are unknown.

Clinical Features

Congenital hypoplastic anemia usually presents in infancy, most often at about 2 to 3 months of age. Approximately 25% are anemic at birth; about 10% are diagnosed after 1 year of age. About half of children with CHA have associated physical anomalies such as craniofacial anomalies (cleft or high-arched palate, widely spaced eyes, and flat nasal bridge), abnormalities of the thumbs, growth retardation, and deafness.

Laboratory

The anemia is moderate to severe (hemoglobin 2–10 g/dL) and is often macrocytic. The reticulocyte count is <1%. The proportion of fetal hemoglobin is increased, and the cells have increased expression of the fetal form of the I/i antigen group. Erythrocyte adenosine deaminase levels are increased. The bone marrow shows an absence of recognizable erythroid precursors in most cases, although occasional proerythroblasts may be present in a few cases.

Differential Diagnosis

The common types of childhood anemia (iron deficiency, hemoglobinopathy) must be excluded. Thereafter, the most important differential diagnosis is CHA versus *transient erythroblastopenia of childhood* (**TEC**). The most useful distinguishing features include age at onset, presence of a family history of anemia starting in infancy, and presence of associated physical anomalies (Table 8–5).

Table 8–5
Congenital Hypoplastic Anemia versus Transient Erythroblastopenia of Childhood

Characteristic	CHA	TEC
Age at Onset	Usually <1 year	Usually >1 year
Family History	Sometimes present	Absent
MCV	Frequently elevated	Normal
RBC precursors in bone marrow	Absent or decreased	Absent or decreased
Fetal hemoglobin*	Increased	Normal
RBC i antigen*	Present	Absent
RBC adenosine deaminase activity	Elevated	Normal

*These features are useful only in the reticulocytopenic child; RBCs may have fetal characteristics during recovery phase of TEC.
Adapted from Hoffman R, Benz EJ, Shattil SJ, et al, editors. Hematology: basic principles and practices. 3rd ed. New York: Churchill Lievingstone; 2000. p. 347.

Treatment

The primary treatment for CHA is corticosteroids. Prednisolone (or equivalent) is started at a dose of 2 mg/kg/day. The reticulocyte count usually begins to increase within 2 weeks, and the hemoglobin begins to rise within 1 month. The corticosteroid dose is then tapered to determine the minimum effective dose, given on an alternate-day schedule. Up to 70% of children respond to corticosteroids, but often the best hemoglobin level that can be achieved is 8 to 9 g/dL. About 40 to 50% of children require chronic transfusions because of failure to respond or unacceptable side effects from corticosteroids. Iron overload becomes a significant problem, and iron chelation therapy is required to prevent the development of cirrhosis and other complications of excess iron.

Bone marrow transplantation has been effective in a small number of children with severe CHA unresponsive to corticosteroids. Erythropoietin, cyclosporin A, interleukin-3, and androgens have also been tried in CHA, but results in general have been disappointing.

Transient Erythroblastopenia of Childhood

Transient erythroblastopenia of childhood is an acquired self-limited red cell aplasia occurring in previously healthy children. There is spontaneous recovery, and recurrence is unusual. The most likely etiology is a transient immune-mediated suppression of erythropoiesis related to a preceding viral infection. A few cases appear to be related to parvovirus B19, but no specific virus has been implicated in the majority of cases.

Clinical Features

Transient erythroblastopenia of childhood usually occurs between the ages of 1 and 5 years, with the majority of cases presenting around 2 years. Transient erythroblastopenia of childhood may occur in children less than 1 year old, and thus the age range may overlap with CHA. There is often a history of a preceding viral infection. Symptoms include a gradual onset of fatigue and decreased activity.

The physical examination is unremarkable except for pallor. Physical anomalies seen in CHA are absent.

The anemia is normocytic. Neutropenia is common; the platelet count is usually normal. Hemoglobin F is not increased, and the erythrocytes express the adult I antigen. The erythrocyte adenosine deaminase is normal.

The bone marrow is normocellular; there is an absence or marked decrease in recognizable erythroid progenitors.

No treatment is usually required. Reticulocytosis usually begins within 1 month of onset, and recovery is complete within 4 to 8 weeks. Red cell transfusions are sometimes needed for severe anemia. These should be guided by the presence of symptoms rather than by the hemoglobin level.

Acquired Pure Red Cell Aplasia

Acquired pure red cell aplasia (PRCA) can be divided into **primary** (idiopathic) and **secondary** types. The classification and causes of acquired PRCA bear a strong similarity to those of acquired aplastic anemia (Table 8–6). Most cases of primary acquired PRCA appear to be caused by an IgG antibody that inhibits proliferation and/or maturation of erythroid progenitor cells.

Causes of secondary acquired PRCA include the following:

- **Thymoma:** Approximately 5% of patients with thymoma develop red cell aplasia, and thymoma is found in approximately 10 to 15% of patients with PRCA. Pure red cell aplasia may precede the diagnosis of thymoma or appear years after its resection. The anemia will resolve in about 30 to 40% of patients after resection of the thymoma.
- **Hematologic Malignancies:** PRCA has been seen in association with a wide variety of hematologic neoplasms, but the strongest association is with *chronic lymphocytic leukemia* (CLL). Most cases are associated with typical B-CLL, but occasional cases are associated with leukemia of large granular lymphocytes or T-cell leukemia.

- **Parvovirus B19:** Parvovirus B19 is the cause of transient aplastic crises in patients with chronic hemolytic anemias, such as sickle cell anemia, and causes transient erythroid hypoplasia in normal people. Parvovirus B19 can cause chronic red cell aplasia in immunocompromised patients, such as patients with HIV. Administration of intravenous immunoglobulin results in recovery of erythropoiesis.
- **Other Infections:** Pure red cell aplasia may also be seen with other infections, most often viral hepatitis, EBV, mumps, cytomegalovirus (CMV), HIV, and *Mycoplasma pneumoniae*. However, PRCA is a rare complication of these infections.
- **Autoimmune Hemolytic Anemia:** Pure red cell aplasia occurs in a small number of cases of immune hemolytic anemia. In these cases, it is

Table 8–6
Causes of Pure Red Cell Aplasia

Congenital and Childhood Variants

Congenital hypoplastic anemia (Diamond-Blackfan anemia)

Transient erythroblastopenia of childhood

Acquired

Primary

Secondary

   Thymoma

   Hematologic malignancies: chronic lymphocytic leukemia, non-Hodgkin's lymphomas, Hodgkin's disease, others

   Non-hematologic malignancies

   Infections: parvovirus B19, HIV, EBV, adult T-cell lymphocytotrophic virus I, hepatitis, mumps, cytomegalovirus (CMV), *Mycoplasma pneumoniae*

   Autoimmune hemolytic anemia

   Collagen vascular diseases: systemic lupus erythematosus, rheumatoid arthritis

   Drugs and chemicals

   Pregnancy

   Severe renal failure

   Severe malnutrition

   Miscellaneous

Red cell aplasia with myelodysplastic features

Adapted from Hoffman R, Benz EJ, Shattil SJ, et al, editors. Hematology: basic principles and practices. 3rd ed. New York: Churchill Livingstone; 2000. p. 343.

believed that the antibody reacts with erythroid progenitors in the marrow, as well as more mature erythrocytes.

- **Drugs and Chemicals:** A long list of drugs and chemicals has been associated with PRCA (Table 8–7). The strongest associations are with diphenylhydantoin (Dilantin), azathioprine, chlorpropamide, and isoniazid. In most cases, erythropoiesis recovers after the drug is stopped.
- **Pregnancy:** Pure red cell aplasia is a rare complication of pregnancy (not to be confused with the mild dilutional decrease in hemoglobin that is normally present in the third trimester). Erythropoiesis usually recovers after delivery. Recurrence with subsequent pregnancies is unusual.

Clinical Features

Most patients with acquired PRCA are adults, with the peak age of onset in the fifth to seventh decades. The typical picture is a gradual onset of fatigue and weakness. The physical examination is usually unremarkable, except for pallor, in cases of idiopathic PRCA, but may show the changes of the primary illness in secondary PRCA.

Laboratory

The anemia is normocytic and may be quite severe. The white cell and platelet counts are normal. The blood smear shows unremarkable RBC

Table 8–7
Drugs and Chemicals Associated with Pure Red Cell Aplasia

Allopurinol	Fenoprofen	Sulfasalazine
α-Methyldopa	FK506 (tacrolimus)	Sulindac
Aminopyrine	Gold compounds	Thiamphenicol
Azathioprine	Halothane	Tolbutamide
Benzene	Isoniazid	Rifampin
Carbamazepine	Dapsone-pyrimethamine	Valproic acid
Cephalothin	Methazolamide	Zidovudine
Chloramphenicol	Penicillin	
Chlorpropamide	D-Penicillamine	
Trimethoprim-sulfamethoxazole	Phenobarbital	
Diphenylhydantoin (Dilantin)	Phenylbutazone	
Estrogens	Procainamide	

Adapted from Hoffman R, Benz EJ, Shattil SJ, et al, editors. Hematology: basic principles and practices. 3rd ed. New York: Churchill Livingstone; 2000. p. 344.

morphology. The reticulocyte count is depressed. The serum lactic dehydrogenase, bilirubin, and haptoglobin are all normal.

The bone marrow is normocellular, with an absence or marked decrease in recognizable erythroid precursors (<1% of marrow cells). Granulocyte precursors and megakaryocytes are present and show normal maturation. There should be no morphologic abnormalities in any cell lines. Lymphocytes may be increased in number, and lymphoid aggregates may be present on biopsy. The presence of proerythoblasts with vacuolated cytoplasm raises a possibility of parvovirus B19 infection or severe malnutrition. In occasional cases, PRCA may be preceded by a period of dyserythropoiesis, with erythroid hyperplasia in the marrow and maturation arrest at the proerythroblast or basophilic erythroblast stage.

Cytogenetic analysis performed on the bone marrow is usually normal. The presence of a clonal cytogenetic abnormality suggests a myelodysplastic syndrome.

Evaluation

The evaluation is generally similar to that of aplastic anemia. A complete past medical history is required, with particular attention to any family history of anemia and a complete list of medications. A computed tomographic (CT) scan of the chest should be obtained to detect or exclude thymoma. Cobalamin (vitamin B_{12}) and folate levels should be determined. Serologic studies for hepatitis viruses, parvovirus B19, HIV, systemic lupus erythematosus, and other autoimmune diseases should be obtained. Lymphocytosis in the blood or marrow should be studied by flow cytometry to detect or exclude chronic lymphocytic leukemia. Any suggestions, from the history or physical examination, of an illness that could cause secondary PRCA should be evaluated appropriately.

Treatment

All possible medications should be discontinued, and any infections should be treated. Any other type of secondary PRCA should be treated appropriately. If no cause of secondary PRCA is found and erythropoiesis fails to recover within 1 month, the patient is considered to have primary PRCA.

The treatment for idiopathic PRCA (or secondary PRCA not responding to treatment of the primary illness) is immunosuppressive therapy, starting with corticosteroids. Prednisone (1 mg/kg/day or equivalent) is given and the reticulocyte count and hemoglobin are monitored weekly or biweekly. About 40% of patients show improvement within 1 month; patients who will respond usually do so within 2 to 3 months. Once the hematocrit level reaches 35%, the dose can be slowly decreased over 3 to 4 months and then discontinued. Alternative therapies for patients who fail to respond to corticosteroids include cytotoxic agents such as cyclophosphamide or azathioprine, cyclosporine, antithymocyte globulin, and intra venous immunoglobulin. Combination of a cytotoxic agent or cyclosporine with a corticosteroid may be more beneficial than single agents used alone Plasmapheresis may be helpful in patients with an IgG inhibitor who fail to respond to immunosuppressive medications. Splenectomy has been used a a final measure in patients who fail to respond to any of the immunosup pressive regimens.

Overall, approximately two-thirds of patients respond to immunosup pressive therapy. Relapses are common in patients who respond to therapy (up to 80%), but most patients respond to repeat immunosuppressive ther apy. Occasional patients may require low-dose maintenance immunosup pressive therapy for 1 to 2 years.

Spontaneous remissions have been reported to occur in about 5 to 10% of patients.

Red Cell Aplasia with Myelodysplastic Features

Pure red cell aplasia may rarely be the initial presenting feature of myelodysplastic syndrome (MDS). Such patients eventually develop pancy topenia, with obvious dysplastic features. In some patients, this evolves into an acute myelogenous leukemia; others die of bone marrow failure. Patient with dysplastic changes in the blood or bone marrow at diagnosis are a higher risk for transformation, as are patients with a clonal cytogenetic abnormality on cytogenetic analysis.

Patients having PRCA with myelodysplastic features should be tried on immunosuppressive therapy, as above. Most fail to respond and will even tually require chronic transfusion therapy.

CONGENITAL DYSERYTHROPOIETIC ANEMIAS

The *congenital dyserythropoietic anemias* (**CDA**) are an uncommon group of inherited conditions characterized by anemia with morphologic abnormal ities of erythroid precursors in the bone marrow. Three distinct types have been recognized. Unlike CHA or other types of red cell aplasia, the CDAs are characterized by *erythroid hyperplasia in the bone marrow*, with ineffec tive erythropoiesis. The anemia in many cases is mild and may not be detected for years, possibly not until adulthood.

The three described types are as follows:

- **Congenital dyserythropoietic anemia type I** appears to be inherited as an autosomal recessive disorder. The anemia is usually mild to moderate (hemoglobin 8–11 g/dL) with mild macrocytosis, anisocytosis, and poikilocytosis. Splenomegaly is present. The bone marrow is hypercellular with increased erythroid precursors. A characteristic feature is internuclear bridges between erythroblasts. The cause is unknown.

- **Congenital dyserythropoietic anemia type II** is also known as HEMPAS (**H**ereditary **E**rythroblastic **M**ultinuclearity with a **P**ositive **A**cidified **S**erum test). It is the most common type of CDA. Inheritance is autosomal recessive. Most patients have mild to moderate anemia; however, severe anemia is occasionally present. Erythrocytes are usually normocytic or mildly macrocytic. Acanthocytes and other bizarre cells may be seen. The characteristic feature is that acidified serum from approximately 30% of normal people lyses CDA type II cells. Unlike paroxysmal nocturnal hemoglobinuria (PNH), the patient's own serum does not cause hemolysis. The bone marrow shows erythroid hyperplasia; many late erythroid precursors are binucleate, with occasional multinucleate cells. On electron microscopy there are two layers to the cell membrane.

- **Congenital dyserythropoietic anemia type III** is the rarest of the CDAs. Most cases are inherited in an autosomal dominant fashion. There is usually a mild macrocytic anemia. There may be an element of intravascular hemolysis, with consequent iron loss. The bone marrow aspirate shows striking multinuclearity of erythroblasts (up to 12 nuclei per cell).

Treatment

The anemia in many cases of CDA is mild and does not require specific therapy. Occasional patients with severe anemia require chronic red cell transfusions. Iron overload may develop due to increased gastrointestinal absorption, even without transfusions, and iron chelation therapy may be required.

Additional Readings

Ball SE, Gordon-Smith EC. Failure of red cell production. In: Lilleyman JS, Hann IM, Blanchette VS, editors. Pediatric hematology. 2nd ed. London: Churchill-Livingstone; 1999. p. 65–81.

Horowitz MH. Current status of allogeneic bone marrow transplantation in acquired aplastic anemia. Semin Hematol 2000;37:30–42.

Young NS. Hematopoietic cell destruction by immune mechanisms in acquired aplastic anemia. Semin Hematol 2000;37:3–14.

Erythrocytosis and Polycythemia

A decrease in the hemoglobin or hematocrit (anemia) is a common clinical problem. An *increase* in the hemoglobin is much less common. An increase in the hemoglobin is designated *erythrocytosis* or *polycythemia*.

Erythrocytosis is defined as an increase in red cells (or blood hemoglobin) *per unit volume*. **Polycythemia** (also called **absolute erythrocytosis**) indicates an absolute increase in *red cell mass* and reflects an increase in red blood cell (RBC) production. Since the red cell count given on the complete blood count (CBC) reflects a ratio of red cells per unit volume, it is possible to have an increase in the RBC count (or hemoglobin or hematocrit) due to either an increase in the red cell mass (polycythemia) or a decrease in the plasma volume (*relative erythrocytosis*). Polycythemia can be a response to some other condition causing hypoxemia (*secondary polycythemia*), can result from inappropriate erythropoietin secretion due to renal disease or some neoplasms, or can represent an autonomous neoplastic condition (*polycythemia vera*). Polycythemia vera (sometimes called *polycythemia rubra vera*) is a chronic myeloproliferative disorder and is discussed in Chapter 14.

RELATIVE ERYTHROCYTOSIS

Relative erythrocytosis represents a decrease in the intravascular plasma volume rather than an increase in the red cell mass. Acutely, it may result from decreased fluid intake; increased fluid loss from sweating, vomiting, or diarrhea; increased urine output due to diuretics or osmotic diuresis; severe burns; or a shift of fluid into the extravascular space ("third spacing"). It may also occur at high altitude. In most conditions, the cause will usually be obvious.

Patients with chronic relative erythrocytosis have been described as having *Gaisböck syndrome*, *stress erythrocytosis*, *spurious polycythemia*, or *pseudopolycythemia*. The classic patient is a middle-aged male, often overweight, hypertensive, and a cigarette smoker. The existence of Gaisböck syndrome as a true clinical entity has been challenged; these patients may represent the extreme end of the normal population rather than a syndrome.

Relative erythrocytosis can be confirmed by determining the red cell mass and plasma volume by radioisotope dilution studies. The red cell mass is normal, but the plasma volume is decreased.

It is controversial whether patients with relative erythrocytosis should be treated with phlebotomy to rapidly lower the hemoglobin. The increased hemoglobin does increase blood viscosity and may increase the risk of stroke or other thrombotic event; however, phlebotomy has not been shown to provide a definite benefit. The hemoglobin can often be decreased by controlling weight and blood pressure and discontinuing smoking. Cytotoxic drugs like hydroxyurea should be avoided.

POLYCYTHEMIA (ABSOLUTE ERYTHROCYTOSIS)

Absolute erythrocytosis can be divided into *primary* (idiopathic polycythemia or polycythemia vera) and *secondary* types. Secondary polycythemia is due to increased erythropoietin effect, which may be either *physiologically appropriate* (due to decreased tissue oxygenation) or *physiologically inappropriate* (due to neoplasms, renal cysts, exogenous erythropoietin, androgen excess).

- **Physiologically appropriate** absolute erythrocytosis is due to hypoxemia. The kidneys respond to decreased oxygen supply by increasing erythropoietin production. Causes include living at high altitude, chronic pulmonary disease with hypoxemia, heart disease with right to left shunt, hypoventilation syndromes, abnormal hemoglobin with decreased oxygen delivery to tissues (high-oxygen-affinity hemoglobins, methemoglobins), and carboxyhemoglobin due to cigarette smoking.
- **Physiologically inappropriate** absolute erythrocytosis is due to increased erythropoietin effect that is not due to tissue hypoxemia. This can occur with (1) renal disease of various types, including cysts and renal artery stenosis; (2) neoplasms, particularly renal cell carcinomas, hepatocellular carcinomas, and cerebellar hemangioblastomas (less often uterine leiomyomas, meningiomas, and others); (3) androgens; and (4) exogenous erythropoietin ("blood doping").

Rare cases of **familial polycythemia** have been reported, many with autosomal dominant inheritance.

Table 9–1 summarizes the causes of erythrocytosis and polycythemia.

Evaluation of Erythrocytosis

The first goal of evaluation is to distinguish relative erythrocytosis from true polycythemia. In patients with true polycythemia, it is necessary to distinguish patients with polycythemia vera from secondary polycythemia and to detect medically important (and possibly correctable) causes of secondary polycythemia.

Evaluation of a patient with erythrocytosis begins with a history and physical and selected laboratory tests and imaging studies (Table 9–2).

Table 9–1
Causes of Erythrocytosis and Polycythemia

Relative Erythrocytosis	Polycythemia (True Erythrocytosis)
Hemoconcentration: • Copious sweating • Severe vomiting or diarrhea • Increased urine output: diuretics, osmotic diuresis • Burns • Shift into extravascular space ("third spacing") Spurious polycythemia (Gaisböck syndrome)	Secondary to decreased tissue oxygenation (physiologically appropriate): • High altitude • Pulmonary disease with hypoxemia • Cyanotic congenital heart disease • Hypoventilation syndromes: Pickwickian syndrome, sleep apnea • Abnormal hemoglobins: high-oxygen-affinity hemoglobins, methemoglobins • Carboxyhemoglobin (cigarette smoking) Secondary to abnormal erythropoietin production or response (physiologically inappropriate): • Renal disease: cysts, hydronephrosis, renal artery stenosis, focal glomerulonephritis • Neoplasms: renal cell carcinoma, hepatocellular carcinoma, cerebellar hemangioma, others • Androgen abuse • Erythropoietin abuse ("blood doping") Idiopathic polycythemia Familial polycythemia Polycythemia rubra vera

Adapted from Lee RG, Foerster J, Lukens J, et al, editors. Wintrobe's clinical hematology. 10th ed. Baltimore: Williams & Wilkins; 1999. p. 1542.

Table 9–2

Tests to Consider in Patients with Erythrocytosis

Initial Studies	Subsequent Studies
Room air arterial blood gas (PaO$_2$ and SaO$_2$)	Red cell mass and plasma volume studies
Chest radiograph	Serum erythropoietin level (sensitive assay)
Urinalysis	Carboxyhemoglobin level
	Hemoglobin electrophoresis
	Hemoglobin-oygen dissociation curve (P$_{50}$)
	Abdominal CT scan

History

It is important to ask about previous CBCs to determine if the patient has ever had an abnormal hemoglobin. Check for any symptoms of cardiac or pulmonary disease that might be associated with hypoxemia. Other things to consider include (1) living at high altitude; (2) snoring (sleep apnea); (3) medications, particularly diuretics and androgens; (4) occupational exposure to carbon monoxide; (5) cigarette smoking; and (6) a family history of blood disease.

Examination

The patient should be examined for cyanosis and clubbing of the fingertips. Careful examination of the cardiac and respiratory systems is critical. Palpate the abdomen for masses. Carefully check the spleen size; the presence of splenomegaly suggests polycythemia vera or another myeloproliferative disorder.

Laboratory Studies

The presence of leukocytosis or thrombocytosis suggests polycythemia vera or another myeloproliferative disorder. The blood smear should be examined for immature granulocytes, giant platelets, or other abnormal cells; the presence of any of these would suggest a myeloproliferative disorder. Routine serum chemistries should be tested, particularly urea nitrogen and creatinine. A careful urinalysis is critical. A **room air arterial blood gas** (partial pressure of oxygen [PaO$_2$] and oxygen saturation [SaO$_2$]) should be done.

 Red cell mass and **plasma volume** studies are the next step if no cause for the erythrocytosis has been detected with the simple screen. Red cell mass is measured by removing some of the patient's red cells, labeling them with a known amount of radioactive chromium or other isotope, injecting them back into the patient, and then determining the radioactive content of a second aliquot of blood after the cells have been allowed to equilibrate. Plasma volume is determined by injecting albumin labeled with another radioactive isotope, allowing it to equilibrate, and then measuring the proportion of the isotope contained in a blood sample.

⇨ It has been suggested that any man with a hematocrit over 60% or woman with hematocrit over 50% *must* have an expanded red cell mass and that red cell mass studies are unnecessary in such patients.

If the patient is found to have a decreased plasma volume and a normal red cell mass (relative erythrocytosis), it is then necessary to determine the cause of the decreased plasma volume. If no cause is found, the patient is presumed to have Gaisböck syndrome.

If the patient is found to have an increased red cell mass, polycythemia vera or another myeloproliferative disorder must be excluded. The features that favor polycythemia are listed in Table 9–3. A **serum erythropoietin (EPO) level**, using a sensitive assay, may help in this distinction: a patient with polycythemia vera has erythrocyte production that is independent of erythropoietin, and thus the EPO level is usually decreased. A normal or elevated erythropoietin level suggests that the erythrocytosis is driven by EPO and thus is presumably secondary. It is important to note that the EPO level may return to the normal range if the increased hemoglobin compensates for the decreased tissue oxygen supply. A normal EPO level does not exclude erythropoietin-dependent polycythemia.

A test for **blood carboxyhemoglobin level** should be done, particularly in cigarette smokers. If the patient has a family history of erythrocytosis, a hemoglobin electrophoresis and hemoglobin-oxygen dissociation curve should also be done. The **hemoglobin electrophoresis** will detect methe-

Table 9–3
Features That Favor Polycythemia Vera

Leukocytosis and/or thrombocytosis

Splenomegaly

Decreased serum erythropoietin level

Increased serum cobalamin level

Increased leukocyte alkaline phosphatase (LAP) score

Endogenous erythroid colony growth

No detectable primary cause

moglobinemias and some cases of high-oxygen-affinity hemoglobins. However, the **hemoglobin-oxygen dissociation curve** is needed to detect most high-oxygen-affinity hemoglobin variants. A decrease in the partial pressure at which hemoglobin is 50% saturated with oxygen (P_{50}) indicates a high-oxygen-affinity hemoglobin variant.

An **abdominal CT scan** should be considered to look for intra-abdominal neoplasms (renal cell carcinomas, hepatocellular carcinomas) and to accurately measure the spleen size.

Other tests that can be done include a leukocyte alkaline phosphatase (LAP) score and serum cobalamin levels. Both are often increased in polycythemia vera. A bone marrow examination with cytogenetic analysis can sometimes be helpful. The bone marrow in patients with polycythemia vera usually has hyperplasia of all cell lineages (including granulocytic progenitors and megakaryocytes) and an absence of stainable iron and may have fibrosis and cytogenetic abnormalities. Bone marrows from patients with erythroid hyperplasia of other causes usually have pure erythroid hyperplasia (without increased granulocyte precursors or megakaryocytes). As well, fibrosis is absent, stainable iron is more often present, and cytogenetic abnormalities are absent. A more sophisticated test that is occasionally helpful is the assay of bone marrow cells for *endogenous erythroid colony growth*. Erythroid progenitors from patients with polycythemia vera demonstrate growth in culture independent of added erythropoietin. This test is not widely available but not usually needed.

Treatment of Erythrocytosis

Treatment of polycythemia vera is discussed in Chapter 14.

Control of blood pressure and a reduction in weight will often decrease the hemoglobin in patients with Gaisböck syndrome. If they are experiencing symptoms due to the increased hemoglobin (transient ischemic attacks, cerebrovascular accidents, congestive heart failure, digital ischemia), a program of phlebotomy should be undertaken to decrease the hematocrit to about 45% and maintain it at that level. Approximately 250 to 500 mL of blood can be withdrawn once or twice per week as needed. Saline may need to be given to compensate for the decrease in blood volume.

Primary causes of secondary polycythemia (chronic pulmonary disease, cardiac disease, renal cell carcinoma) should be treated appropriately. If the patients are having symptoms from hyperviscosity, phlebotomy should be used to rapidly lower the hematocrit.

Familial polycythemia usually does not require treatment.

10

Disorders of Leukocyte Function and Number

This chapter presents the disorders of neutrophil function and causes of increased or decreased white blood cell counts (excluding hematologic malignancies such as leukemia). Immune deficiencies of lymphocytes will not be discussed as they are more in the field of immunology rather than hematology.

NEUTROPHIL FUNCTION

Polymorphonuclear neutrophil leukocytes (PMNs) are the most common granulocytes and the primary defense against bacterial infection. Although we call them white *blood* cells (WBCs), their primary site of action is the extravascular spaces. In order to function properly, PMNs must complete several sequential steps. A deficiency in any one of these steps results in increased susceptibility to infection. The sequential steps are as follows:

- **Chemotaxis:** Neutrophils must move toward *chemotactic agents* released by bacteria or inflammatory processes. Chemotactic agents include bacterial products (small peptides), complement components (C5a), leukotrienes (LTB4), and others. In order to do this, the neutrophils must have cell surface receptors to detect the chemotactic agents, and they must be able to move toward the site of infection.
- **Adherence to and passage through the endothelium:** Adherence to the endothelium is mediated by cell adhesion molecules (CAMs) on PMNs that recognize other CAMs on the endothelial surface. The "stickiness" of the CAMs is increased by inflammatory mediators, increasing the tendency of PMNs to adhere to the endothelium. There are several fam-

ilies of CAMs and their receptors. One family that is important in leukocyte function is the *integrin* family. The integrins are dimers consisting of an α chain and a β chain; there are many different α and β chains that form various combinations. Three integrins that combine the β_2 **subunit** (**CD18** in the Cluster Designation [CD] system) with three different α chains are particularly important in neutrophil function: C11a/CD18 (also called LFA-1), CD11b/CD18 (Mac1), and CD11c/CD18. Together these are sometimes called the *leukocyte integrins*.

- **Phagocytosis:** This is stimulated by *opsonins* on the surface of the microorganisms. Important opsonins include immunoglobulins, particularly IgG, and complement components, particularly C3b.
- **Microbial killing:** Neutrophils have several killing mechanisms, including oxygen-dependent mechanisms, reactive nitrogen intermediates generated through the nitric oxide pathway, and nonoxidative mechanisms ("defensins").

The oxygen-dependent killing mechanisms are a critical part of microbial killing. Activation of these mechanisms is indicated by a brief increase in oxygen consumption, described as the "respiratory burst." The system starts with generation of superoxide (O_2^-) by the enzyme *NADPH oxidase* (also called the *respiratory burst oxidase*), which requires NADPH (the reduced form of nicotinamide adenine dinucleotide phosphate). Superoxide is converted to hydrogen peroxide (H_2O_2) by the enzyme superoxide dismutase or is converted to hydroxyl radical ($OH^\bullet$) in the presence of iron. Hydrogen peroxide is converted to hypochlorous acid (HOCl), a potent antimicrobial agent, by the enzyme *myeloperoxidase* (MPO). The NADPH required for generation of superoxide is generated by the hexose monophosphate shunt (see Figure 3–1). The NADPH oxidase is a complex enzyme with multiple subunits. One of the key subunits is *cytochrome* b. The gene for one part of cytochrome *b* (*CYBB*) is on the X chromosome; the genes for the other subunits of the enzyme are on autosomal chromosomes.

Neutrophil Kinetics

The total body neutrophil pool is divided into three compartments: the *bone marrow storage compartment*, the *blood compartment*, and the *extravascular compartment*. The bone marrow storage compartment contains $\sim$2 $\times$ 10^9 cells/kg. The blood compartment contains $\sim$0.7 $\times$ 10^9 cells/kg, approximately half circulating (the circulating pool) and half adhering to or rolling along endothelial cells (the marginating pool). The size of the extravascular pool is not known.

DISORDERS OF NEUTROPHIL FUNCTION

Disorders of neutrophil function can be classified into **congenital** versus **acquired** disorders. They can further be classified into disorders of **chemotaxis, decreased phagocytosis due to impaired opsonization**, and **defects in microbial killing**. Some of the inherited disorders are associated with morphologic abnormalities in neutrophils, with or without associated abnormalities in neutrophil number.

Manifestations of Neutrophil Function Disorders

The most common manifestation of neutrophil function disorders is recurrent infections, predominantly due to bacteria. There may also be an increase in some fungal infections, predominantly *Candida* and *Aspergillus* species. The most common sites of infection are the skin, mouth and oropharynx, and respiratory tract.

Congenital Disorders of Neutrophil Function

Congenital disorders of neutrophil function are uncommon. The most common *clinically significant* inherited disorder of neutrophil function is **chronic granulomatous disease**. **Myeloperoxidase deficiency** is actually more common, but the majority of patients with MPO deficiency are asymptomatic. In some cases, there are morphologic abnormalities in neutrophils but without functional defects (Table 10–1).

Chronic Granulomatous Disease

The incidence of chronic granulomatous disease (**CGD**) is ~1 in 500,000 in the United States. Most cases result from a deficiency of NADPH oxidase, with loss of the respiratory burst and oxygen-dependent killing mechanisms. The majority of cases (~65–75%) are due to mutations in the *CYBB* gene for cytochrome *b*, on the X chromosome; inheritance is therefore X-linked in most cases. The X-linked forms are occasionally associated with the McLeod phenotype (absence of the Kell blood group antigens on erythrocytes), retinitis pigmentosa, and Duchenne's muscular dystrophy. The genes for these diseases are all located close to the *CYBB* gene on the X chromosome.

The primary manifestation of CGD is recurrent and intractable infections by microorganisms that possess the enzyme catalase, with granulomatous inflammation (histiocytes and lymphocytes) at the sites of infection. Common pathogens associated with CGD are listed in Table 10–2. The majority of cases are clinically severe and usually become evident within the first year of life; milder cases may not present clinically until adolescence or even later. The neutrophils are able to kill organisms lacking the

Table 10–1
Congenital Disorders of Neutrophil Function

Disorder	Deficiency	Inheritance	Manifestations
Chronic granulomatous disease (CGD)	NADPH oxidase; cytochrome *b* subunit	Majority X-linked (~75%); remainder autosomal recessive	Recurrent infections with catalase-positive organisms; granulomatous inflammation at site of infections
Myeloperoxidase (MPO) deficiency	Myeloperoxidase	Autosomal recessive	May have disseminated *Candida* or other fungal infections, particularly in diabetics; majority of patients have no increase in infections
Leukocyte adhesion deficiency type 1	β₂ integrin chain (CD18)	Autosomal recessive	Recurrent pyogenic infections (gingivitis, periodontitis) without neutrophil response; persistent neutrophilia
Chédiak-Higashi syndrome	Granule fusion	Autosomal recessive	Partial oculocutaneous albinism; large lysosomal granules in PMNs, monocytes, melanocytes and other cells; increased susceptibility to pyogenic infections; may terminate as lymphoma-like accelerated phase
Specific granule deficiency	Absence of secondary granules	Autosomal recessive	Recurrent skin and sinus infections, predominantly with staphylococci
Alder-Reilly anomaly	Incomplete degradation of mucopolysaccharides	Autosomal recessive	Large purple granules in PMNs, lymphocytes, and monocytes; normal neutrophil function, with no increased susceptibility to infection; associated with mucopolysaccharidoses (Hunter's and Hurler's syndromes)
May-Hegglin anomaly		Autosomal dominant	Large pale blue granules in PMNs resembling Döhle's bodies; thrombocytopenia with giant platelets; defects in platelet function; no increase in infections
Pelger-Huët anomaly		Autosomal dominant	Majority of PMNs have bilobed nuclei ("pince nez" cells), with a few trilobed nuclei; coarse nuclear chromatin; no increase in susceptibility to infection

Table 10–2
Common Pathogens in Chronic Granulomatous Disease

Staphylococcus aureus

Streptococcus viridans

Gram-negative enterics: *Serratia, Klebsiella, Salmonella*, others

Pseudomonas species

Burkholderia cepacia

Fungi: *Candida, Aspergillus, Paecilomyces*

Nocardia

Mycobacteria

catalase enzyme since the organisms supply H_2O_2 for the neutrophils to generate hypochlorous acid; however, catalase-positive organisms degrade any H_2O_2 produced, and subsequently PMNs cannot generate hypochlorous acid. The most common types of infection in patients with CGD are pneumonitis, lymphadenitis, cutaneous infections, and impetigo. Other infections are listed in Table 10–3.

The defect in CGD effects eosinophils, monocytes, and histiocytes (macrophages), as well as neutrophils. The white cell count is normal and increases appropriately in response to infection. Leukocytes have no morphologic abnormalities and have normal chemotaxis and phagocytosis. However, after ingesting the organisms, they are unable to kill them. Neutrophils initially aggregate at sites of infection but are unable to kill the microorganisms; they are followed by an accumulation of histiocytes, which

Table 10–3
Common Infections in Chronic Granulomatous Disease

Pneumonitis

Lymphadenitis

Cutaneous infections, impetigo

Perirectal abscesses

Osteomyelitis

Hepatic abscesses

Septicemia

Urinary tract infections

ingest the microorganisms but are also unable to kill them. The result is chronic granulomatous inflammation, with persistence of the infection until it is surgically drained and treated with appropriate antibiotics.

The diagnostic test for CGD is the **nitroblue tetrazolium test** (**NBT test**). Nitroblue tetrazolium is a colorless compound that is reduced by normal neutrophils to a blue-black pigment. Neutrophils from patients with CGD are unable to reduce NBT to the colored pigment. Female carriers of X-linked CGD show a mixed reaction: half of their neutrophils are able to reduce NBT and produce the pigment, the other half are unable to reduce the NBT and remain colorless.

Treatment of CGD involves aggressive surgical drainage and antibiotic therapy for any infections. Prophylactic trimethoprim-sulfamethoxazole, with or without dicloxacillin, reduces the frequency of infections. Recently, γ-interferon has been shown to improve microbial killing and decrease the number of serious infections in patients with CGD (the mechanism for this is unknown). The disorder used to be uniformly fatal in childhood for severe cases, but supportive therapy and prophylactic antibiotics have improved the outlook in recent years.

Mutations in other enzymes in the respiratory burst pathway can also cause CGD, including glutathione peroxidase, glutathione synthetase or reductase, and catalase, but these are all uncommon. Rare patients with severe glucose-6-phosphate dehydrogenase (G6PD) deficiency also have features of CGD.

Myeloperoxidase Deficiency

Myeloperoxidase deficiency is the most common inherited enzyme deficiency in neutrophils, occurring in ~1 in 2,000 individuals, but the majority of cases have little or no increase in infections. Inheritance is autosomal recessive. Neutrophils with MPO deficiency have a strong prolonged respiratory burst; they are able to kill most organisms, although killing may be slower than in normal PMNs. However, PMNs are unable to kill *Candida* and some other fungi, and some patients with MPO deficiency (particularly diabetics) may suffer from disseminated candidiasis or other infections.

The diagnosis can be made by a slide staining reaction for the presence of myeloperoxidase.

Leukocyte Adhesion Deficiency Type 1

Leukocyte adhesion deficiency type 1 (LAD-1) is due to an inability to synthesize the β_2 chain (CD18) of the leukocyte integrins. Because the common β chain cannot be synthesized, there is a deficiency of all three of the leukocyte integrins (CD11a/CD18, CD11b/CD18, and CD11c/CD18). Leukocyte adhesion deficiency type 1 neutrophils have defects in motility, phagocytosis, granule secretion, and respiratory burst activity. Patients with LAD-1 have recurrent bacterial infections starting in infancy. The infections most often involve the skin and subcutaneous tissues, the mouth, the middle ear, and the oropharynx. The severity is variable; patients with severe LAD-1 deficiency have a high death rate in childhood, whereas patients with milder disease can survive into their twenties and thirties. Neutrophils are morphologically normal on blood smear, but the white cell count is usually elevated (12,000–100,000/μL), even between episodes of infection. The diagnosis can be made by demonstrating the absence of the leukocyte integrins on PMNs by flow cytometry. There is no specific therapy.

There is a second type of leukocyte adhesion deficiency, designated *leukocyte adhesion deficiency type 2 (LAD-2)*. LAD-2 is due to an inability to synthesize the sialyl-Lewis X moieties on the ligands for CAMs in the selectin family (E-selectin and P-selectin). Clinically, it resembles LAD-1. It is extremely rare.

Disorders with Morphologic Abnormalities in Neutrophils

There are several disorders associated with morphologic abnormalities in PMNs, including the Chédiak-Higashi syndrome, the May-Hegglin anomaly, the Alder-Reilly anomaly, and the Pelger-Huët anomaly. The Chédiak-Higashi syndrome is associated with functional disorders of PMNs and an increased susceptibility to infection; the others are largely laboratory curiosities, with no functional consequences (see Table 10–1).

Chédiak-Higashi Syndrome

The Chédiak-Higashi syndrome is associated with partial oculocutaneous albinism, increased susceptibility to bacterial infections, large granules in PMNs and other granule-containing cells including melanocytes, and a bleeding tendency due to abnormal platelet function. The cause is believed to be abnormal fusion and function of granule membranes; however, the molecular basis for the disorder is unknown. It is inherited as an autosomal recessive disorder.

The skin is pale, and the hair is a characteristic silvery gray. Photophobia is present. Large basophilic granules resembling abnormal lysosomes are present in PMNs, melanocytes, hair, pigmented cells of the eye, and others. The granules may also be present in monocytes and lymphocytes. The granules in PMNs stain positively for peroxidase.

Children with Chédiak-Higashi syndrome have an increased susceptibility to pyogenic bacteria, particularly staphylococci and other gram-positive bacteria. The most common infections are in the respiratory tract and skin. Many patients die of infection in infancy or early childhood; others may survive into their twenties and thirties. Most of those that survive eventually develop an accelerated phase characterized by lymphadenopathy, hepatosplenomegaly, peripheral neuropathy, anemia, neutropenia, and tissue infiltration by mononuclear cells. This has sometimes been considered to represent a malignant lymphoma but may actually represent a reactive lymphohistiocytic process. There is no specific treatment.

Acquired Disorders of Neutrophil Function

Acquired disorders in neutrophil function can be divided into *defects in chemotaxis* and *decreased phagocytosis due to impaired opsonization* (Table 10–4). The clinical features are often dominated by the primary illness, and the neutrophil dysfunction is secondary. The main therapy is to treat the primary disease. Any infections that occur should be treated with appropriate antibiotic therapy.

Evaluation of Patients with Possible Disorders of Neutrophil Function

The possibility of a disorder of neutrophil function should be considered in any patient with recurrent pyogenic infections or infections that do not appear to respond to appropriate therapy.

Table 10–4
Acquired Neutrophil Dysfunction

Defects in Chemotaxis	Decreased Phagocytosis due to Impaired Opsonization
Autoimmune disorders: SLE, rheumatoid arthritis, polymyositis	Multiple myeloma
Diabetes mellitus	Acquired hypogammaglobulinemia
Sarcoidosis	Asplenism
Leprosy	
Hodgkin's disease	
Severe malnutrition	
Hemodialysis	
Severe hypophosphatemia	
Graft-versus-host disease	
Treatment with antithymocyte globulin (ATG)	

The evaluation should begin with a history and physical examination. Onset in childhood or a family history of recurrent infections increases the likelihood of an inherited disorder of granulocyte function. In adults, consider diseases that can be associated with defects in neutrophil function such as diabetes mellitus, autoimmune diseases, and malignancies.

A complete blood count (CBC) and differential should be performed (Table 10–5). Neutropenia should be excluded by calculating the absolute neutrophil count (proportion of mature neutrophils [segmented + band neutrophils] multiplied by the absolute leukocyte count). A normal absolute neutrophil count is ≥1,500 μL for Caucasians and ≥1,200 μL for African Americans. Review the blood smear for morphologic abnormalities in neutrophils and other cells. If the neutrophil number is normal and no morphologic abnormalities are found, the evaluation should proceed with an NBT test and stain for MPO. If these are normal, expression of CD18, CD11a, CD11b, or CD11c should be tested by flow cytometry. If these tests are normal, the patient may need to be referred to a specialized center for immune disorders for more complex testing, such as neutrophil motility, phagocytosis, and bacterial killing assays.

ABNORMALITIES OF LEUKOCYTE NUMBER

Abnormalities in leukocyte number can be divided into increases and decreases in each of the different cell types. The discussion of leukocytosis will be restricted to non-neoplastic causes; leukemias and other hematologic malignancies are discussed elsewhere.

Many people think of leukocyte number in terms of the traditional leukocyte count and differential; thus, a differential showing 60% lymphocytes is considered to indicate an increase in blood lymphocytes (lymphocytosis). It is more accurate to think in terms of *absolute number* of a specific cell type rather than a percentage. For example, a differential showing 60% lymphocytes with a total leukocyte count of 10,000/μL represents an *absolute lymphocytosis* (10,000/μL × 0.60 = 6,000 lymphocytes/μL; normal ≤4,000/μL). On the other hand, 60% lymphocytes with a total leukocyte count of 4,000/μL represents a *relative* (but not absolute) *lymphocytosis*

Table 10–5
Laboratory Evaluation of Possible Neutrophil Disorder

Complete blood count and differential
Review of blood smear
Nitroblue tetrazolium test and stain for myeloperoxidase
Expression of CD18, CD11a, CD11b, or CD11c by flow cytometry

$(4,000/\mu L \times 0.60 = 2,400/\mu L)$. In the latter instance, the abnormality could be a decrease in the number of neutrophils (neutropenia) rather than an increase in lymphocytes.

The possibility of *factitious leukocytosis* due to laboratory error should always be kept in mind. Possible causes of factitious leukocytosis include cryoglobulinemia and platelet clumps; the aggregated immunoglobulins or clumped platelets may form particles about the same size as leukocytes. Always repeat the CBC and review the blood smear before embarking on an extensive evaluation of an abnormal WBC count.

Leukemoid Reaction

A leukemoid reaction is a marked elevation of the white cell count resembling leukemia but due to a benign condition. The lower WBC limit for a leukemoid reaction is $\geq 50,000$ cells/μL ($\geq 30,000$ cells/μL in some series). A leukemoid reaction can be predominantly granulocytic, lymphocytic, or occasionally monocytic. Granulocytic leukemoid reactions occur in both children and adults; lymphocytic leukemoid reactions predominantly occur in childhood.

Causes of leukemoid reactions include any *severe infection, burns, malignancies* (especially with bone marrow metastases), *myelofibrosis, hemorrhage* or *hemolysis, eclampsia,* and others. Tuberculosis may cause granulocytic, lymphocytic, or monocytic leukemoid reactions. *Bordetella pertussis* ("whooping cough") is notorious for causing lymphocytic leukemoid reactions in children; the lymphocytes are predominantly small and appear mature, but many have prominent nuclear folds (descriptively called "buttock cells").

Features that help distinguish leukemoid reactions from leukemia include the total white count (usually higher in leukemia), the presence of immature leukocytes or nucleated erythrocytes on smear, and the presence of lymphadenopathy or splenomegaly (Table 10–6). However, none of these features are absolute, and clinical judgment is often required.

Neutrophilia

Causes

Neutrophilia is defined as an absolute neutrophil count greater than $\sim 7,000/\mu L$ in the adult (Figure 10–1). In most instances, neutrophilia is caused by an infection, some other type of inflammation, acute stress, tissue damage, or necrosis (Table 10–7). In most cases, the cause is obvious.

Stress neutrophilia represents a shift of neutrophils from the marginating pool into the circulating pool and results from physical exertion, other

Table 10–6
Features That Distinguish Leukemoid Reactions from Leukemia

Feature	Leukemoid Reaction	Leukemia
WBC count	Usually ≤75,000/μL	Often ≥75,000/μL
Immature cells	Usually absent	Often present
Nucleated RBCs	Usually absent	Sometimes present
Thrombocytopenia	Usually absent	Often present
Lymphadenopathy, splenomegaly	Usually absent	May be present
Serum cobalamin (vitamin B_{12}) level	Normal	Often increased in chronic myelogenous leukemia (CML) and other myeloproliferative disorders
Cytogenetic abnormalities	Absent	Often present
Leukocyte alkaline phosphatase (LAP) score	Increased	Decreased in CML; may be increased in other chronic myeloproliferative disorders

types of stress, and epinephrine injection. The effect is transient and does not involve increased bone marrow granulocyte production. The percent of band neutrophils is not increased.

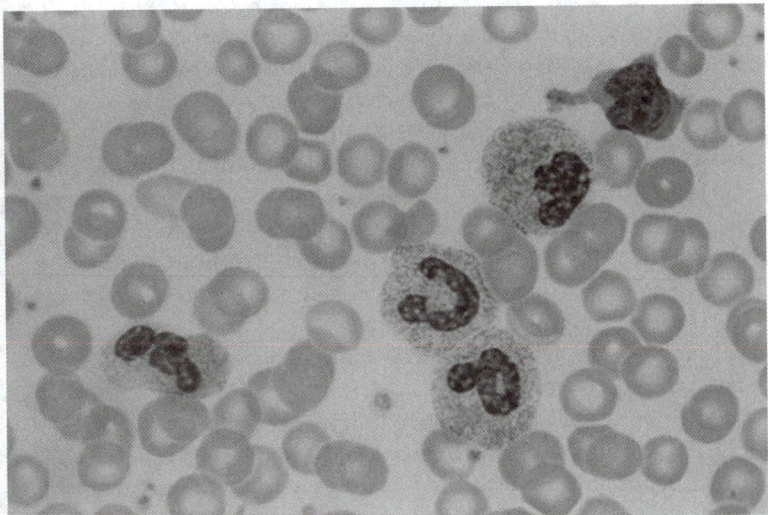

Figure 10–1 Neutrophilia. The neutrophils show heavy granular staining ("toxic granulation").

Table 10–7
Causes of Neutrophilia

Infections

Tissue damage or necrosis: surgery, burns, trauma, myocardial infarction, other tissue necrosis, hyperthermia

Inflammatory disorders: rheumatoid arthritis, other autoimmune diseases, gout, others

Acute stress or physical exertion, seizures

Acute hemorrhage

Hemolysis: acute or chronic

Metabolic disorders: diabetic ketoacidosis

Hodgkin's disease

Non-hematologic malignancies

Medications: lithium, corticosteroids, epinephrine, hematopoietic growth factors

Chronic idiopathic neutrophilia

Hereditary neutrophilia

Infection is the most common cause of sustained neutrophilia. Bacterial infections, particularly *Streptococcus pneumoniae* and staphylococci, are generally associated with the most striking neutrophilia, but neutrophilia can also occur with fungal infections, some viral infections, rickettsial infections, and others. The proportion of band neutrophils is often, although not invariably, increased.

Any process associated with *tissue injury* or *necrosis* results in neutrophilia. Thus, neutrophilia is seen after surgery, myocardial infarction, damage to other tissues, heat stroke, or hyperthermia. Neutrophilia is also seen with *inflammatory disorders*, such as rheumatoid arthritis, acute gouty arthritis, acute glomerulonephritis, serum sickness, and others.

Malignancies can also cause neutrophilia. Hodgkin's disease may be associated with neutrophilia and eosinophilia. Non-hematologic malignancies (lung carcinoma, for example) can cause neutrophilia; this is probably due to necrosis of the tumor in most cases, but production of hematopoietic growth factors such as granulocyte colony-stimulating factor (G-CSF) by tumor cells has been shown.

Acute hemolysis is associated with neutrophilia; chronic hemolytic anemias such as sickle cell anemia are associated with chronic neutrophilia, with total white cell counts of 12,000 to 15,000/μL.

Medications are a common cause of neutrophilia. *Epinephrine* causes a shift of neutrophils from the marginating pool into the circulating pool. *Glucocorticoids* such as prednisone can cause neutrophilia by blocking neutrophil exit from the blood into tissues and by increasing neutrophil proluction by the marrow. *Lithium* has been shown to cause neutrophilia through increased bone marrow production of granulocytes and has been used therapeutically for patients with neutropenia. *Hematopoietic growth factors* such as G-CSF and granulocyte-macrophage colony-stimulating factor (GM-CSF) cause neutrophilia by stimulating bone marrow production.

Rare cases of *chronic idiopathic neutrophilia* and *hereditary neutrophilia* have been described. In general, these are not associated with significant complications.

Differential Diagnosis

The differential diagnosis includes all the causes of neutrophilia noted above. In general, the most important differential diagnosis is a chronic myeloproliferative disorder, particularly chronic myelogenous leukemia (CML), or some other hematologic malignancy.

Evaluation

In most cases, the cause of neutrophilia will be evident based on the patient's symptoms, physical examination, and routine diagnostic studies. If there is no obvious explanation, careful review of the blood smear is indicated to look for immature granulocytes, nucleated erythrocytes, or other abnormalities; if any are found, a bone marrow aspirate and biopsy are indicated. A *leukocyte alkaline phosphatase* (*LAP*) *score* (sometimes called a *neutrophil alkaline phosphatase* or *NAP* score) should be done; this is characteristically decreased in CML but increased in leukemoid reactions and chronic myeloproliferative disorders other than CML. A serum cobalamin (vitamin B_{12}) may be helpful; it is usually increased in CML and other chronic myeloproliferative disorders but normal in leukemoid reactions and other causes of neutrophilia. Finally, a bone marrow aspirate and biopsy with cytogenetic analysis may occasionally be required.

Neutropenia

Neutropenia is defined as an **absolute neutrophil count** (segmented + band neutrophils) **less than ~1,500/μL for Caucasians** and **less than ~1,200/μL for African Americans**. The term *agranulocytosis* is sometimes used to indicate severe neutropenia.

Calculation of Absolute Neutrophil Count (ANC)

ANC = WBC $\times$ (Segs [%] + Bands[%]) $\times$ 0.01

Example: WBC = 6,000/μL; 50% Segs, 10% Bands

$$ANC = 6,000/μL \times (50 + 10) \times 0.01$$
$$= 3,600/μL$$

Neutropenia and Risk of Infection

Severe neutropenia may predispose the patient to serious, possibly life-threatening infections. In general, a patient with an ANC ≥1,000/μL is at little risk of severe infection; fever, if present, could be managed on an outpatient basis. A patient with an ANC of 500 to 1,000/μL has a slightly increased risk of serious infection; hospitalization and broad-spectrum antibiotics may be indicated. A patient with an ANC <500/μL is at significant risk of serious infection and should almost always be hospitalized and given broad-spectrum antibiotics. However, the presence or absence of an adequate bone marrow granulocyte reserve may be more important than ANC per se; some patients with chronic severe neutropenia but a normal bone marrow granulocyte pool have few problems or symptoms. A patient with a similar ANC but a hypoplastic marrow with few mature granulocytes may be in serious trouble. The most common sites of infections in patients with neutropenia are the oral and mucosal surfaces, skin, perirectal and genital areas, respiratory tract, and gastrointestinal tract, as well as bacteremia. The most common organisms are *Staphylococcus aureus* and gram-negative enteric bacilli. Patients with severe prolonged neutropenia may develop fungal infections (particularly *Candida* species and *Aspergillus*), nosocomial infections, and infections due to unusual bacteria such as *Nocardia*.

Causes of Neutropenia

Neutropenia can be divided into *congenital* (*inherited*) and *acquired* types (Table 10–8).

- **Kostmann's syndrome** (**severe congenital neutropenia**) is characterized by severe neutropenia (usually <200/μL) starting in early infancy. Children suffer from infections of the umbilical cord, skin, otitis media, pneumonia, gingivitis, and urinary tract infections. The most common organisms are *S. aureus*, *Escherichia coli*, and *Pseudomonas*. Inheritance is autosomal recessive. The bone marrow shows granulocyte maturation arrest, with no cells maturing past the myelocyte stage. Without treatment, the disease is usually lethal in childhood. Treatment with G-CSF increases the neutrophil count and decreases infections but must be continued indefinitely. Development of acute myelogenous leukemia has been reported in a few patients treated with G-CSF.
- **Cyclic neutropenia** is characterized by periodic severe neutropenia (often <200/μL) occurring in regular 21- to 30-day cycles. Platelets, monocytes, eosinophils, and reticulocytes may also cycle in parallel with neutrophils. The disease usually begins in infancy or childhood, but occasional adult-onset cases occur. The disease may be sporadic or inherited; familial cases have an autosomal dominant pattern of inheritance. Periods of severe neutropenia may be associated with mucosal

Table 10–8
Causes of Neutropenia

Inherited (Congenital) or Chronic	Acquired
Severe congenital neutropenia (Kostmann's syndrome)	Infection related: • Viral: hepatitis B virus, EBV, HIV • Bacterial: gram-negative septicemia, brucellosis • Rickettsial: Rocky Mountain spotted fever, typhus fever • Protozoal • Fungal • Any severe infection
Cyclic neutropenia	
Chronic benign neutropenia	
Idiopathic chronic severe neutropenia	
Neutropenia associated with congenital immune deficiencies (cellular or humoral): • X-linked agammaglobulinemia • Hyper-IgM syndrome • Familial	Drug related: • Expected • Idiosyncratic
	Immune neutropenia: • Isoimmune neonatal neutropenia • Chronic immune neutropenia • Miscellaneous immunologic neutropenia
Neutropenia associated with phenotypic abnormalities: • Shwachman syndrome: metaphyseal chondroplasia, dwarfism, pancreatic insufficiency, and neutropenia • Dyskeratosis congenita • Barth's syndrome: X-linked recessive cardioskeletal myopathy and neutropenia	Felty's syndrome: severe rheumatoid arthritis, splenomegaly, and neutropenia
	Nutritional: severe cachexia, cobalamin or folate deficiency, copper deficiency
	T-γ lymphocytosis (large granular lymphocyte leukemia)
	Hairy cell leukemia
	Myelodysplasia, acute leukemia, aplastic anemia*

*Usually associated with abnormalities in other cell lines (anemia, thrombocytopenia).
Adapted from Lee RG, Foerster J, Lukens J, et al, editors. Wintrobe's clinical hematology. 10th ed. Baltimore: Williams & Wilkins; 1999. p. 1864.

ulcerations, fever, and malaise; patients are asymptomatic between episodes of neutropenia. Severe infections are uncommon, probably due to the brief duration of severe neutropenia. Adult-onset cases may respond to corticosteroids or cyclosporine; G-CSF is the treatment of choice for pediatric cases. Treatment with G-CSF raises the absolute neutrophil count and decreases the frequency of infections, however, it does not eliminate the cycling of the neutrophil count.

- **Chronic benign neutropenia** is a heterogeneous group of conditions characterized by *severe neutropenia* but *no serious infections*. It may be either inherited or acquired and may occur at any age. Patients may have mild skin or oral cavity infections. The bone marrow is cellular and contains all stages of granulocyte precursors up to the band stage; the blood neutrophil count increases appropriately in response to infections. In pediatric cases, the neutropenia usually resolves by age 4 years. The neutropenia responds to G-CSF, but treatment is not needed in the absence of serious complications.

- **Idiopathic chronic severe neutropenia** is characterized by severe neutropenia with onset in late childhood or adulthood, significant infections, and no obvious underlying cause. Immune neutropenia must be excluded. Treatment with specific growth factors is required.

- **Infections** *are probably the most common cause of acquired neutropenia.* Transient neutropenia of variable severity is often seen during many viral infections. Hepatitis B virus, Epstein-Barr virus (EBV), and HIV are prone to cause prolonged severe neutropenia. A variety of bacterial infections can cause neutropenia, particularly sepsis with gram-negative organisms. Other organisms that can be associated with neutropenia include tuberculosis, fungi (*Histoplasma*), rickettsia (Rocky Mountain spotted fever), and protozoa (malaria, leishmaniasis).

- **Drugs** *are probably the second most common cause of neutropenia.* There are two main types of drug-related neutropenia, analogous to drug-related anemia: an expected dose-related effect that will occur in all patients given sufficiently high doses (for example, chemotherapy drugs) and an idiosyncratic reaction that occurs in only a small proportion of patients given the medication, which is often not dose related. In most cases, the expected type causes pancytopenia rather than selective neutropenia. A wide variety of medications can cause the idiosyncratic type of reaction (Table 10–9); many of these can also cause anemia.

  Mechanisms of drug-induced neutropenia include (1) *immune-mediated destruction of neutrophils* or granulocyte precursors, characteristic of penicillins, propylthiouracil and other antithyroid agents, gold, and quinidine; (2) *dose-dependent inhibition of granulocytopoiesis,* characteristic of β-lactam antibiotics, carbamazepine, and valproic acid; and (3) *direct damage to the bone marrow environment or granulocyte precursors by the drug or metabolites,* characteristic of sulfasalazine, captopril, and phenothiazines. The drugs that have the highest risk for agranulocytosis include *antithyroid drugs, macrolide antibiotics, procainamide, trimethoprim-sulfamethoxazole, carbamazepine, indomethacin,* and *sulfonylureas.* The time of onset of neutropenia may vary dramatically; immune-mediated mechanisms often occur within a few days.

Table 10–9

Drugs Associated with Neutropenia

Heavy metals: Gold

Analgesics and anti-inflammatory agents: indomethacin, ibuprofen, acetylsalicylic acid (aspirin), diflunisal, sulindac, tolmetin

Antipsychotics, antidepressants, neuropharmacologic agents: phenothiazines, clozapine, tricyclic antidepressants (imipramine, desipramine), diazepam (Valium), chlordiazepoxide (Librium), amoxapine, haloperidol

Anticonvulsants: valproic acid, phenytoin, trimethadione, mesantoin, ethosuximide, carbamazepine

Antithyroid drugs: propylthiouracil, methimazole, carbimazole

Cardiovascular drugs: procainamide, captopril, aprindine, propranolol, hydralazine, methyldopa, quinidine, diazepoxide, nifedipine, propafenone, ticlopidine, vesnarinone

Antihistamines: H_1-blockers: tripelennamine, brompheniramine; H_2-blockers: cimetidine, ranitidine

Antimicrobials: penicillins, cephalosporins, vancomycin, chloramphenicol, gentamicin, clindamycin, doxycycline, flucytosine, nitrofurantoin, griseofulvin, metronidazole, rifampin, isoniazid, streptomycin, mebendazole, levamisole, pyrimethamine, sulfonamides, antimalarials (chloroquine, hydroxychloroquine, quinacrine), ethambutol, dapsone, ciprofloxacin, trimethoprim, imipenem/cilastin, antivirals (zidovudine, fludarabine, acyclovir)

Thiazide diuretics: hydrochlorothiazide

Oral hypoglycemic agents: chlorpropamide, tolbutamide

Miscellaneous: quinine, allopurinol, cochicine, famotidine, flutamide, tamoxifen, penicillamine, retinoic acid, metoclopramide, phenindione, ethacrynic acid, ethanol, spironolactone, methazolamide, acetazolamide, levodopa

Adapted from Lee RG, Foerster J, Lukens J, et al, editors. Wintrobe's clinical hematology. 10th ed. Baltimore: Williams & Wilkins; 1999. p. 1866.

of starting the medication, particularly in patients who have previously received the medication. In contrast, the effects of direct marrow suppression may not appear for several weeks or even months after the medication is started.

- **Immune neutropenia** is analogous to immune hemolytic anemia: antibodies against neutrophils cause destruction of neutrophils by splenic sequestration or direct complement-mediated lysis. Immune neutropenia can occur in several different settings:
  - **Isoimmune neonatal neutropenia** is analogous to Rh hemolytic disease of the newborn (*erythroblastosis fetalis*). The mother develops antibodies against neutrophil antigens present on fetal cells inherited from the father that she herself lacks. The antibodies cross

the placenta and cause destruction of fetal neutrophils. The duration of neutropenia averages about 7 weeks but may last up to 4 months. Neutropenia may be severe, and there is a significant infection risk. Treatment includes antibiotic therapy for infections, plasma exchange, intravenous immunoglobulin, transfusion of maternal leukocytes, and G-CSF, which may be required for severe cases.

- **Chronic immune neutropenia** may occur as an isolated phenomenon or may be seen in association with autoimmune diseases such as systemic lupus erythematosus, rheumatoid arthritis, Graves' disease, or Wegener's granulomatosis. It may also occur with chronic hepatitis. It may occur at all ages, from childhood to adulthood. Patients may have skin and lower respiratory tract infections, but severe infections are relatively uncommon. Treatment depends on the severity of complications; if the patient is not having serious infections, no treatment may be needed. The underlying cause (if any) should be treated.

- **Felty's syndrome** is the triad of *rheumatoid arthritis* (usually severe), *splenomegaly,* and *neutropenia*. Patients often have a high titer rheumatoid factor and may have vasculitis. Treatment of the underlying rheumatoid arthritis with gold compounds, D-penicillamine, or other immunosuppressive agents may help raise the neutrophil count. Splenectomy increases the neutrophil count in the majority of patients, although relapse may occur. Splenectomy should be reserved for cases in which other treatments fail.

- **Nutritional** neutropenia may be seen with severe cachexia or starvation deficiencies of cobalamin (vitamin B_{12}) or folic acid (usually in association with hypersegmentation of neutrophils, macrocytic anemia, and megaloblastic changes in the marrow), and copper deficiency.

- **T-γ lymphocytosis (large granular lymphocyte leukemia)** is an uncommon proliferation of large lymphocytes with azurophilic (reddish-purple) granules. Two different variants occur. The common variant in the United States is an indolent proliferation of natural killer–like T cells associated with neutropenia, rheumatoid arthritis, and a variety of autoantibodies. The second type, which is common in the Far East but rare in the United States, is an aggressive leukemia of true NK cells. A diagnosis of T-γ lymphocytosis is suspected if numerous large granular lymphocytes appear on the blood smear and is confirmed by flow cytometry.

- **Hairy cell leukemia** (HCL) is an uncommon but interesting variant of chronic B-cell leukemia, characterized by neutropenia, marked splenomegaly, and lymphocytes with fine filamentous cytoplasmic projections ("hairy cells") on a blood smear. The diagnosis can be suspected if the characteristic hairy cells appear on the blood smear and is confirmed by demonstrating a positive acid phosphatase reaction after preincubation with tartaric acid (TRAP stain). Hairy cell leukemia is discussed further in Chapter 16.

- **Aplastic anemia, myelodysplasia, and acute leukemia** are conditions usually associated with abnormalities of multiple cell lines and are discussed in other chapters.

Evaluation

The first step is a careful history and physical. The patient should be asked about past previous infections, including frequency, severity, onset, and type of infections. Onset in childhood would suggest congenital or inherited neutropenia, such as Kostmann's syndrome. Check for a pattern of cyclical infections and, if present, determine the time period. Also determine if there is a family history of severe infections. Particular attention should be paid to a detailed medication history, including over-the-counter medications, diet supplements, and herbal medicines. On physical examination, look for signs of skin or perianal infections, lymphadenopathy, and splenomegaly.

On laboratory evaluation, carefully examine the CBC. Abnormalities in the hemoglobin, mean corpuscular volume, or platelet count suggest a multilineage hematopoietic disorder rather than pure neutropenia. Carefully examine the blood smear for immature or abnormal granulocytes, hypersegmented neutrophils, or abnormalities in erythrocyte or platelet morphology. Look for an increased number of "hairy" or large granular lymphocytes. Check the hepatic transaminases (alanine aminotransferase, aspartate aminotransferase) for evidence of hepatitis; if they are elevated, check serologies for hepatitis viruses. Consider assays for antinuclear antibodies (ANAs) and other autoantibodies. If there are abnormalities in erythrocytes or platelets that are not explained by the history, physical, or other laboratory tests, a bone marrow examination should be performed to look for evidence of myelodysplasia, leukemia, or some other hematologic disease.

Treatment

After the initial evaluation, the critical question is whether immediate further evaluation and treatment are required or whether the patient may simply be followed and observed. If the patient appears stable, there are no signs of serious infection, and there are no other major abnormalities on CBC or other laboratory tests, then the patient can probably be observed without treatment. The WBC and differential should be monitored to see if there is recovery of the ANC. If the patient has a severely decreased ANC

($\leq$500/μL) and is febrile, he or she should be admitted, cultured, and started on broad-spectrum antibiotics pending results of the cultures.

All medications that could be associated with neutropenia should be stopped, and any primary illnesses that can cause neutropenia should be treated appropriately. A trial of corticosteroids may be indicated for patients with immune neutropenia.

If the patient has severe neutropenia, particularly in the presence of infection, treatment with G-CSF may be beneficial.

Eosinophilia

Eosinophils are typically reported as percent of leukocytes, with the normal range being approximately 0 to 7%. Any eosinophil count >7% is often considered eosinophilia. However, eosinophilia is better defined based on the *absolute number* of eosinophils in the blood rather than as a percent of white cells. Therefore, **eosinophilia is defined as >700 eosinophils per microliter** (>0.7 $\times$ 10^3/μL or >0.7 $\times$ 10^9/L). Eosinophilia is sometimes divided into mild (0.7–1.5 $\times$ 10^3/μL), moderate (1.5–5.0 $\times$ 10^3/μL), and marked (>5.0 $\times$ 10^3/μL) eosinophilia. A marked elevation in eosinophils (of any etiology) can cause tissue damage by various mechanisms; prominent among these are the eosinophil major basic protein (MBP), eosinophil peroxidase, eosinophil cationic protein, and eosinophil-derived neurotoxin. Consequences of a sustained marked elevation in eosinophils can include endomyocardial fibrosis, thromboemboli, strokes, peripheral neuropathy, skin lesions (angioedema, urticaria), and others. A sustained eosinophil count >1,500/μL, with associated tissue damage, characterizes the uncommon *hypereosinophilic syndrome* (see next section, page 185). In most cases of eosinophilia, however, there is only a mild increase in eosinophils, and the significance lies in the underlying cause rather than the eosinophilia itself.

Causes

The most common causes of eosinophilia are *parasitic infections*, *allergic reactions*, and *atopic skin diseases*. Eosinophilia can also be seen with other infections, neoplasms, autoimmune (collagen vascular) diseases, and in a variety of other conditions.

Mnemonic for Causes of Eosinophilia: NAACP

N—Neoplasms
A—Allergies (including drug reactions) and asthma
A—Addison's disease
C—Collagen vascular diseases
P—Parasitic (and other) infections

- **Parasitic infections**: Eosinophilia is typically associated with parasites that invade tissues. It is less often seen with intestinal parasites that do not invade tissue. The most common parasitic infections associated with eosinophilia in the United States are *Toxocara canis* and *T. catis* ("visceral larva migrans"), ascariasis, trichinosis, hookworm, and strongyloidiasis. Other examples include *Clonorchis sinensis* (liver fluke) and schistosomiasis. Tropical eosinophilia is most often associated with filariasis.
- **Other infections**: Eosinophilia is occasionally seen with a variety of other infections, including mycobacteria (tuberculosis), fungi (*Coccidioides immitis*), bacteria (scarlet fever, brucellosis), rickettsia, and viruses (particularly herpes).
- **Allergic reactions**: Eosinophilia is commonly seen in allergic reactions such as bronchial asthma, allergic rhinitis (hay fever), and angioneurotic edema. It can also be seen as a reaction to medications. The eosinophilia associated with allergic reactions is typically mild but can be marked.
- **Drug reactions**: Virtually any medication can be associated with eosinophilia, usually manifesting as an allergic reaction. The drugs most frequently associated with eosinophilia include antibiotics (especially penicillins and cephalosporins), antifungal and antituberculous agents, gold compounds, phenothiazines, nonsteroidal anti-inflammatory agents, anticonvulsants, oral hypoglycemic agents, anticoagulants, chemotherapy agents, and others. Striking eosinophilia can be seen with interleukin-2. Skin rashes, interstitial nephritis, pulmonary infiltrates, and hepatitis may be present, in addition to the eosinophilia.
- **Skin diseases**: Striking eosinophilia can be seen with dermatitis herpetiformis and pemphigus. Eosinophilia can also be seen with many other skin diseases.
- **Hematologic diseases**: Eosinophilia can be associated with acute myeloid leukemia and chronic myeloproliferative disorders, particularly chronic myelogenous leukemia (CML). Eosinophilia is relatively common in systemic mastocytosis.
- **Neoplasms**: *Hodgkin's lymphoma* is the neoplasm most often associated with eosinophilia; the incidence in Hodgkin's may be up to 20% of cases, but the degree of eosinophilia is usually mild. Eosinophilia can also be seen with other lymphomas and also can occur with carcinomas and other neoplasms. In some cases, eosinophilia may be related to the breakdown of tumor cells. In other cases, the neoplastic cells have been shown to produce factors that stimulate eosinophil production.
- **Autoimmune** ("collagen vascular") **diseases**: Eosinophilia can be associated with severe rheumatoid arthritis, polyarteritis nodosa, and allergic granulomatosis (Churg-Strauss syndrome).

- **Pulmonary diseases**: Eosinophilia can be seen with many pulmonary diseases in addition to asthma, including *Löffler's syndrome* and *pulmonary infiltration with eosinophilia* (**PIE**) *syndrome*. Löffler's syndrome is a self-limited, usually mild illness characterized by pulmonary symptoms, infiltrates on chest radiograph, and eosinophilia; some cases are probably due to undiagnosed infections. The PIE syndrome is a more chronic, relapsing illness characterized by cough, dyspnea, fever, bilateral infiltrates on chest radiograph, and eosinophilia. Again, the PIE syndrome can be associated with many infections, including parasitic infections. It can also be seen with neoplasms, allergic reactions, and collagen vascular diseases. Corticosteroid therapy can be helpful if not contraindicated by the underlying illness.

- **Miscellaneous causes**: Eosinophilia can be associated with a wide variety of other conditions, including pernicious anemia, graft-versus-host disease following bone marrow transplant, and ingestion of contaminated cooking oil (*toxic oil syndrome*) or L-tryptophan (*eosinophilia-myalgia syndrome*). Rare cases of hereditary eosinophilia have been described; the eosinophilia is usually mild, inherited as an autosomal dominant trait, and clinically benign.

Evaluation

The evaluation of possible eosinophilia begins with calculation of the absolute eosinophil count to confirm that it is elevated. Review the blood smear to confirm the presence of eosinophilia, to see if the eosinophils appear morphologically mature, and to detect any other abnormalities (Figure 10–2). Allergic diseases and drug reactions generally result in only mild or moderate eosinophilia. *Marked eosinophilia is usually due to parasitic diseases or the idiopathic hypereosinophilic syndrome* but can be due to any of the causes of eosinophilia.

On history, ask about symptoms of allergic diseases, including hay fever, asthma, and atopic skin diseases. A careful medication history (including over-the-counter or herbal medications and dietary supplements) is required. Ask about alterations in bowel habits that might suggest parasitic infection, as well as consumption of poorly cooked meat or any other unusual foods. Consider the patient's occupation and hobbies, particularly those that might result in exposure to organic products, and consider any recent travel, particularly to areas of endemic parasitic infestations. On physical examination, examine the skin for rashes and the nose and ears for signs of allergic rhinitis. Listen to the lungs for wheezing or evidence of reactive airway disease. Check for hepatosplenomegaly, lymphadenopathy, and abnormal masses. Routine laboratory studies, including liver chemistries and urinalysis, should be done, as well as chest radiography.

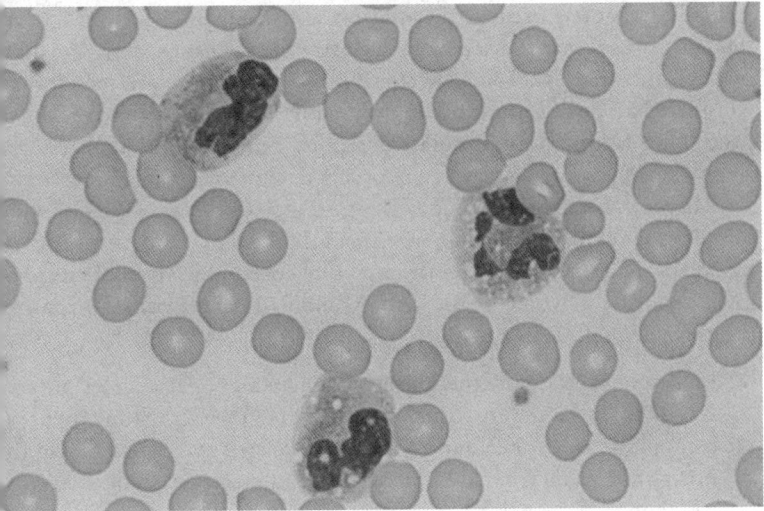

Figure 10–2 Eosinophilia. All three leukocytes in the field are eosinophils. The eosinophil count was 14,000 μL. The patient developed endomyocardial fibrosis. No cause was established.

Further evaluation will depend on the results of the history, physical, and simple laboratory tests. Clues to a possible cause should be appropriately followed. *In the absence of signs or symptoms, extensive evaluation for parasitic disease or neoplasm is probably not warranted.*

Treatment

Mild or moderate eosinophilia per se does not require any treatment; however, any underlying cause should be treated appropriately. The eosinophil count should be followed periodically.

Idiopathic Hypereosinophilic Syndrome

The idiopathic hypereosinophilic syndrome is a rare condition characterized by the following:

- An eosinophil count greater than 1,500/μL (1.5×10^9/L), sustained for at least 6 months
- No apparent cause for the eosinophilia
- Tissue damage due to eosinophilia

The organs most often involved are the *heart*, *central nervous system*, and *peripheral nervous system*. The skin, lungs, gastrointestinal tract, and virtually every other organ in the body can also be involved. It is now know that some cases that previously would have been diagnosed as idiopathi hypereosinophilic syndrome are clonal proliferations and can therefore b considered a type of chronic myeloproliferative disorder. T-cell lymphoma producing factors that stimulate eosinophil production, appear to b responsible for some cases, whereas others remain unexplained.

The leukocyte count usually ranges from ~10,000 to 30,000/μL, with 3 to 70% eosinophils. The eosinophils usually look normal and mature on th blood smear, although occasional immature eosinophils or mild morpho logic abnormalities may be present. Myeloblasts and dysplastic change should be absent.

⇨ It is important to note that the eosinophil count by itself does not dif ferentiate between reactive eosinophilia, the idiopathic hypere osinophilic syndrome, and eosinophilia related to a hematologic (o other) malignancy. In addition, the absolute level does not determin whether end-organ damage will or will not occur.

Cardiac manifestations occur in half or more of the cases. The mos common cardiac abnormalities include endomyocardial necrosis and fibro sis, valvular abnormalities, and mural thrombi. The late manifestation include a restrictive cardiomyopathy and mitral and/or tricuspid valvula insufficiency. *Neurologic signs* occur in approximately half of patients Embolic strokes may occur due to emboli from the endocardial thrombi Altered mental status, confusion, ataxia, and memory loss may be present Peripheral neuropathies may also develop. The *skin* is commonly involved cutaneous manifestations can include angioedema and urticaria, erythe matous papules and nodules, and mucosal ulcerations. Other organs tha are often involved include the lungs (chronic, nonproductive cough), the gastrointestinal tract, and the eyes.

The idiopathic hypereosinophilic syndrome is a diagnosis of exclu sion. The most important diagnostic step is to exclude causes of reactive eosinophilia, particularly parasitic infections. Appropriate studies include stool examination for ova and parasites and serologic studies for *Strongy loides*, *Trichinella*, *Toxocara*, and others as indicated. A bone marrow exam ination with cytogenetic analysis should be performed. Other hematologic diseases or malignancies must also be excluded, including lymphoma, CML and the other chronic myeloproliferative disorders.

The primary **treatment** of a symptomatic patient with the hypere osinophilic syndrome is *corticosteroids* (prednisone starting at approxi mately 1 mg/kg/day for 2 weeks, followed by a slow taper). Hydroxyurea is the first alternative for patients who fail to respond or who are unable to tol erate prednisone. Other alternative therapies that have been used include interferon-α, cyclophosphamide, and cyclosporine. Early series of patients with the hypereosinophilic syndrome showed high mortality rates; recent series show a much improved outcome (≥80% 5-year survival).

▷ Eosinophilia is fairly common, but it is usually modest. In a hospitalized patient, the cause is most likely a reaction to a drug or medication until proven otherwise. In the outpatient setting, an allergic reaction is most likely. In foreign countries or in countries where parasitic infections are common, parasites are the most likely cause.

Basophilia

Basophilia is defined as >**150 basophils/μL** (>0.15 × 10^9/L). Basophilia per se is rarely a clinical problem. It is most common and most striking in CML and is also common in the other chronic myeloproliferative disorders, although it tends to be less striking. It also occurs in a variety of other conditions (Table 10–10). Acute basophilic leukemia has also been described but is exceptionally uncommon. Basophilia can occasionally be associated with urticaria, peptic ulcer disease, or other complications of hyperhistaminemia.

The first step in evaluation of basophilia is to exclude CML or some other chronic myeloproliferative disorder. The presence of other hematologic abnormalities (neutrophilia, increased hemoglobin) suggests a chronic myeloproliferative disorder and should stimulate a leukocyte alkaline phosphatase (LAP) score and/or bone marrow examination with cytogenetics. If there are no hematologic abnormalities, the other conditions listed in Table 10–10 should be excluded.

Basophilia by itself does not require therapy; however, the underlying condition should be identified and treated appropriately.

Monocytosis

Monocytosis is defined as >**1,000 monocytes/μL** (>1.0 × 10^9/L) and can be due to a wide variety of causes (Table 10–11).

Infection is the most common cause of monocytosis. Transient monocytosis is common in many viral infections, usually during the recovery phase. Monocytosis also occurs with tuberculosis, infective endocarditis, syphilis, brucellosis, malaria, trypanosomiasis, and Rocky Mountain spotted fever.

In general, the main problem is to differentiate monocytosis due to acute or chronic leukemia from reactive monocytosis. Check the CBC for other hematologic abnormalities, review the blood smear to see if the monocytes are mature or immature, and look for blasts and other immature or abnormal cells. If there are unexplained abnormalities in the CBC, the

Table 10–10
Causes of Basophilia

Chronic myelogenous leukemia (CML)

Other chronic myeloproliferative disorders: polycythemia vera, essential thrombocythemia, agnogenic myeloid metaplasia (idiopathic myelofibrosis)

Infections: chronic sinusitis, varicella, smallpox

Ulcerative colitis

Lung carcinoma

Miscellaneous: hypothyroidism, iron deficiency, some chronic hemolytic anemias, nephrotic syndrome

monocytes appear immature or blasts or other abnormal cells are noted on the blood smear, then a bone marrow examination with cytogenetic analysis should be done. If not, or if the bone marrow is unremarkable, the other listed causes of monocytosis should be excluded.

Monocytosis per se does not require any treatment. Treatment (if necessary) should be directed against the underlying cause.

Lymphocytosis

Lymphocytosis is defined as a lymphocyte count >**4,000/μL** (>4 × 10⁹/L) for adults and >**9,000/μL** (>9 × 10⁹/L) for children. It is important to distinguish between *absolute lymphocytosis*, which is an increase in the total lymphocyte count, and *relative lymphocytosis*, which is an increase in the lymphocyte percent due to neutropenia, without an increase in the absolute lymphocyte count.

Table 10–11
Causes of Monocytosis

Infections: viruses, tuberculosis, infective endocarditis, syphilis, brucellosis, parasites (malaria, trypanosomiasis), rickettsiae (Rocky Mountain spotted fever)

Acute and chronic leukemias: AML, CML, chronic myelomonocytic leukemia (CMML)

Other hematologic neoplasms: lymphomas, Hodgkin's disease

Carcinomas: breast, ovary, prostate

Granulomatous diseases: sarcoidosis

Inflammatory bowel disease

Collagen vascular diseases

The majority of lymphocytes (~85%) in the peripheral blood are T cells, with T helper (CD4+) generally about twice as common as T cytotoxic/suppressor (CD8+) cells. The majority of reactive lymphocytoses also consist predominantly of T cells. In contrast, the majority of lymphocytic leukemias consist predominantly of B cells.

Causes

There are many possible causes of lymphocytosis (Table 10–12). In children and young adults, lymphocytosis is almost always reactive, due to infections. The main concern is to exclude acute lymphoblastic leukemia. In older adults, *sustained* lymphocytosis is very suggestive of chronic lymphocytic leukemia (CLL), although reactive lymphocytosis can occur at all ages.

- **Viral infections:** These infections are a very common cause of lymphocytosis, particularly in children. Virtually any virus can be associated with lymphocytosis; however; three viruses are particularly prone to cause marked lymphocytosis: *Epstein-Barr virus* (**EBV**), which causes infectious mononucleosis; *cytomegalovirus* (**CMV**), which causes most cases of "Mono spot"-negative infectious mono; and *viral hepatitis*. The lymphocytes associated with mononucleosis are typically large, with abundant pale blue cytoplasm, enlarged nuclei with fine nuclear chromatin, and prominent nucleoli. They are usually called atypical lymphocytes, but I prefer the term "reactive." The reactive lymphocytes often appear to "hug" surrounding erythrocytes. Interestingly, EBV infects B lymphocytes; however, the large lymphocytes seen in the blood are T cells, presumably reacting to the infected B cells.

Table 10–12
Causes of Lymphocytosis

Viral infections, particularly EBV, CMV, viral hepatitis
Bordetella pertussis (whooping cough)
Toxoplasmosis
Brucellosis
Acute infectious lymphocytosis
Tertiary or congenital syphilis
Drug hypersensitivity reactions
Endocrine disorders: thyrotoxicosis, Addison's disease, hypopituitarism
Persistent polyclonal B-cell lymphocytosis
B-cell chronic lymphocytic leukemia and other lymphocytic leukemias

- *Bordetella pertussis*: This is a bacterial infection of infancy and child-hood that causes whooping cough, often associated with striking lym-phocytosis. The white count is typically ~20,000 to 40,000/μL (20–40 × 10^9/L), with a predominance of lymphocytes, but may be >150,000/μL. The lymphocytes have a characteristic appearance: they appear small and mature, with well-condensed nuclear chromatin, but many have striking nuclear grooves (descriptively termed "buttock cells") (Figure 10–3). This appearance is not *diagnostic for* pertussis, but it is extremely characteristic. It can be a clue to isolate the patient and start erythro-mycin while the pertussis workup (nasopharyngeal swab for a fluores-cent antibody stain and culture on appropriate media) is pending.
- **Toxoplasmosis:** *Toxoplasma gondii* is a parasite that is usually acquired from cat feces. It can cause a clinical syndrome resembling mononucle-osis and lymphocytosis of cells resembling the atypical lymphocytes of infectious mononucleosis.
- **Acute infectious lymphocytosis:** This is a syndrome of variable sys-temic symptoms and lymphocytosis, which most often occurs in chil-dren. It is presumed to be due to some infectious agent based on the pattern of transmission and occurrence in epidemics, but no specific agent has been identified. The systemic symptoms can include diarrhea, abdominal pain, cough and dyspnea, fever, headache, and others. The

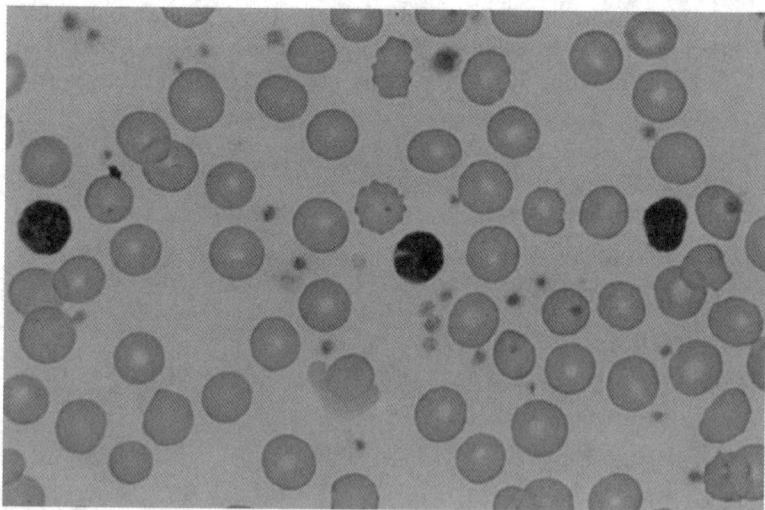

Figure 10–3 Lymphocytosis (*Bordetella pertussis*). Lymphocytosis of small mature lym-phocytes with prominent nuclear grooves ("buttock cells") in a 3-month-old child with respira-tory distress. Immunofluorescent stain on a nasopharyngeal swab demonstrated *Bordetella pertussis*.

lymphocytosis begins within the first week; it usually decreases over the next few weeks but can persist for up to 3 months. The white count is typically ~40,000 to 50,000/μL (40–50 × 10^9/L) with 60 to 97% lymphocytes. The lymphocytes typically appear small and mature. Phenotyping shows that they are predominantly T cells.

- **Persistent polyclonal B-cell lymphocytosis:** This is an uncommon syndrome that usually occurs in young to middle-aged women who are heavy cigarette smokers. The lymphocytosis is usually asymptomatic, but patients may have fever, fatigue, weight loss, lymphadenopathy, and recurrent respiratory infections. The lymphocytes are predominantly B cells and show the normal distribution of kappa and lambda immunoglobulin light chains. The mechanism is unknown.

Evaluation

First, calculate the absolute lymphocyte count to differentiate relative from absolute lymphocytosis. If absolute lymphocytosis is confirmed, the key is to differentiate *reactive lymphocytosis* from a *lymphocytic leukemia*. In children, the main question is reactive lymphocytosis versus acute lymphoblastic leukemia or some other acute leukemia. In adults, the main question is reactive lymphocytosis versus CLL.

Clinical history: Important considerations include the age of the patient and any signs or symptoms of a disease associated with reactive lymphocytosis (ie, infectious mononucleosis, pertussis, viral hepatitis). If the patient has had lymphocytosis previously, determine for how long.

Complete blood count: Look for any abnormalities other than lymphocytosis. Reactive lymphocytosis is usually not associated with either anemia or thrombocytopenia but can be associated with neutropenia. Acute lymphoblastic leukemia is almost always associated with anemia and/or thrombocytopenia and often associated with neutropenia. In CLL, the CBC is usually normal at diagnosis, except for the lymphocytosis.

Blood smear: Check to see if the lymphocytes look small and mature or reactive. Reactive lymphocytes are often large, with abundant basophilic (blue) cytoplasm; the nuclei may appear enlarged and have relatively fine chromatin and nucleoli, but the nuclear-cytoplasm ratio is usually low. Reactive lymphocytes often appear to "hug" erythrocytes. Sometimes distinguishing reactive lymphocytes from blasts can be difficult; a key distinguishing feature is that *reactive lymphocytes* tend to be *variable in appearance* on an individual slide, whereas blasts tend to be much more monotonous. Chronic lymphocytic leukemia is characterized by predominantly small mature-appearing lymphocytes. The nuclear chromatin often appears condensed into chunks or blocks, giving the nuclei a characteristic "soccer ball" appearance. Disintegrating nuclei ("smudge cells") are also commonly present.

Physical examination: Pay particular attention to *lymph nodes* and the *spleen.* Children or young adults with infectious mononucleosis often have splenomegaly and lymphadenopathy (particularly enlargement of posterior cervical lymph nodes). In adults, generalized lymphadenopathy or marked splenomegaly suggests a lymphoproliferative disorder.

If there is any indication of acute leukemia (blasts or other immature cells on the blood smear or unexplained anemia, neutropenia, or thrombocytopenia), a routine bone marrow examination should be done plus flow cytometry, cytogenetics, and possibly other special tests. Hospitalization during the workup should be considered for patients who have fever or other systemic symptoms, evidence of bleeding, severe anemia, neutropenia, or thrombocytopenia.

If the lymphocytosis remains unexplained after all of the above, the next diagnostic step would be immunophenotyping by flow cytometry on the peripheral blood, looking for evidence of a malignant lymphoproliferative disorder. It might be reasonable to observe the patient for a few weeks to see if the lymphocytosis resolves, particularly in children or young adults, before ordering this relatively expensive test. In older adults, particularly those who are asymptomatic and have only mild lymphocytosis and no anemia, thrombocytopenia, or neutropenia, it would also be reasonable to observe the patient for a few weeks or months. If the patient is symptomatic, has significant lymphadenopathy or splenomegaly, or has significant anemia, thrombocytopenia, or neutropenia, then further evaluation including flow cytometry should be performed more quickly.

Flow cytometry: Flow cytometry is useful in distinguishing reactive lymphocytosis from lymphocytic leukemias. It can also determine the lineage of lymphocytic leukemias (B cell versus T cell) and help subclassify lymphocytic leukemias. The immunophenotype of lymphocytic leukemias will be discussed further in Chapter 16.

Figure 10–4 summarizes the evaluation of an elevated WBC count or abnormal leukocytes on a blood smear.

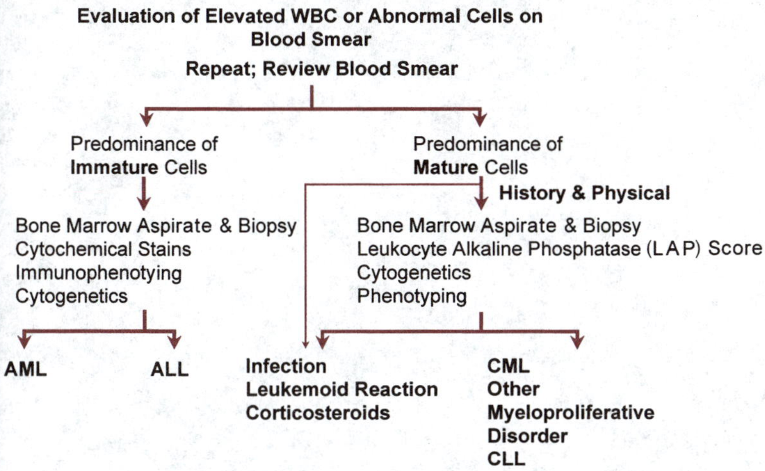

Evaluation of Elevated WBC or Abnormal Cells on Blood Smear
Repeat; Review Blood Smear

Predominance of **Immature** Cells

Predominance of **Mature** Cells

History & Physical

Bone Marrow Aspirate & Biopsy
Cytochemical Stains
Immunophenotyping
Cytogenetics

Bone Marrow Aspirate & Biopsy
Leukocyte Alkaline Phosphatase (LAP) Score
Cytogenetics
Phenotyping

AML   ALL

Infection
Leukemoid Reaction
Corticosteroids

CML
Other Myeloproliferative Disorder
CLL

Figure 10–4 **Evaluation of elevated WBC or abnormal cells on blood smear.**

11

Quantitative Disorders of Platelets: Thrombocytosis and Thrombocytopenia

Immune Thrombocytopenic Purpura, Heparin-Induced Thrombocytopenia, Thrombotic Thrombocytopenic Purpura, and the Hemolytic-Uremic Syndrome

THROMBOCYTOSIS

Thrombocytosis is defined as a platelet count exceeding the upper limit of the reference range. A value of **>400,000 platelets/μL** ($>400 \times 10^9$/L) can be used as a guideline; however, it is recommended that you check the range in your own laboratory. The term **thrombocythemia** is sometimes used synonymously with thrombocytosis, but it should be restricted to the chronic myeloproliferative disorder **primary thrombocythemia** (also known as *essential thrombocythemia*). Primary thrombocythemia will be discussed in more detail in Chapter 14.

Thrombocytosis is usually secondary to some other condition (*reactive thrombocytosis*) and is not associated with an increased risk of thrombosis or other complications. Primary thrombocythemia, on the other hand, may be associated with thrombosis or bleeding. *Reactive thrombocytosis is far more common than primary thrombocythemia.*

Causes of Thrombocytosis

Common causes of reactive thrombocytosis are listed in Table 11–1 and include the following:

- **Infection:** Infections are probably the most common cause of thrombocytosis. Thrombocytosis is common with acute bacterial infections

Table 11–1
Causes of Thrombocytosis

Artifact (pseudothrombocytosis):
- Schistocytes
- Acute leukemia (white cell fragments)
- Cryoglobulinemia
- Microorganisms

Primary (essential) thrombocythemia; other chronic myeloproliferative disorders

Secondary (reactive) thrombocytosis:
- Acute stress or physical exertion
- Inflammation: rheumatoid arthritis, other autoimmune disorders, inflammatory bowel disease
- Infections
- Malignancies
- Acute hemorrhage
- Acute hemolysis
- Iron deficiency
- Surgery
- Post-splenectomy
- Rebound thrombocytosis following thrombocytopenia

and also occurs in chronic infections such as tuberculosis, bacterial endocarditis, and osteomyelitis.

- **Inflammation:** Inflammation of any type is often associated with thrombocytosis. Examples include rheumatoid arthritis and inflammatory bowel disease.
- **Malignancy:** Thrombocytosis is present by definition in primary thrombocythemia but is often present in the other chronic myeloproliferative disorders. Thrombocytosis may also occur with non-hematologic malignancies.
- **Post-splenectomy:** The spleen normally contains about 30% of the total platelet mass, and thrombocytosis is common during the first weeks or months following splenectomy. However, the platelet count gradually returns toward the normal range in most patients.
- **Iron deficiency:** Thrombocytosis is common in patients with iron deficiency anemia.
- **Miscellaneous:** Thrombocytosis is often present in association with acute hemorrhage or trauma, surgery, acute hemolysis, and transiently after an episode of thrombocytopenia (rebound thrombocytosis).

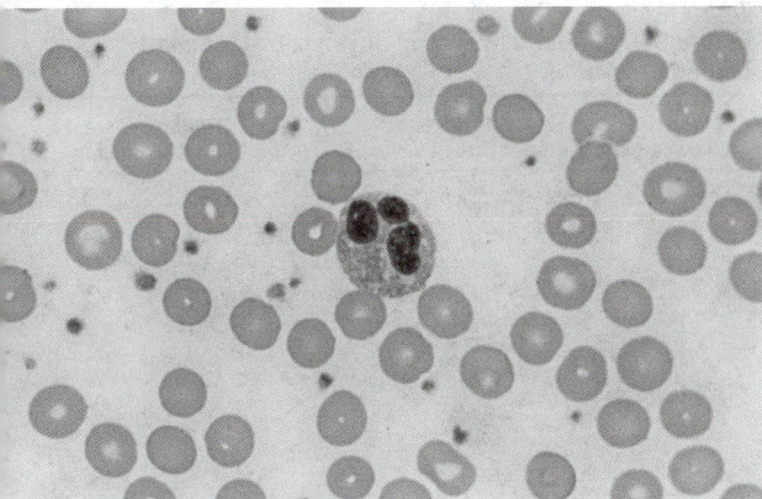

Figure 11–1 **Thrombocytosis (post-splenectomy).** Platelet count of 700,000/µL after splenectomy.

Evaluation of Thrombocytosis

➪ First exclude *artifactual thrombocytosis* (pseudothrombocytosis) and confirm the presence of thrombocytosis by reviewing the blood smear (Figure 11–1).

The most important distinction is between reactive thrombocytosis and primary thrombocythemia. Some features may be helpful in the distinction, but none are absolute (Table 11–2).

Sometimes the only way to be certain is to follow the patient for several months: in reactive thrombocytosis, either the platelet count will drop or the underlying cause will become apparent; in primary thrombocythemia, the platelet count will remain elevated or increase.

Treatment of Thrombocytosis

Reactive thrombocytosis is not associated with increased risk of either thrombosis or hemorrhage, and treatment of the thrombocytosis per se is unnecessary. The underlying cause of thrombocytosis should be identified and treated appropriately.

THROMBOCYTOPENIA

Thrombocytopenia is defined as a platelet count below the reference range for a particular laboratory; **<150,000/µL** can be used as a rough guide.

Table 11–2

Distinction of Reactive Thrombocytosis from Primary Thrombocythemia

Characteristic	Reactive Thrombocytosis	Essential Thrombocythemia
Known cause of reactive thrombocytosis	Present	Absent
Platelet count	Typically 500,000–700,000/μL; *usually* <1,000,000/μL	Almost always >600,000/μL; often >1,000,000/μL
Thrombosis or hemorrhage	No	Often
Splenomegaly	No	Yes
Giant platelets and megakaryocyte fragments in blood	No	Yes
Bone marrow fibrosis	No	Yes
Megakaryocyte clusters on bone marrow biopsy	No	Yes
Abnormal cytogenetic analysis on bone marrow	No	Occasional

Thrombocytopenia is a far more common clinical problem than thrombocytosis.

The consequence of thrombocytopenia is risk of hemorrhage. In general, *assuming normal platelet function*, the risk of hemorrhage correlates with the platelet count. A platelet count >100,000/μL is associated with no risk of hemorrhage, even with surgery. A platelet count <5,000/μL is associated with a significant risk of spontaneous severe hemorrhage (Table 11–3). The relationships between platelet count and risk of hemorrhage may not be valid if the patient has a primary platelet disorder, is on medication that interferes with platelet function, or has other risk factors for bleeding.

Conditions in which thrombocytopenia is the *sole* or *primary* manifestation are discussed in this chapter. Conditions with thrombocytopenia as part of a more generalized blood disorder (ie, myelodysplasia or acute leukemia) will be considered in other chapters. Immune thrombocytopenic purpura (usually called **immune thrombocytopenic purpura, or ITP**), heparin-induced thrombocytopenia, and thrombotic thrombocytopenic purpura and the hemolytic-uremic syndrome (TTP-HUS) will be discussed separately.

Table 11–3
Platelet Count versus Risk of Hemorrhage

Platelet Count*	Risk of Hemorrhage
>100,000/μL	None
50,000–100,000/μL	No risk of spontaneous bleeding; may have bleeding with major trauma or surgery
20,000–50,000/μL	May have minor spontaneous bleeding; major bleeding uncommon except with major trauma or surgery
10,000–20,000/μL	Minor bleeding likely; some risk of major bleeding
<5,000–10,000/μL	Significant risk of severe life-threatening bleeding

Assumes normal platelet function: no primary platelet dysfunction, no other disease that interferes with platelet function, and no medications that interfere with platelet function (eg, aspirin, other nonsteroidal anti-inflammatory drugs).

◇ **It is critical that artifactual thrombocytopenia (*pseudothrombocytopenia*) be excluded before undertaking evaluation or treatment for thrombocytopenia.** Causes of pseudothrombocytopenia include platelet clumping (Figure 11–2), platelet satellitism around neutrophils (Figure 11–3), hereditary giant platelet syndromes, a clotted specimen, or an old specimen. The most common cause of pseudothrombocytopenia is *platelet clumping*.

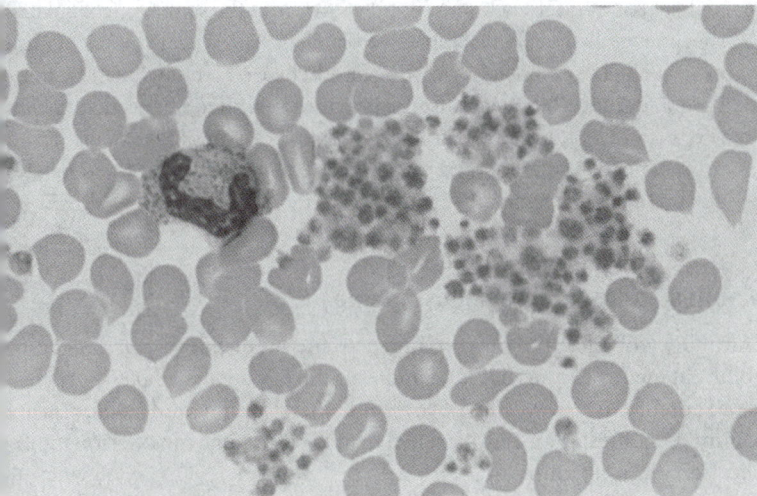

Figure 11–2 Platelet clumping (pseudothrombocytopenia). Large platelet clumps on the blood smear from a 21-year-old asymptomatic woman. The hematology analyzer reported a platelet count <11,000/μL. Specimen anticoagulated with citrate showed a normal platelet count.

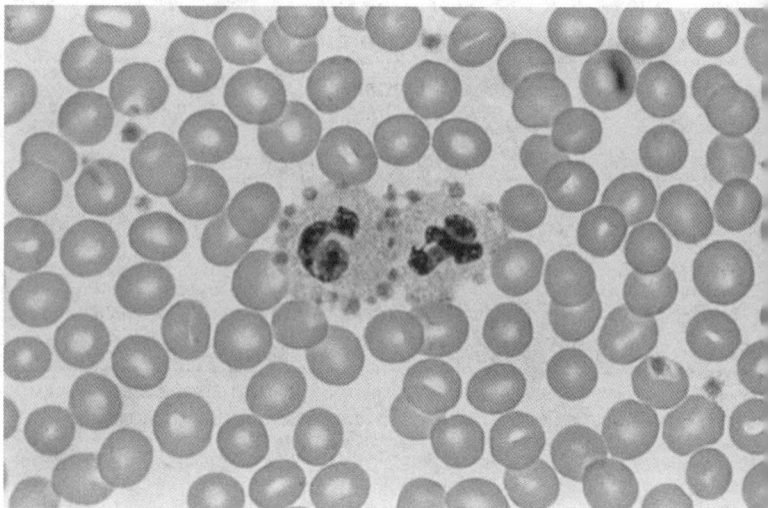

Figure 11–3 Platelet satellitism. Platelets adhering to the surface of a neutrophil. In this case, the reported platelet count was only slightly decreased.

⇨ **Platelet Clumping:** Approximately 1 in 1,000 people have an antibody that induces platelet clumping in blood samples anticoagulated with ethylenediaminetetraacetic acid (EDTA). The clumped platelets are not counted as platelets by hematology analyzers; therefore, the reported platelet count is falsely low. A blood smear from the same anticoagulated specimen will show large clumps of platelets. An accurate platelet count can usually be obtained by drawing another specimen into a citrate anticoagulant tube. **Platelet clumping is a purely in vitro phenomenon that is clinically insignificant.** Patients with platelet clumping actually have a normal platelet count (unless there is some other reason for them to have an abnormal platelet count) and have **no** increased risk of bleeding.

Manifestations of Thrombocytopenia

Thrombocytopenia presents with **mucocutaneous bleeding**: *petechiae* (pinpoint cutaneous hemorrhages), *cutaneous purpura, gingival bleeding, epistaxis* (nosebleeds), *menorrhagia, gastrointestinal bleeding,* and *hematuria* are common manifestations. Intracranial hemorrhage is the most serious complication but is uncommon.

⇨ Deep visceral hematomas, hemarthroses, or muscle hematomas are uncommon with thrombocytopenia and suggest a defect in the coagulation cascade.

Causes of Thrombocytopenia

Thrombocytopenia can occur via three general mechanisms: **impaired platelet production**, **increased platelet utilization or destruction**, or **platelet sequestration in the spleen**. Causes of thrombocytopenia can be divided into *inherited thrombocytopenic syndromes, congenital but not inherited* causes, *acquired immune-related* causes, and *acquired non-immune* causes (Table 11–4):

1. **Inherited thrombocytopenic syndromes:** Inherited defects in platelet production are uncommon. Examples include the following:

   - **Thrombocytopenia–absent radii (TAR) syndrome:** This syndrome is a congenital thrombocytopenia with decreased marrow megakaryocytes and absent radii. Other skeletal, cardiac, and renal anomalies may sometimes occur. It is inherited as autosomal recessive.
   - **Wiskott-Aldrich syndrome:** This syndrome includes severe thrombocytopenia with small platelets, eczema, and increased susceptibility to infections. It is inherited in an X-linked recessive manner.
   - **May-Hegglin anomaly:** This includes thrombocytopenia with giant bizarre platelets and inclusions in the white cells. It is inherited as autosomal dominant.
   - **Bernard-Soulier syndrome (BSS):** This syndrome includes mild thrombocytopenia with large platelets and platelet function defects. It is due to a deficiency of platelet glycoprotein Ib-IX/V (the receptor for von Willebrand's factor) and is inherited as autosomal recessive.
   - **Gray platelet syndrome:** This includes thrombocytopenia with hypogranular platelets. It is inherited as autosomal dominant and may be associated with severe bleeding.
   - **Miscellaneous:** Many inherited thrombocytopenia syndromes have thrombocytopenia alone, with normal platelet structure and function. Inheritance is variable.

2. **Congenital but not inherited thrombocytopenia:**

   - **Intrauterine viral infection:** Rubella, cytomegalovirus, hepatitis, varicella, and other viruses may cause thrombocytopenia in the neonate.
   - **Maternal drugs or medications:** Thiazide diuretics, oral hypoglycemic agents, ethanol, steroids (adrenal corticosteroids, estrogens), quinine, and quinidine taken during pregnancy may result in transient thrombocytopenia in the newborn.
   - **Maternal immune thrombocytopenic purpura:** Maternal ITP or other immunologic diseases (such as systemic lupus erythematosus) may be associated with thrombocytopenia in the newborn due

Table 11–4
Causes of Thrombocytopenia

Pseudothrombocytopenia (artifactual)
- Platelet clumping
- Platelet satellitism

Inherited
- Thrombocytopenia–absent radii (TAR) syndrome
- Wiskott-Aldrich syndrome
- May-Hegglin anomaly
- Bernard-Soulier syndrome
- Gray platelet syndrome

Congenital non-inherited
- Intrauterine viral infection
- Maternal drugs or medications: thiazide diuretics, oral hypoglycemic agents, ethanol, steroids, quinine, and quinidine
- Maternal ITP or other immunologic diseases
- Neonatal alloimmune thrombocytopenia

Acquired
Immune:
- Idiopathic
- Infections: viruses (EBV, CMV, HIV), bacteria, riskettsiae, *Mycoplasma*, others
- Drugs: quinidine, quinine, gold, rifampin, trimethoprim-sulfamethoxazole, others
- Lymphoproliferative disorders
- Autoimmune (collagen vascular) diseases
- Post-transfusion purpura
- Other

Non-immune:
- Infections
- Disseminated intravascular coagulation (DIC)
- Thrombotic thrombocytopenic purpura (TTP)
- Hemolytic-uremic syndrome (HUS)
- Preeclampsia/eclampsia and the HELLP syndrome
- Massive transfusion
- Gestational thrombocytopenia

Platelet sequestration in the spleen
- Hypersplenism: usually associated with anemia and/or leukopenia

to transplacental passage of antiplatelet antibodies. However, *serious complications in the newborn are rare*. There is a tendency for the infant's platelet count to be lower with more severe maternal thrombocytopenia. The infant's platelet count may be fine at birth but drop a few days later; therefore, the platelet count should be monitored for several days after delivery.

- **Neonatal alloimmune thrombocytopenia:** Neonatal alloimmune thrombocytopenia (**NAIT**) may occur if fetal platelets have an antigen inherited from the father that is absent on the mother's platelets, usually the PLA[1] antigen. Approximately 98% of the population has the PLA[1] antigen; therefore, ~1 in 50 pregnancies is at risk for NAIT. However, the actual incidence is much less (1:1,000 to 1:5,000 pregnancies). It may occur during the first pregnancy, unlike erythroblastosis fetalis due to Rh incompatibility, which usually occurs only in second or later pregnancies. Neonatal alloimmune thrombocytopenia is associated with a significant risk of fetal injury or death due to intracranial hemorrhage, which may occur prenatally. Treatment consists of giving PLA[1]-negative platelets (the mother's are usually the easiest to get, if she is a suitable donor!), and/or exchange transfusion.

3. **Immune thrombocytopenias:** Immune thrombocytopenia may develop when antibodies or immune complexes attach to platelets and the platelets are subsequently phagocytized and destroyed by macrophages, predominantly in the spleen. Idiopathic autoimmune thrombocytopenic purpura (ITP) and heparin-induced thrombocytopenia (HIT) will be discussed separately. Causes of immune thrombocytopenia include the following:

   - **Infections:** Thrombocytopenia may occur in a variety of infections, including viruses (Epstein-Barr virus [EBV], CMV, human immunodeficiency virus [HIV]), bacteria, mycoplasma, rickettsia, mycobacteria, and protozoa (malaria). The patient infected with HIV deserves special attention.
   - **Drugs:** Many drugs have been associated with thrombocytopenia. The most common are heparin, quinine, quinidine, gold compounds used to treat rheumatoid arthritis, trimethoprim-sulfamethoxazole, and rifampin. Others include antibiotics (penicillins and cephalosporins), H_2-blockers, antiepileptics (phenytoin, carbamazepine, valproic acid), thiazide diuretics, and furosemide. Monoclonal antibodies against the platelet IIb/IIIa glycoprotein (abciximab; ReoPro), used during angioplasty to prevent thrombosis of the vessels, also cause thrombocytopenia.
   - **Lymphoproliferative disorders:** Chronic lymphocytic leukemia (CLL) and occasionally other lymphoproliferative disorders may be associated with immune thrombocytopenia.
   - **Autoimmune diseases:** Thrombocytopenia may develop in autoimmune diseases, particularly systemic lupus erythematosus (SLE). Thrombocytopenia may be the initial sign of SLE and may precede other manifestations of SLE by several months or years.

- **Post-transfusion purpura:** Post-transfusion purpura is characterized by **severe thrombocytopenia 3 to 14 days after transfusion**. It
usually occurs in multiparous women but may occur in anyone who
has previously received transfusions. It occurs when a person who
lacks the PLA[1] (HPA-1) platelet antigen is given blood products
containing PLA[1]-positive platelets and subsequently develops anti-
PLA[1] antibodies. It is unclear why the patient's own platelets, which
lack the PLA[1] antigen, are destroyed. Thrombocytopenia usually
lasts ~2 weeks to 2 months. The usual treatment is intravenous
immunoglobulin (~2 mg/kg given over 2 days); plasma exchange
may be required. Platelet transfusions are not helpful, even transfusion of PLA[1]-negative platelets.

4. **Acquired non-immune thrombocytopenia:**

- **Infections:** Thrombocytopenia due to non-immune mechanisms is
common in a wide variety of infections. Transient bone marrow
suppression is probably the most common mechanism.
- **Disseminated intravascular coagulation (DIC):** Thrombocytopenia is common in DIC due to increased platelet consumption.
- **Preeclampsia/eclampsia and the HELLP syndrome:** Preeclamp-
sia/eclampsia is characterized by hypertension and proteinuria during pregnancy. Thrombocytopenia occurs in approximately 15 to
20% of women with preeclampsia. A subset of women with severe
preeclampsia develop a microangiopathic hemolytic anemia with
elevated liver enzymes and thrombocytopenia, designated the
HELLP syndrome (*h*emolysis, *e*levated *l*iver enzymes, and *l*ow
*p*latelets). The mechanism of thrombocytopenia in preeclampsia is
unclear. Control of hypertension and delivery of the fetus usually
result in recovery of the platelet count. There is a higher incidence
of maternal and fetal complications with the HELLP syndrome.
- **Massive transfusion:** Thrombocytopenia may occur in patients
receiving massive red cell transfusions (usually ≥20 units of packed
red cells) due to dilution. Platelet transfusions should be given if
severe thrombocytopenia with bleeding develops.
- **Gestational thrombocytopenia:** Mild thrombocytopenia occurs in
up to 5% of pregnant women during the third trimester. This is due
at least in part to dilution from the expanded blood volume. The
platelet count remains above 70,000/μL (70 × 10⁹/L), there are no
maternal or fetal complications, and no treatment is indicated.
More severe thrombocytopenia, or thrombocytopenia occurring
earlier in pregnancy, raises the possibility of ITP. Thrombocytopenia associated with hypertension, proteinuria, or schistocytes on
the blood smear suggests preeclampsia or the HELLP syndrome.

5. **Platelet sequestration in the spleen (hypersplenism):** Normally, approximately 30% of total platelets are sequestered in the spleen. If the spleen is enlarged, this may increase to as much as 90% and result in mild thrombocytopenia. In most cases, thrombocytopenia due to hypersplenism will be accompanied by anemia and/or leukopenia.

Evaluation of Thrombocytopenia

⇨ *The first step in evaluation of thrombocytopenia is to review a blood smear to exclude platelet clumping or other cause of pseudothrombocytopenia.* In the process, carefully examine the smear for fragmented red cells (schistocytes), blasts or other abnormal leukocytes, a marked increase in small lymphocytes, or other abnormalities that might suggest a specific cause of thrombocytopenia.

⇨ *Always think about the possibility of HIV infection in any young patient with thrombocytopenia or any person with risk factors for HIV.* Thrombocytopenia may be the first manifestation of HIV and may occur early in the infection.

⇨ *Consider the clinical setting.* A patient in the intensive care unit could have many possible causes of thrombocytopenia, such as medications (including heparin), sepsis, and disseminated intravascular coagulation. Thrombocytopenia in a pregnant woman raises a completely different differential, including preeclampsia, HELLP syndrome, or gestational thrombocytopenia.

Further evaluation of thrombocytopenia includes the following:

- **History:** Ask how long the patient has had bleeding symptoms. Determine if the patient has had a previous platelet count and whether the count was normal or decreased. Also ask if there is any family history of thrombocytopenia (a long history of thrombocytopenia or thrombocytopenia in family members raises the question of congenital or inherited thrombocytopenia). Ask about recent symptoms of infection, skin rashes, arthritis, and other symptoms of SLE or other autoimmune diseases.
- **Medication history:** A *careful medication history is critical.* Ask about over-the-counter medications, dietary supplements, and dietary and herbal supplements, particularly quinine.
  - A surprising number of people take quinine at night to prevent leg cramps. Quinine in tonic water ("gin and tonics") can also cause thrombocytopenia in someone who is sensitized to quinine. Quinine may be listed as *cinchona* in dietary supplements.

- **Physical examination:** Look for petechiae, purpura, and other signs c bleeding. Carefully palpate for lymphadenopathy or a palpable spleer
- **Laboratory:**
  - **CBC:** Abnormalities in the white cell count or anemia (other tha mild) raise the possibility of a more serious hematologic disorde such as acute leukemia or myelodysplasia.
  - **Blood smear:** Look for schistocytes, blasts, or other immature o abnormal cells. The presence of schistocytes suggests thromboti thrombocytopenic purpura or one of the other microangiopathi hemolytic anemias.
  - **Serum chemistries:** Liver enzymes should be checked to exclud viral hepatitis.
  - **Serologies for autoimmune disease:** If there is any suggestion o autoimmune diseases on history or physical, an assay for anti nuclear antibodies should be done.
  - **HIV test:** Serologies for HIV should be checked in any patient a risk (some people suggest that new-onset thrombocytopenia in *any one* is a reason to check HIV serologies).
  - **Bone marrow:** A bone marrow examination is probably no necessary in the absence of other hematologic abnormalities, but one should be performed if other hematologic abnormalities are present

Treatment of Thrombocytopenia

- Any precipitating cause should be treated appropriately.
- All possible medications should be discontinued, including heparin, quinine, and other drugs known to be associated with thrombocytope- nia.
- Drugs that might interfere with platelet function (ie, aspirin) should be avoided.
- If the thrombocytopenia is not severe and there is no evidence of bleed- ing, the patient may be observed to see if the thrombocytopenia resolves spontaneously.
- Corticosteroids or intravenous immunoglobulin may be given for sus- pected immune thrombocytopenia.
- If the patient is severely thrombocytopenic and there is evidence of bleeding, platelet transfusions can be given.

The decision to treat a patient for thrombocytopenia should depend on the clinical condition of the patient, *not* the platelet count. A patient with no evidence of significant bleeding might not require any treatment, even with a platelet count as low as 20,000 to 30,000/μL. Conversely, a patient with significant bleeding should be treated, even with a platelet count above that level. Most experts would probably consider hospitalization and treatment for ewly diagnosed patients with a platelet count ≤5,000 to 10,000/μL even without bleeding to prevent intracranial hemorrhage.

DIOPATHIC AUTOIMMUNE THROMBOCYTOPENIC PURPURA*

diopathic autoimmune thrombocytopenic purpura (ITP) is immune hrombocytopenia occurring without a recognizable cause. Idiopathic utoimmune thrombocytopenic purpura can be divided into *acute* and *hronic* types. Acute ITP is much more common in children, chronic ITP is nore common in adults.

Acute Idiopathic Autoimmune Thrombocytopenic Purpura

Acute ITP usually occurs in children between 2 and 6 years of age. There is relatively sudden onset of petechiae, often beginning a few weeks after a viral infection. Acute ITP may also follow vaccinations. The thrombocytopenia can be severe, but bleeding manifestations are usually mild. Spontaneous recovery occurs in up to 90% of cases. The duration of illness varies from a few days to 6 months, with an average of 4 to 6 weeks. No treatment is required in most cases, and recurrence is unusual.

⇨ A clue to acute ITP in childhood: *the child looks much better than the platelet count.*

Chronic Idiopathic Autoimmune Thrombocytopenic Purpura

Chronic ITP is most common in adults, although a small number of children demonstrate a chronic course. The onset is usually insidious, with a several-month history of gradually worsening epistaxis, gingival bleeding, and menorrhagia in women. There is no history of preceding infection. It occurs more often in women than in men (~3:1), and most cases occur in young adults (~70% below age 40 years). The course tends to be fluctuating, with episodes of thrombocytopenia lasting a few weeks or months. Multiple recurrences are common, and spontaneous long-term remissions are rare.

Diagnosis

Idiopathic autoimmune thrombocytopenic purpura is largely a diagnosis of exclusion. The diagnosis of ITP is based predominantly on *history, physical*

---

*A panel of experts from the American Society of Hematology (ASH) put together a practice guideline for the diagnosis and treatment of ITP, published in the July 1, 1996, issue of *Blood*. This discussion largely follows those guidelines.

examination, *CBC*, and *blood smear*. The history should exclude other possible causes of thrombocytopenia (drugs, HIV or other infections, autoimmune disorders). The physical examination in ITP should be unremarkable except for perhaps a palpable spleen tip; the presence of lymphadenopathy or more than mild splenomegaly suggests an underlying lymphoproliferative disorder. The blood smear should confirm thrombocytopenia. Platelets often appear slightly large, and the mean platelet volume (MPV) may be increased. There may be a mild microcytic anemia if the patient has iron deficiency due to chronic blood loss. *There should be no evidence of other hematologic diseases* such as acute leukemia, CLL, myelodysplasia, or thrombotic thrombocytopenic purpura. **If there is no other cause for thrombocytopenia detected by history, physical, CBC, and blood smear, then the patient probably has ITP and should be treated as such**. In most cases, no further diagnostic tests are necessary.

- Assays for antiplatelet antibodies analogous to the direct antiglobulin (Coombs') test for erythrocytes have been developed but have not become widely accepted. Recent assays detecting antibodies specific for platelet glycoproteins (GP IIb-IIIa, GP Ib-IX/V) appear to be relatively specific (a patient with an elevated level *probably* has immune-mediated thrombocytopenia) but are not yet adequately sensitive for clinical use (a negative assay does not *exclude* ITP).

- A bone marrow examination should be considered in older patients (over ~60 years) or before splenectomy is performed. It should also be performed if there are any abnormalities on CBC or blood smear other than thrombocytopenia. A bone marrow examination is usually not needed in young patients with no evidence of other hematologic diseases.

- Idiopathic autoimmune thrombocytopenic purpura may be associated with autoimmune thyroid diseases. It has therefore been suggested that thyroid hormone levels be checked prior to splenectomy to detect or exclude occult thyroid disease.

Treatment

The decision to treat ITP should be based on signs of bleeding, not just the platelet count. However, most experts would probably start treatment if the platelet count is <30,000/μL in newly diagnosed patients even without bleeding, or at a higher platelet count if there is significant bleeding. Treatment options include the following:

- **Corticosteroids:** Corticosteroids are the standard initial therapy for ITP. Prednisone or equivalent is started at ~1 to 2 mg/kg per day, maintained at that dose for ~3 to 4 weeks, and then slowly tapered over 1 to 4 months. The platelet count usually begins to rise within 1 week and reaches a maximum by 2 to 4 weeks. Signs of bleeding often begin to improve within a few days, even before the platelet count begins to increase. High-dose parenteral corticosteroids (methylprednisolone 1 g daily for 3 days) may be useful to rapidly increase the platelet count in patients with very low counts and significant bleeding. Approximately 65 to 85% of patients respond to corticosteroids.

- **Intravenous immunoglobulin (IVIG):** Intravenous immunoglobulin is useful to rapidly increase the platelet count. The mechanism of action is probably blockade of the reticuloendothelial system, preventing phagocytosis of platelets. The dose is 0.5 to 1 g/kg daily for 2 or 3 days, repeated every 10 to 21 days as needed. The platelet count usually begins to rise within 2 to 4 days. The rapid response makes IVIG useful in emergency situations. A combination of IVIG and high-dose corticosteroids may increase the response rate. Intravenous immunoglobulin is well tolerated but very expensive. Some patients may become refractory after multiple courses.

- **Anti-Rh$_o$ (D) antibody (WinRho SDF):** WinRho SDF is a polyclonal antibody preparation against the Rh$_o$ (D) red cell antigen, which may be useful in Rh$_o$ (D)-positive patients (~85% of the population). WinRho SDF is well tolerated and less expensive than IVIG. Patients often develop a mild immune hemolytic anemia, with a drop of 1 to 2 g/dL in the hemoglobin, but this is usually well tolerated. Approximately 50% of patients respond to this treatment.

- **Platelet transfusions:** Platelet transfusions do not increase the platelet count (the transfused platelets are destroyed as quickly as the patient's own platelets) and, as a rule, should be avoided. However, they should be given if the patient has severe bleeding, in which case, they may be beneficial even in the absence of an increase in the count. It may be helpful to give platelets following IVIG and bolus intravenous corticosteroids.

- **Splenectomy:** Splenectomy removes the primary site of platelet destruction and also a site of antibody production. Approximately 65% of patients have a complete response, and an additional 15% have a partial response. Unfortunately, approximately 15% of responders relapse. Relapse usually occurs within a few months but may not occur for several years. The main side effect of splenectomy is the risk of overwhelming sepsis; fortunately, this is uncommon in patients who have a splenectomy as adults.

- **Other therapies:** Other therapies that are used in refractory patients, or those that relapse after splenectomy, include vincristine, cyclophosphamide, other cytotoxic agents, and danazol.

⇨ It is wise to anticipate the eventual need for splenectomy in most adult patients and prepare for it by vaccinating patients against *Streptococcus pneumoniae, Haemophilus influenzae*, and meningococcus as soon as the diagnosis of ITP is made.

Disease Course

Most cases of chronic ITP have a waxing and waning course, but long-term remissions are uncommon. The majority of patients respond to corticosteroids initially but relapse after the medication is discontinued. Splenectomy is the mainstay of therapy for patients who relapse after corticosteroids; ~30% of patients require some type of therapy after splenectomy, usually low-dose alternate-day corticosteroids.

- *The goal of therapy in patients with chronic ITP is to* **prevent serious bleeding**, *not to normalize the platelet count.* Patients with chronic ITP may tolerate astonishingly low platelet counts with no or minimal bleeding, and the side effects from therapy may be more burdensome than the low platelet count itself.

HEPARIN-INDUCED THROMBOCYTOPENIA

Approximately 20 to 30% of patients given heparin develop thrombocytopenia, making it the drug that most often causes thrombocytopenia in hospitalized patients. Heparin-induced thrombocytopenia has been divided into two types (type I and type II). Paradoxically, the major risk in type II HIT is thrombosis rather than hemorrhage.

Type I Heparin-Induced Thrombocytopenia

The majority of patients have type I HIT. This appears to result from non-immunologic activation of platelets, with subsequent removal of platelets by the reticuloendothelial system. Type I HIT usually develops during the *first days* of heparin therapy, is relatively mild (platelet count >100,000/μL), and has no adverse clinical consequences. It may resolve spontaneously, even if the heparin is continued. *Type I HIT does not require discontinuation of heparin.*

Type II Heparin-Induced Thrombocytopenia

Type II HIT occurs in ~3 to 5% of patients receiving unfractionated heparin; it is less common in patients receiving low-molecular-weight heparin ($\leq$1%). It is caused by an IgG antibody that reacts with a complex of heparin bound to platelet factor 4 (PF4), which activates the platelet. The antibody-heparin-PF4 complex also injures endothelial cells. The combination of platelet activation plus endothelial cell damage probably accounts for the occurrence of thrombosis in type II HIT.

- Type II HIT usually occurs after *5 to 14 days of therapy* with unfractionated heparin, later than type I HIT. However, type II HIT can occur more rapidly in patients who have received heparin within 3 to 4 months prior to the current heparin therapy.

- The platelet count is typically ~50,000 to 70,000/μL, with a ≥50% drop in the platelet count from the initial value. However, *the drop in platelet count may be modest, and the platelet count may remain in the normal range.*
- The risk of type II HIT is much greater with unfractionated heparin than with low-molecular-weight heparin and appears to be dose related. However, *type II HIT has been reported with all types of heparin preparations and with all doses of heparin.* Even subcutaneous "mini-dose" heparin and heparin flushes for indwelling vascular catheters may be associated with type II HIT.
- Although the risk of type II HIT appears to be much lower if low-molecular-weight heparin is used initially, low-molecular-weight heparin is not safe once the patient has developed the HIT antibody.
- Thrombotic events in type II HIT can include deep venous thrombosis and pulmonary embolism, arterial or venous gangrene of limbs, myocardial infarcts and strokes, and skin necrosis.

Diagnosis

The diagnosis of type II HIT is largely clinical and requires a high degree of suspicion. There are no laboratory tests that have been widely accepted in the evaluation of HIT. The serotonin release assay is considered the "gold standard" test but is technically difficult and not widely available. An enzyme-linked immunosorbent assay (ELISA) test for the IgG HIT antibody is more widely available but has a significant false-negative rate; therefore, a negative ELISA does not exclude HIT. In addition, many patients develop positive ELISA after exposure to heparin, without either thrombocytopenia or thrombotic complications.

Treatment

Type I HIT does not require therapy, and heparin can be continued. Therapy is required for type II HIT due to the risk of thrombosis. *The first step in treatment of type II HIT is to stop heparin.* Unfortunately, patients may develop thrombosis after heparin is discontinued, and patients may have life-threatening thrombotic disorders that require anticoagulation. Anticoagulation with warfarin is not considered safe because venous gangrene has been observed with warfarin in this setting.

- **Danaparoid** (Orgaran) is a synthetic mixture of heparin-like compounds, which has been successfully used in this circumstance; however, up to 10% of patients have cross-reactivity between heparin and danaparoid, and progression of thrombosis has been observed.
- Two thrombin inhibitors have recently been approved for use in this circumstance: **hirudin** (lepirudin [Refludan]) and **Argatroban** (Novastan). These can be monitored using the standard partial thromboplastin time (PTT) clotting assay. Lepirudin is renally excreted, and the dose

must be adjusted for patients with renal insufficiency. Argatroban is metabolized by the liver.

The risk of HIT can be reduced by using low-molecular-weight heparin instead of unfractionated heparin or by restricting the use of unfractionated heparin to 5 days or less. A platelet count should be obtained prior to starting heparin and every 2 to 3 days afterwards, as long as the patient remains on the drug.

THE THROMBOTIC MICROANGIOPATHIES: THROMBOTIC THROMBOCYTOPENIC PURPURA AND THE HEMOLYTIC-UREMIC SYNDROME

Thrombotic thrombocytopenic purpura (TTP) and hemolytic-uremic syndrome (HUS) are characterized by **microangiopathic hemolytic anemia** (mechanical fragmentation of erythrocytes, indicated by schistocytes on blood smear), **thrombocytopenia**, and **thrombi composed primarily of platelets and von Willebrand's factor in different organs**. Thrombotic thrombocytopenic purpura usually occurs in adults and frequently has prominent neurologic involvement. Hemolytic-uremic syndrome typically occurs in children and is characterized by predominant renal involvement. They have often been grouped together as **TTP-HUS** because of significant clinical overlap and frequent difficulty in distinguishing between them.

Distinction between HUS and TTP is based on age, a history of bloody diarrhea preceding the onset of HUS, the occurrence of HUS in epidemics, and the tendency for predominance of renal manifestations in HUS versus neurologic manifestations in TTP (Table 11–5). However, there is overlap between the two conditions, and the distinction is not always clear.

A variety of conditions can be associated with a microangiopathic hemolytic anemia and thrombocytopenia, from which TTP and HUS must be distinguished (Table 11–6).

Table 11–5
Distinction of HUS from TTP

Feature	HUS	TTP
Age	Predominantly children	Predominantly adults
Renal manifestations*	Dominant	Less common
Neurologic manifestations*	Less common; less severe	Common; severe

*Some series have found no differences in the incidence of renal and neurologic manifestations between TTP and HUS in adults.

Table 11–6
Causes of Microangiopathic Hemolytic Anemia

Hemolytic-uremic syndrome (HUS):
- Toxin associated (epidemic)
- Sporadic

Primary thrombotic thrombocytopenic purpura (TTP):
- Congenital
- Single episode
- Intermittent

Secondary TTP:
- Drug related: mitomycin C, quinine, cyclosporin, oral contraceptives, ticlopidine, clopidogrel
- HIV related
- Bone marrow transplant

Disseminated intravascular coagulation (DIC)

Infection:
- Rickettsiae
- Hemorrhagic viruses (hantavirus)

Pregnancy related:
- Preeclampsia/eclampsia
- HELLP syndrome

Scleroderma
Systemic lupus erythematosus
Malignant hypertension

Hemolytic-Uremic Syndrome

Hemolytic-uremic syndrome is most common in children under the age of 5 years, although cases also occur in older children and adults. The majority of cases follow an episode of gastroenteritis caused by toxin-producing *Escherichia coli* strain **O157:H7** or sometimes *Shigella dysenteriae*. This is designated *typical* or *epidemic HUS* (sometimes called D+ HUS for "diarrhea associated"). *Escherichia coli* O157:H7 is usually acquired by eating poorly cooked meat. Most cases occur during the spring or summer. Epidemics of HUS have been traced to poorly cooked hamburgers served at fast-food restaurants. Hemolytic-uremic syndrome occurs in only ~5% of individuals infected with toxigenic *E. coli*. Two groups of people are at highest risk of HUS related to *E. coli* O157:H7: young children and older adults.

The responsible toxin has been designated **verocytotoxin** or **Shiga toxin**. The toxin binds to specific receptors on endothelial cells, damaging the cell. The endothelial cell damage predisposes to the formation of platelet thrombi.

Clinical Features

Signs of renal disease usually begin approximately 2 to 14 days (median ~7) after the onset of bloody diarrhea. There may be hematuria, oliguria, or anuria, and up to 60% of patients require temporary dialysis support. Other systems can also be involved, including the heart (myocarditis and pericardial effusion) and the central nervous system. Neurologic symptoms are present in ~30 to 50% of cases, most commonly irritability and somnolence; confusion, paresis, and seizures are less common. *The severity of thrombocytopenia and microangiopathic hemolytic anemia is variable and may be mild.*

Diagnosis

A diagnosis of HUS is suspected by a history of bloody diarrhea preceding the onset of renal disease. The blood smear shows schistocytes and thrombocytopenia, although these may be subtle. The prothrombin time (PT) and PTT are normal. The direct antiglobulin (Coombs') test is negative. Stool should be cultured for the *E. coli* O157:H7 strain and sent for an assay to detect the Shiga toxin. Because of the risk of HUS, all patients with bloody diarrhea should have stool specifically cultured on selective media for *E. coli* O157:H7, such as sorbitol-containing MacConkey's agar (SMAC). The stool culture and toxin assay may be negative in cases presenting ≥7 days after the onset of diarrhea; in this situation, acute and convalescent serologies for the O157 lipopolysaccharide or the Shiga toxin can be useful. A ≥4-fold rise in titer in the convalescent specimen confirms the diagnosis.

A kidney biopsy is usually not necessary for diagnosis. If performed, the typical finding is bland-appearing (hyaline) thrombi in glomerular capillaries and arterioles, which are composed predominantly of platelets. Occasionally, there is predominant involvement of larger arteries, with less involvement of glomerular capillaries and small arterioles; this suggests a higher likelihood of residual renal impairment.

Treatment of HUS in children is predominantly supportive, with control of blood pressure and dialysis as needed for azotemia. Plasma exchange therapy (as used for TTP) does not appear to be beneficial in diarrhea-associated HUS in children. The majority of children recover spontaneously, although some may have or develop residual chronic renal insufficiency.

Hemolytic-uremic syndrome occurring in adults has a significant risk of mortality or residual renal insufficiency, particularly in adults over 65 years. It is often difficult to distinguish HUS from TTP in adults, and some authorities consider microangiopathic hemolytic anemia of unknown etiology in adults as TTP-HUS without trying to distinguish between them. Since the prognosis of HUS is adults is relatively poor and the distinction between HUS and TTP is often not clear, therapeutic plasma exchange should be considered in adults who appear to have HUS. Some studies have suggested that plasma exchange may be beneficial in adult HUS linked to *E. coli* O157:H7.

Sporadic HUS (not associated with *E. coli* O157:H7) has a worse prognosis, with a smaller number of patients having complete recovery of renal function. The cause of sporadic HUS is not known; it may relate to deficiencies in complement regulatory proteins.

Thrombotic Thrombocytopenic Purpura

Thrombotic thrombocytopenic purpura was first described in 1924. For many years, it was considered a rare and mysterious disease, with a very high mortality rate. Thrombotic thrombocytopenic purpura is now being diagnosed with greater frequency, partly due to an increased awareness of the disease, but partly because there appears to be an absolute increase in its incidence. It now appears that there are several syndromes within the spectrum of TTP, including familial forms (chronic relapsing TTP), single-episode TTP, and intermittent TTP. Thrombotic thrombocytopenic purpura may also be associated with other conditions, including medications (mitomycin C, quinine, oral contraceptives, ticlopidine), pregnancy, SLE and other autoimmune disorders, infections (particularly HIV), malignancies, and following bone marrow transplantation. These can be grouped together as *secondary TTP*. **In most cases, however, there is no obvious precipitating factor**.

The first breakthrough in understanding the pathophysiology of TTP was the discovery of unusually large multimers of von Willebrand's factor (ULvWF) in the plasma of patients with recurring TTP, between episodes of disease. Endothelial cells normally produce these very large vWF multimers, but they are cleaved into the normal vWF multimer sizes by a plasma enzyme known as *vWF metalloproteinase* or *vWF cleaving enzyme*. A deficiency of the vWF metalloproteinase results in persistence of the unusually large vWF multimers. Unusually large multimers of von Willebrand's factor are able to spontaneously agglutinate platelets under conditions of high shear stress. The identification of the ULvWF multimers and the vWF metalloproteinase has explained some of the different types of TTP. However, the specificity of vWF metalloproteinase deficiency and ULvWF multimers for TTP is unclear. Some studies have found ULvWF in patients with a variety of conditions other than TTP and occasionally even in normal individuals.

- Chronic relapsing TTP is caused by an inherited deficiency in the vWF metalloproteinase. The disease begins in childhood and is characterized by recurrent episodes of illness occurring at intervals of approximately 3 to 4 weeks. Inheritance appears to be autosomal recessive. Episodes of illness can be prevented by periodic infusions of plasma, which supply the deficient enzyme.
- Most cases of idiopathic TTP in adults are due to an acquired inhibitor of the vWF metalloproteinase. The inhibitor has been identified as an IgG antibody. It is not known why the inhibitor develops or why some patients have only a single episode of illness whereas others have recurrent episodes.

- Some cases of secondary TTP, such as TTP following bone marrow transplantation, do not appear to be related to the presence of ULvWF multimers or deficiencies in the vWF metalloproteinase.

Endothelial cell injury appears to be an important additional factor in TTP; serum from patients with TTP can cause apoptosis of endothelial cells. The mechanism of endothelial cell injury is unclear.

Epidemiology

Thrombotic thrombocytopenic purpura can occur at any age but is most common in young adults (median age ~40 years). It is approximately twice as common in women than men. Thrombotic thrombocytopenic purpura was originally described as a pentad of findings, including *fever, thrombocytopenia, microangiopathic hemolytic anemia,* and *neurologic* and *renal abnormalities (Table 11–7)*. However, the full pentad is now relatively uncommon, occurring in less than half of patients. At least 75% of patients have a combination of microangiopathic hemolytic anemia, thrombocytopenia, and neurologic abnormalities.

⇨ **Current diagnostic criteria for presumptive TTP have been reduced to a dyad: microangiopathic hemolytic anemia and thrombocytopenia occurring in the absence of other causes of microangiopathic hemolytic anemia**.

Signs and Symptoms

Approximately 10 to 40% of patients have symptoms of an upper respiratory tract infection within 2 weeks prior to the onset of illness. The most common presenting symptoms are purpura and neurologic abnormalities. Neurologic symptoms can vary from headache and confusion to somnolence, seizures, aphasia, stroke, or coma. Renal involvement is less common

Table 11–7
Thrombotic Thrombocytopenic Purpura: Manifestations

Microangiopathic hemolytic anemia
Thrombocytopenia
Neurologic signs and symptoms
Renal insufficiency
Fever

Less than half of patients have all five findings; ≥75% have the combination of microangiopathic hemolytic anemia, thrombocytopenia, and neurologic abnormalities.

and less prominent than in HUS; signs of renal involvement include olig-uria and azotemia.

Diagnosis

Diagnosis of TTP requires a high degree of suspicion and exclusion of other causes of microangiopathic hemolytic anemia (Table 11–8). In general, *a patient with microangiopathic hemolytic anemia, thrombocytopenia, a negative direct antiglobulin (Coombs') test, and no evidence of DIC or any other cause for microangiopathic hemolytic anemia is presumed to have TTP.* There are no widely available tests for confirming the diagnosis. The unusually large vWF multimers are usually not present in the plasma during acute episodes, and assays for the inhibitor to the vWF metalloproteinase are not widely available.

Laboratory

Laboratory abnormalities in TTP include anemia, thrombocytopenia, schis-tocytes on the peripheral blood smear (Figure 11–4), and elevated serum lactic dehydrogenase. The PT and PTT are usually normal or only mildly abnormal, and fibrin degradation products are not significantly elevated.

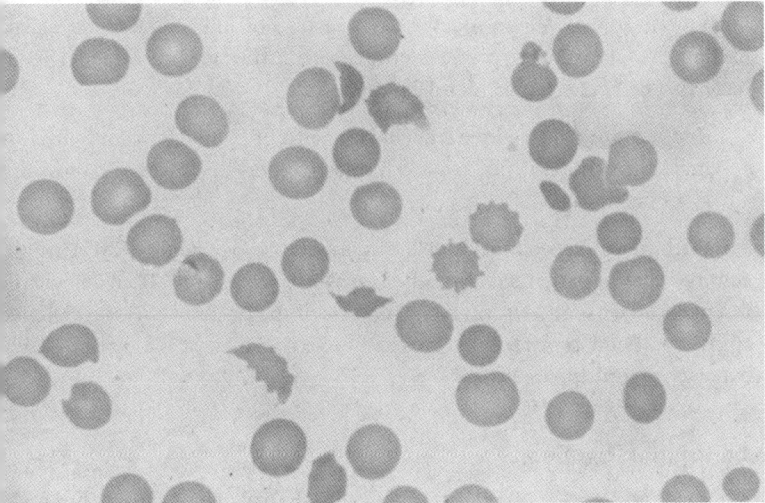

Figure 11–4 Thrombotic thrombocytopenic purpura (TTP). Numerous schistocytes and decreased platelets.

Table 11–8
Differential Diagnosis of TTP

Disseminated intravascular coagulation (DIC)

Systemic lupus erythematosus, scleroderma

Septic or tumor emboli

Immune complex vasculitis

Malignant hypertension

Infection: rickettsiae, hemorrhagic viruses

Cryoglobulinemia

Hemolytic-uremic syndrome (HUS)

Treatment

The treatment for TTP is plasma exchange: plasmapheresis with replacemen of the patient's plasma with fresh frozen plasma (FFP). This removes th ULvWF and replaces the deficient vWF metalloproteinase. At least on plasma volume should be exchanged daily, and plasmapheresis should b continued for several days after the platelet count has returned to norma and then tapered off. Most patients respond to plasmapheresis within sev eral days. Patients who are refractory to daily plasma exchange can be trie on replacement with cryosupernatant ("cryopoor plasma"; plasma that ha been depleted of vWF and factor VIII) instead of FFP. Twice-daily plasm exchanges, splenectomy, corticosteroids, vincristine, and antiplatelet agent have also been tried in refractory patients.

⇨ **Replace the removed patient plasma with *FFP*.** Replacement with nor mal saline or albumin, as used in plasmapheresis for other condition is ineffective in TTP.

With plasma exchange, ≥90% of patients survive acute TTP. A signifi cant number of patients relapse after recovery (relapse rate 10 to 36% in dif ferent series), usually within a few months of the original episode. Splenec tomy has been reported to prevent recurrence in some patients wh experience multiple relapses.

Additional Readings

Allford SL, Machin SJ. Current understanding of the pathophysiology of thromboti thrombocytopenic purpura. J Clin Pathol 2000;53:497–501.

Caiola E. Heparin-induced thrombocytopenia: how to manage it, how to avoid i Cleve Clin J Med 2000;67:621–4.

orge JN. How I treat patients with thrombotic thrombocytopenic purpura-hemolytic-uremic syndrome. Blood 2000;96:1223–9.

orge JN. Platelets. Lancet 2000;355:1531–9.

orge JN, Raskob GE, Shah SR. Drug-induced thrombocytopenia: a systematic review of published case reports. Ann Intern Med 1998;129:886–90.

orge JN, Woolf SH, Raskob GE, et al. Idiopathic thrombocytopenic purpura: a practice guideline developed by explicit methods for the American Society of Hematology. Blood 1996;88:3–40.

ote: A periodically updated list of case reports of drugs associated with thrombo-openia is available at: http://moon.ouhsc.edu/jgeorge.

12

Classification of Hematopoietic and Lymphoid Neoplasms: An Overview

Classification of hematopoietic and lymphoid neoplasms can seem overwhelming. This chapter is an overview of classification; the individual diseases will be discussed in later chapters. Classification can be reasonably straightforward if you keep a few major characteristics in mind.

MAJOR CHARACTERISTICS

All hematopoietic and lymphoid neoplasms can be described according to *three major characteristics*:

- **Aggressiveness:** *Acute* versus *Chronic*
- **Lineage:** *Lymphoid* versus *Myeloid*
- **Predominant Site of Involvement:** *Blood and Bone Marrow* versus *Tissue*

If you remember these three simple characteristics and put them into the various possible combinations, you can figure out the basic classifications for hematologic neoplasms. After that, it's just a matter of filling in the details.

Aggressiveness: Acute versus Chronic

Hematologic neoplasms can be divided into **acute** and **chronic** types based on two characteristics: **survival** and **maturation**.

Survival

- **Acute:** Survival measured in *weeks or a few months* (without effective therapy)
- **Chronic:** Survival measured in *years*

With effective therapy for many of the acute neoplasms, the survival difference between acute and chronic neoplasms has been greatly diminished or eliminated.

Maturation

- **Acute:** Predominance of *immature cells* (blasts)
- **Chronic:** Predominance of *mature cells*

Lineage: Lymphoid versus Myeloid

This division relates to the first step in differentiation of the hematopoietic stem cell into the CFU-L (colony-forming unit-lymphoid) and the CFU-GEMM (colony-forming unit-granulocyte-erythrocyte-megakaryocyte-macrophage). Neoplasms derived from the CFU-L are designated lymphoid; those derived from the CFU-GEMM are myeloid. (It seems a little odd for a neoplasm of erythroid cells to be termed "myeloid," but that is the way it goes.)

Lymphoid malignancies can be divided into B-cell, T-cell, and plasma cell neoplasms. Immature lymphoid tumors are often designated *lymphoblastic*.

Myeloid tumors can be divided into granulocytic, monocytic, megakaryocytic, and erythroid types.

Predominant Site of Involvement: Blood and Bone Marrow versus Tissue

Neoplasms with predominant **blood and bone marrow** involvement are called **leukemias**. Neoplasms with predominant **tissue** involvement are called **lymphomas** if composed of lymphocytes and **granulocytic sarcomas** (sometimes called *chloromas* or *extramedullary myeloid tumors*) if composed predominantly of myeloid cells.

The distinction between lymphocytic leukemias and lymphomas is not always straightforward; sometimes the distinction becomes rather arbitrary. Fortunately, for purposes of treatment and prognosis, it usually does not matter which label is applied.

The Leukemias: Putting It All Together

Table 12–1
Classification of Leukemias

	Acute	**Chronic**
Lymphoid	Acute Lymphoblastic Leukemia (ALL)	Chronic Lymphocytic Leukemia (CLL)
Myeloid	Acute Myeloid Leukemia (AML)	Chronic Myeloproliferative Disorders

Each of these major categories has several subcategories.

Variations on a Theme (1): Lymphomas, Hodgkin's Disease, and Myelomas

Primary tumors of lymph nodes are divided into **non-Hodgkin's lymphomas** and **Hodgkin's disease** (also called **Hodgkin's lymphoma**). Non-Hodgkin's lymphomas are derived from lymphocytes, either B cells or T cells. Hodgkin's disease is distinguished by the presence of a characteristic cell called the *Reed-Sternberg cell*. The cell of origin of Hodgkin's disease was unknown for a long time, but it now appears that Hodgkin's disease is also a malignancy of lymphocytes.

Tumors of plasma cells (the last stage of life of B lymphocytes) are called **myelomas** or **plasmacytomas**. The term myeloma is used for plasma cell tumors in the bone marrow; plasmacytoma is usually used for plasma cell tumors outside the bone marrow.

Variations on a Theme (2): The Chronic Myeloproliferative Disorders

In Table 12–1, it may seem that Chronic Myeloproliferative Disorders are listed where you would expect to find Chronic Myeloid Leukemia. There is a disease called chronic myelogenous leukemia, but it is only one of several diseases in the category of chronic (ie, mature) malignancies derived from myeloid cells. These represent clonal proliferations of early hematopoietic precursors in which regulation of proliferation is lost, but maturation and differentiation are retained. There are chronic myeloproliferative disorder variants corresponding to different cell lineages derived from the CFU-GEMM:

- **Chronic myelogenous leukemia** (also called **chronic granulocytic leukemia**): Granulocytes

- **Polycythemia vera** (also called **polycythemia rubra vera**): Erythrocytes
- **Primary thrombocythemia** (also called **essential thrombocythemia**): Megakaryocytes (platelets)
- **Idiopathic myelofibrosis** (**agnogenic myeloid metaplasia**): Neoplastic population of megakaryocytes that drives fibroblasts to make reticulin fibers, resulting in bone marrow fibrosis

Variations on a Theme (3): The Myelodysplastic Syndromes

The myelodysplastic syndromes are clonal disorders of hematopoietic stem cells, associated with impaired maturation and differentiation. The myelodysplastic syndromes are characterized by *ineffective hematopoiesis*. The bone marrow is cellular, but many cells die in the bone marrow and do not make it into the peripheral blood. The result is a decreased number of cells having an abnormal appearance (*dysplastic*) and possibly impaired function. In some patients, myelodysplasia evolves into acute leukemia, and thus the myelodysplastic syndromes were once called *preleukemia* or *smoldering acute leukemia*; however, the majority of patients die of bone marrow failure without evolving into acute leukemia. The myelodysplastic syndromes are subclassified into several types, based largely on the number of myeloblasts present:

- **Refractory Anemia**
  —With ringed sideroblasts (**RARS**)
  —Without ringed sideroblasts (**RA**)
- **Refractory Cytopenia with Multilineage Dysplasia** (**RCMD**)
- **Refractory Anemia with Excess Blasts** (**RAEB**)

Variations on a Theme (4): The Myelodysplastic/ Myeloproliferative Disorders

Some conditions have features of both chronic myeloproliferative disorders and myelodysplasia and have been put into a bridge category of myelodysplastic/myeloproliferative disorders. The diseases in this category are

- **Atypical Chronic Myelogenous Leukemia** (**aCML**)
- **Juvenile Myelomonocytic Leukemia** (**JMML**)
- **Chronic Myelomonocytic Leukemia** (**CMML**)

Chronic myelomonocytic leukemia was previously classified as a myelodysplastic syndrome and is listed as such in most textbooks.

A Note on Classification Systems

There are many classification systems used for hematopoietic neoplasms, and there have been several new classification systems recently proposed

(Table 12–2). The newer systems incorporate information gained from new diagnostic methods (cytogenetics, immunophenotyping, and molecular tests) and are thus more biologically accurate. They also have greater relevance for prognosis and treatment than the old classification systems. Although it can be difficult to keep up with the changes in classification, the newer systems are evolving toward a consensus, which should eventually result in a single classification system. The different classification systems will be discussed in more detail in later chapters.

Table 12–2
Classification Systems for Hematopoietic Diseases

	Older Classification Systems	Newer Classification Systems
Non-Hodgkin's Lymphomas	• Rappaport • Working Formulation • Updated Kiel	• Revised European American Lymphoid Classification (REAL) • WHO*
Hodgkin's Lymphoma	• Rye	• WHO
Acute Leukemias (AML & ALL)	• French-American-British (FAB)	• WHO
Chronic Leukemias	• French-American-British (FAB) • Polycythemia Vera Study Group	• WHO

*World Health Organization.

13

The Acute Leukemias

The acute leukemias are characterized by *uncontrolled proliferation of hematopoietic precursor cells*, with *loss of maturation and differentiation*. The malignant cells (blasts or minimally differentiated precursors) take over the bone marrow and suppress normal hematopoiesis. Before the development of effective chemotherapy, survival of patients with acute leukemia was usually only a few weeks or months. With effective chemotherapy and improved supportive care, there have been significant advances in the prognosis of acute leukemia, particularly in childhood. Unfortunately, many patients with acute leukemia (particularly older adults) cannot be cured with current treatment.

The acute leukemias can be divided into **acute lymphoblastic leukemia** (**ALL**; sometimes called *acute lymphocytic leukemia*), derived from the CFU-L (colony-forming unit-lymphoid), and **acute myeloid leukemia** (**AML**; sometimes called *acute myelogenous leukemia* or *acute nonlymphocytic leukemia* [**ANLL**]), derived from the CFU-GEMM (colony-forming unit-granulocyte-erythrocyte-megakaryocyte-macrophage).

⇨ **Distinction of ALL from AML is the first critical step in the evaluation of acute leukemia** since treatment and prognosis are very different.

In some cases, the distinction between AML and ALL is obvious based on morphologic appearance, but in many cases, special stains or immunophenotyping by flow cytometry are required to make a definitive diagnosis. The only morphologic feature that unequivocally indicates lineage is the presence of linear reddish or maroon structures known as **Auer rods**, which are diagnostic of myeloid lineage. Auer rods consist of linear stacks of primary granules and are often found in blasts in AML.

There are recurring chromosomal alterations associated with some types of acute leukemia, usually reciprocal translocations, and the genes involved in many of these translocations have been identified. Certain chromosomal alterations are associated with distinct types of acute leukemias, and some cytogenetic abnormalities have major prognostic implications. Treatment protocols are beginning to use these recurring cytogenetic alterations in selection of specific therapies.

The acute leukemias have been traditionally classified by the **FAB** (French-American-British) **classification system**. The FAB classification is based largely on morphology and a few cytochemical stains and has limited significance in terms of prediction of prognosis and choice of therapy. A new classification system has recently been proposed under the auspices of the World Health Organization (**WHO**), and the WHO classification will probably replace the FAB classification in the future. However, the FAB system is still used in most textbooks, and it is used in treatment protocols in cooperative trials.

COMPLICATIONS OF ACUTE LEUKEMIA

The main complications of acute leukemia of any type are due to *suppression of normal hematopoiesis*. *Metabolic complications* also occur and can be life-threatening. Occasionally, a very high blast count can cause an increase in blood viscosity (*hyperleukocytosis with leukostasis*). Disseminated intravascular coagulation (DIC) may occur. In addition, sometimes leukemic cells may infiltrate tissues and form a mass, which may impair organ function.

- **Suppression of normal hematopoiesis**: Normal hematopoiesis is almost invariably suppressed. Consequences include *increased risk of infection* due to granulocytopenia and *hemorrhage* due to thrombocytopenia.
- **Metabolic complications**: The high cell turnover of the malignant cells may result in hyperuricemia, hyperphosphatemia, and hyperkalemia. A *tumor lysis syndrome* with acute renal failure (due to urate crystals depositing in renal tubules) may occur with chemotherapy. Intravenous hydration and allopurinol are started, and the urine is alkalinized prior to chemotherapy to prevent this.
- **Hyperleukocytosis and leukostasis syndrome**: A very high blast count, particularly myeloblasts, may increase the blood viscosity. Patients may develop a *leukostasis syndrome* characterized by altered mental status, respiratory failure, and congestive heart failure. Leukostasis can occur with blast counts $\geq$50,000/μL, and the risk increases significantly with blast counts $\geq$100,000/μL. Symptoms include dyspnea, headache, confusion, and stupor. Intraocular hemorrhages may be present. Chest

radiography may show diffuse infiltrates, and arterial blood gases may show hypoxemia. Leukostasis is most common with AML, particularly cases with monocytic differentiation, but can also be seen with ALL, chronic myelogenous leukemia (CML), and, rarely, chronic lymphocytic leukemia (CLL). **Hyperleukocytosis with leukostasis is a medical emergency; the blast count *must* be lowered as soon as possible**. *Leukapheresis* (removal of white cells by an apheresis machine) is used to rapidly reduce the blast count if there is evidence of leukostasis.

LABORATORY DIAGNOSIS OF ACUTE LEUKEMIA

Commonly used diagnostic tests in acute leukemia include the following:

- Complete blood count and careful examination of a well-prepared blood smear
- Bone marrow aspirate (and biopsy in adults) for morphology and special tests
- Cytochemical stains on bone marrow aspirate smears or peripheral blood:
  - Myeloperoxidase (MPO): Positive in most cases of AML
  - Sudan black B (SBB): Positive in most cases of AML
  - Naphthol ASD chloroacetate esterase (specific esterase): Positive in some cases of AML, particularly more differentiated forms; indicates granulocytic differentiation
  - α-Naphthyl butyrate esterase (nonspecific esterase): Positive in some cases of AML; indicates monocytic lineage
  - PAS (periodic acid–Schiff): Positive in some cases of ALL, with a "chunky" or "block" staining pattern; diffuse cytoplasmic PAS reactivity or block positivity may be seen in some cases of AML
- Immunophenotyping by flow cytometry
- Cytogenetic (chromosomal) analysis
- Molecular diagnostic tests

COMPLICATIONS OF THERAPY FOR ACUTE LEUKEMIA

Therapy for acute leukemia generally consists of combination chemotherapy with cytotoxic agents, which, in the process of killing the malignant cells, causes bone marrow aplasia with resultant cytopenias. Thus, the therapy for acute leukemia exacerbates the problems caused by the disease itself. The treatment can be associated with significant morbidity and mortality, predominantly due to infections and hemorrhage.

- **Infections:** Empiric broad-spectrum antibiotics are started immediately if the patient becomes febrile while granulocytopenic (absolute

neutrophil count <500/μL) and are continued until the neutropen
has resolved. Possible antibiotic regimens include (1) ceftazidime pl
ticarcillin/clavulinic acid plus an aminoglycoside; (2) cefoperazone
ceftazidime plus an extended-spectrum penicillin; or (3) a fluoro
quinolone plus an extended-spectrum penicillin or antipseudomon
cephalosporin. Organisms that commonly cause infection in chemo
therapy patients include *Escherichia coli*, *Klebsiella pneumonia*
Pseudomonas species, *Staphylococcus aureus*, and *Streptococcus* specie
Nosocomial organisms can also be a significant risk. Fungal infectio
are a threat in patients who have prolonged neutropenia, and antifu
gal agents are given empirically if the patient remains febrile despi
broad-spectrum antibiotics. Viral infections, predominantly herpe
viruses (*herpes simplex*, *varicella-zoster*, and *cytomegalovirus*), can als
be problematic.

- **Hemorrhage:** Thrombocytopenia is common during therapy, and pro
phylactic platelet transfusions are given to maintain the platelet cou
≥10,000 to 20,000/μL.

- **Other side effects:** Nausea, vomiting, mucositis, and alopecia are con
mon side effects of chemotherapy that are not life-threatening but a
distressing to patients. Infertility is an additional complication, a pa
ticular concern in young patients with ALL.

- **Specific drug side effects:** Individual chemotherapy drugs may hav
specific side effects, in addition to the general effects noted above. Fc
example, cytosine arabinoside in high doses causes cerebellar dysfunc
tion, and the anthracycline drugs, such as daunorubicin or doxorubicir
may cause cardiomyopathy.

An additional concern, particularly in children with ALL, is the deve
opment of **therapy-related AML** or other malignancies.

ACUTE LYMPHOBLASTIC LEUKEMIA (ALL)

Pathophysiology and Classification

Acute lymphoblastic leukemia represents a clonal proliferation of immatur
lymphocyte precursors. The cells may be B-cell precursors (~80 to 85% of case
or T-cell precursors (~15 to 20% of cases). In rare cases, the lineage is unclear.

The **FAB classification** divides ALL into three groups (**L1, L2, and L3**
based strictly on morphology (Table 13–1). The L1 versus L2 FAB types d
not correspond to phenotype (ie, precursor B cell versus precursor T cell
or to cytogenetic abnormalities and have limited prognostic significance. L
has a slightly better prognosis than L2, but this may be largely due to age
The L3 type consists of *mature* B cells (not precursors) and corresponds t
blood involvement by Burkitt's lymphoma.

Table 13–1
AB Classification of ALL

L1:	Most common type in childhood. Monomorphic, small to intermediate-sized blasts that have round nuclei, scant cytoplasm (high nucleus to cytoplasm [n–c] ratio), homogeneous nuclear chromatin, and inconspicuous nucleoli.
L2:	Most common type in adults. Larger, more variable cells with more abundant cytoplasm (lower n–c ratio), irregular nuclear contours, and more prominent nucleoli.
L3:	Rare (~1–3% of ALL). The cells are characterized by deeply basophilic (blue) cytoplasm with prominent clear cytoplasmic vacuoles containing lipid.

The new **WHO classification** differentiates subtypes based on phenotype (precursor B cell versus precursor T cell) and cytogenetic abnormalities. The FAB L1 and L2 designations are not used, and L3 is considered to be a leukemic phase of Burkitt's lymphoma (Table 13–2).

Epidemiology

Acute lymphoblastic leukemia is the most common malignancy in childhood and represents ~85% of childhood acute leukemias. Acute lymphoblastic leukemia also occurs in adults but is uncommon (~15% of adult acute leukemias). The highest incidence of ALL is between 1 and 5 years of age. There is a slight male predominance overall.

There is a marked increase in risk of ALL in children with **trisomy 21 (Down syndrome)**. Other inherited anomalies predisposing to ALL include Bloom syndrome, Fanconi's anemia, and ataxia-telangiectasia. There is also an increased risk following exposure to ionizing radiation. However, *in the majority of cases, there is no known predisposing factor.* There has been much

Table 13–2
WHO Classification of ALL

Precursor B-cell ALL:
Cytogenetic subgroups (with oncogenes involved):
    t(9;22)(q34;q11); *BCR/ABL* (the *Philadelphia chromosome*)
    t(v;11q23); *MLL* rearranged (*MLL = myeloid-lymphoid leukemia* gene)
    t(1;19)(q23;p13); *E2A/PBX1*
    t(12;21)(p12;q22); *TEL/AML1*
Precursor T-cell ALL
Burkitt-cell leukemia

discussion recently about an association between living near high-voltage electric power lines and ALL. Although this question remains unsettled, most evidence at present does not support such an association.

Clinical Features

Signs and symptoms of ALL usually relate to bone marrow infiltration and suppression of normal hematopoiesis. Common signs and symptoms may include the following:

- **Pallor** and **fatigue**
- **Petechiae** or **other bleeding signs**
- **Fever:** Fever is present in approximately half of patients. This may be due to infection, but, in many cases, no infection can be identified.
- **Bone or joint pain:** Bone or joint pain is common, probably due to expansion of the medullary cavity by the malignant cells. The initial symptom in young children may be limping or reluctance to walk.
- **Hepatosplenomegaly** and **lymphadenopathy**
- **CNS involvement:** ALL can involve the central nervous system (*leukemic meningitis*). Leukemic meningitis is uncommon at original diagnosis, but the spinal fluid may be a site of relapse after treatment. The blood-brain barrier decreases penetration of chemotherapy into the cerebrospinal fluid, providing a "pharmacologic sanctuary" for the leukemic cells.

The testes in males may also be a site of relapse. Testicular involvement presents as painless enlargement of the testes. Testicular relapse is usually followed by bone marrow relapse within a short time, unless systemic treatment is given.

A large mediastinal mass may be present in precursor T-cell ALL. Respiratory distress due to compression of the trachea may be the presenting complaint.

Hyperleukocytosis with leukostasis is less common in ALL than AML but may occur.

Laboratory

Anemia and thrombocytopenia are almost always present. The white cell count is variable: it may be high, normal, or occasionally decreased. Blasts are usually present on blood smear (Figure 13–1) but may be absent or hard to find in up to 5% of cases (*aleukemic leukemia*). Serum uric acid and lactic dehydrogenase may be increased.

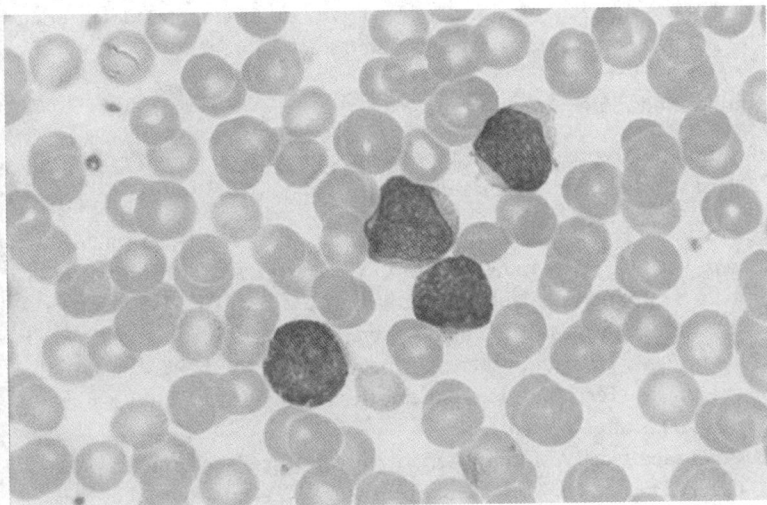

Figure 13–1 **Acute lymphoblastic leukemia (ALL) blood smear.**

Bone Marrow

The bone marrow in ALL usually shows a monomorphic population of blasts, with marked decrease in normal hematopoietic precursors of all types (Figure 13–2). "Block" PAS reactivity may be present, although this

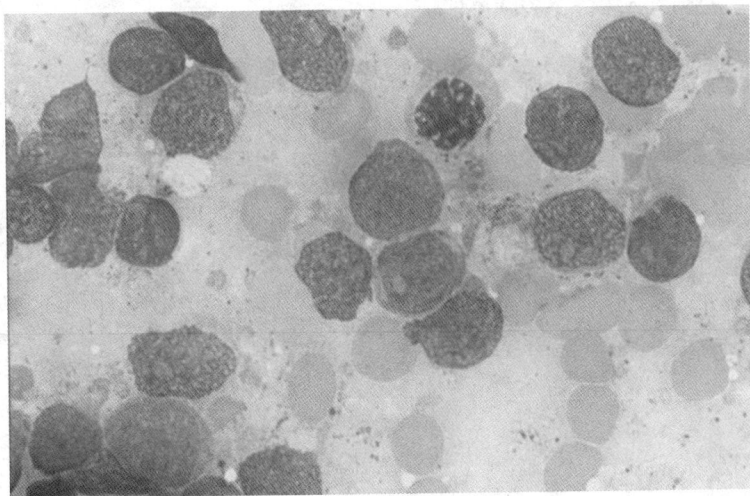

Figure 13–2 **Acute lymphoblastic leukemia (ALL) bone marrow aspirate.**

occurs in less than half of ALL cases. Reactivity for myeloperoxidase, Sudan black B, and specific and nonspecific esterases are absent.

Immunophenotype

Immunophenotyping is usually performed by flow cytometry on either blood or a bone marrow aspirate.

- **Precursor B-cell ALL** characteristically expresses B-cell–associated antigens such as CD19 and CD20. Most cases express **CD10** (the common acute lymphoblastic leukemia antigen or **cALLA**); CD34 (human progenitor cell antigen) is frequently expressed; *cell surface immunoglobulin expression is absent*, but there may be mu (μ) heavy chain present in the cytoplasm. **Terminal deoxynucleotidyl transferase (TdT, a nuclear marker)** is often present.

- **Precursor T-cell ALL** characteristically expresses T-cell antigens such as CD2, CD5, and CD7. CD1a may be present; CD4 and CD8 (the T helper and T suppressor subset antigens) are characteristically either both absent or both expressed. CD3 may be present in the cytoplasm but is absent from the cell surface. Terminal deoxynucleotidyl transferase is usually present.

- **Mature B-cell ALL** (**Burkitt-cell leukemia**) (Figure 13–3) is characterized by the presence of *cell surface immunoglobulin*, with light chain restriction (either kappa *or* lambda light chain, but not a normal mixture of both) and B-cell antigens such as CD19 and CD20. CD10 (cALLA) may be present or absent.

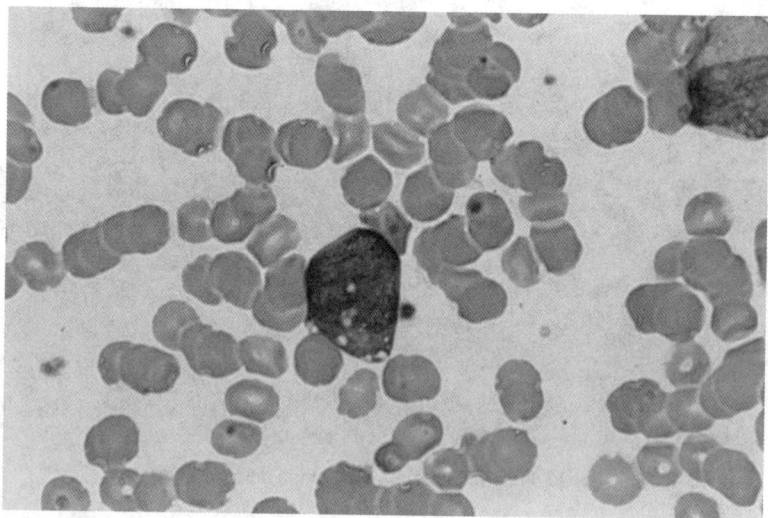

Figure 13–3 Burkitt-cell leukemia (FAB ALL-L3). Basophilic cytoplasm and prominent clear cytoplasmic vacuoles are present.

Expression of myeloid antigens (CD13, CD15, CD33, and others) occurs in 30 to 50% of cases of ALL, more often in children than adults. In most cases, there is only a single myeloid antigen expressed. Myeloid antigen expression does not appear to have any independent prognostic significance in children but may be an adverse prognostic factor in adults.

Cytogenetics

Cytogenetic analysis has become critical for prediction of outcome and selection of therapy in ALL. Chromosomal alterations are present in ≥75% of cases. There may be abnormalities in chromosome number (Table 13–3) or structural alterations in chromosomes, usually reciprocal translocations (Table 13–4).

Molecular Diagnostic Tests

The presence of clonal rearrangements of the lymphocyte antigen receptor genes (immunoglobulin genes for B cells, the T-cell receptor genes for T cells) can be used as evidence of lymphocyte malignancy and can also be used to suggest lineage. Molecular tests can also be used to detect chromosomal abnormalities not detected on standard cytogenetics.

Differential Diagnosis

The differential diagnosis of ALL includes the following:

- **Reactive lymphocytosis:** Reactive lymphocytosis is often seen with viral infections such as infectious mononucleosis (Epstein-Barr virus), viral hepatitis, cytomegalovirus, and others. The lymphocytes usually appear variable, with abundant cytoplasm. Pertussis (whooping cough) may be associated with a striking lymphocytosis; the lymphocytes usually look small and mature, with prominent nuclear folds ("buttock cells"). The

Table 13–3
Numerical Chromosome Abnormalities in ALL

Hyperdiploidy	51 to 65 chromosomes; most common abnormality in chromosome number; associated with a favorable outcome
Near tetraploidy	82 to 94 chromosomes; associated with an unfavorable outcome
Hypodiploidy	Less than 46 chromosomes; associated with an unfavorable outcome
Pseudodiploidy	46 chromosomes with structural alterations; associated with an unfavorable outcome

Table 13–4
Recurring Translocations in ALL

Trans-location	Frequency	Genes Involved	Significance
t(12;21)	25% of pediatric precursor B-cell ALL	*TEL/AML1* (*ETV6/CBFα2*)	Favorable outcome; usually missed on standard cytogenetic analysis and must be detected by molecular methods
t(9;22) (Philadelphia chromosome)	≤5% of pediatric ALL; ~30% of adult ALL	*BCR/ABL*	Highly unfavorable outcome; often associated with myeloid antigen expression
t(1;19)	~5% of pediatric ALL; precursor B-cell phenotype	*E2A/PBX1*	Previously associated with unfavorable outcome; less significant with aggressive therapy
t(v;11q23)	4–8% of pediatric ALL	*MLL*; numerous partners	Common in infant ALL (<1 year); highly unfavorable outcome; often CD10⁻, CD15⁺ phenotype
t(8;14); t(2;8); t(8;22)	<5% of pediatric ALL	c-*MYC* oncogene; immunoglobulin genes	Associated with Burkitt-cell leukemia; formerly highly unfavorable outcome, less significant with aggressive therapy

hemoglobin and platelet count are usually normal in patients with reactive lymphocytosis, and there may be symptoms related to the primary illness.

- **Immune thrombocytopenic purpura (ITP):** ITP presents with petechia or other signs of bleeding, mimicking a common presentation of acute leukemia. In ITP, the hemoglobin and white blood count are usually normal, and the patients otherwise appear healthy.
- **Aplastic anemia:** Aplastic anemia presents with anemia, thrombocytopenia, and leukopenia and clinically may resemble aleukemic leukemia. Hepatosplenomegaly is usually absent. The diagnosis is based upon a hypocellular bone marrow without a predominance of lymphoblasts.
- **Chronic lymphocytic leukemia (CLL):** CLL is characterized by a predominance of small mature-appearing lymphocytes instead of blasts. Flow cytometry of CLL demonstrates a mature B-cell phenotype rather than the immature phenotype seen in ALL. Chronic lymphocytic leukemia is characteristically a disease of adults, whereas ALL is more common in children.

- **Acute myeloid leukemia:** AML, particularly minimally differentiated AML (M0 and M1 in the FAB classification), can be morphologically indistinguishable from ALL. Cytochemical stains and immunophenotyping usually permit distinction.

Treatment

Treatment of ALL is usually separated into three phases: *remission induction, intensification (consolidation),* and *continuation (maintenance).* Treatment includes several drugs that have different mechanisms of action. The total duration of therapy is 2 to 3 years. Treatment of the central nervous system (CNS) is an essential part of therapy, even in the absence of overt CNS involvement, to prevent CNS relapse.

- **Induction:** Typical induction regimens include a corticosteroid (prednisone or dexamethasone) and vincristine, plus L-asparaginase (in children) or an anthracycline (in children with high-risk disease and in adults). This phase lasts approximately 4 to 6 weeks and is designed to reduce the leukemic burden to clinically undetectable levels (ie, induce a complete remission [CR]).
- **Intensification (consolidation):** Intensification regimens can include higher doses of the drugs used to induce remission or a combination of different drugs. Examples of consolidation regimens include (1) methotrexate with or without 6-mercaptopurine, (2) high-dose L-asparaginase, (3) an epipodophyllotoxin such as VP16 with cytosine arabinoside (cytarabine; ara-C), or (4) a combination of vincristine, dexamethasone, L-asparaginase, doxorubicin, and thioguanine with or without cyclophosphamide. This phase typically involves repeated cycles of therapy over approximately 6 months (longer in high-risk patients).
- **Continuation (maintenance):** This phase typically includes weekly methotrexate (orally or by intramuscular injection) and daily oral 6-mercaptopurine. This phase typically lasts approximately 2 to 2$\frac{1}{2}$ years.
- **CNS therapy:** Prophylactic CNS therapy is required in order to prevent CNS relapse. Intrathecal chemotherapy with methotrexate or cytosine arabinoside is used, together with high doses of drugs that cross the blood-brain barrier such as dexamethasone, methotrexate, or cytosine arabinoside. Craniospinal irradiation is used in patients with CNS involvement at diagnosis and in some patients considered at high risk for CNS relapse.

Complications of Treatment

Complications of therapy can be divided into *immediate* and *long-term* complications.

- **Immediate complications:** Immediate complications include nause vomiting, and alopecia. Infection due to granulocytopenia and hemo rhage due to thrombocytopenia may also occur.
- **Long-term complications:** The majority of children treated for ALL ha few or no major long-term effects. *Avascular necrosis of the femoral hea* may occur due to corticosteroids. Methotrexate therapy may result *leukoencephalopathy* and impaired intellectual performance. Short statu and impaired intellectual performance may occur in patients given cra iospinal irradiation; the growth impairment appears to be at least pa tially related to endocrine dysfunction and can often be improved wi growth hormone. A rare complication linked to craniospinal irradiatic is the development of brain tumors, occurring at a median of 10 yea after therapy. These are characteristically aggressive gliomas, and surviv is usually short. Another uncommon complication is the development acute myeloid leukemia, which is linked to chemotherapy with alkylatir agents and topoisomerase II inhibitors (epipodophyllotoxins and anthra cyclines). The AML often passes through a brief myelodysplastic phase; tends to be poorly responsive to therapy, and survival tends to be bri (see **Therapy-Related AML**, on page 252).

Prognosis

The prognosis of childhood ALL has improved dramatically. Over 95% children achieve a complete response, and over 80% of children have long term disease-free survival and are presumed cured. The prognosis in adul is less optimistic; less than 40% of adults are cured. Efforts have been mad to stratify treatment based on prognosis: patients with favorable prognos tic factors can be treated less aggressively, whereas patients with advers prognostic factors may be treated more aggressively from the time of diag nosis. Nearly all adults with ALL are considered high risk.

The initial risk stratification in children is based on age and WBC coun and then readjusted after cytogenetic results are available. An anthracyclin is added to the induction regimen in children considered at high risk, an the intensity of therapy during the consolidation phase is increased. Patient at particularly high risk (such as those with a Philadelphia chromosome may be considered for allogeneic bone marrow transplant (BMT) in firs CR. Prognostic factors of ALL are summarized in Table 13–5.

Special Types of Acute Lymphoblastic Leukemia

Some types of ALL deserve special mention:

- **ALL in infants (<1 year old):** ALL in infancy is associated with translo cations involving the mixed-lineage leukemia (MLL) gene on chromo

Table 13–5

Prognostic Factors in ALL

Factor	Favorable	Unfavorable
Age	2 to 10 years	Below 2 years or above 10 years
WBC count	Low WBC count at diagnosis	WBC >50,000/μL
Phenotype	Precursor B cell	Precursor T cell* Mature B cell*
Chromosome number or DNA Index	Hyperdiploidy DNA Index >1.16	Pseudodiploidy Hypodiploidy Near tetraploidy
Chromosome abnormalities	t(12;21) Trisomy 4 and trisomy 10	c-*MYC* alterations [t(8;14); t(2;8); t(8;22)]* *MLL* alterations (11q23), t(9;22) (Philadelphia chromosome), t(1;19)*
Sex	Female	Male
Ethnicity	Caucasian	African American, Hispanic
Time to complete remission	Short (<7–14 days)	Prolonged time to remission or failure to achieve complete remission

*Prognostic significance of these factors may vary with therapy.

some 11q23 [most often t(4;11)], a very high white cell count, and a highly adverse outcome. The immunophenotype frequently shows expression of CD15 and lack of CD10 (cALLA).

· **Philadelphia chromosome–positive ALL:** The Philadelphia chromosome [t(9;22); *bcr/abl* rearrangement] is present in ~20 to 30% of adult ALL cases but <5% of pediatric cases. The cells usually have a precursor B-cell phenotype, but there is often expression of myeloid antigens such as CD13, CD15, or CD33. Response to therapy is poor; the complete response rate is lower, and remissions tend to be brief.

· **Precursor T-cell ALL:** Precursor T-cell ALL has a predisposition to occur in *young or adolescent males*. The white count is often very high (>100,000/μL), and CNS involvement is common. Patients often have a *mediastinal mass*, probably reflecting origin in the thymus, and may present with respiratory symptoms due to tracheal compression or pleural effusions. T-lineage ALL was thought to have a worse prognosis than precursor B-cell ALL, but with aggressive therapy, the differences have decreased. It has even been suggested that precursor T-cell phenotype may be a favorable prognostic factor in adult ALL (at least in young males).

- **Burkitt-cell leukemia:** Burkitt-cell leukemia (ALL-L3 in the FAB classification) is currently considered to be a leukemic phase of Burkitt's lymphoma. It is associated with translocations involving the c-*MYC* oncogene and one of the immunoglobulin genes, most often t(8;14) (c-*MYC* and the immunoglobulin heavy chain gene). Patients often have bulky mass lesions, most frequently in the abdomen. This type of ALL was formerly considered to have a very poor outcome, but survival in children is significantly improved with use of intensive chemotherapy regimens designed for Burkitt's lymphoma. The outcome for adults with Burkitt-cell leukemia remains poor.

ACUTE MYELOID LEUKEMIA

Pathophysiology and Classification

Acute myeloid leukemia (also known as *acute myelogenous leukemia* and *acute nonlymphocytic leukemia*) is highly heterogeneous, even more so than ALL. Acute myeloid leukemia can show differentiation along any of the lineages derived from the CFU-GEMM, granulocytic, erythroid, megakaryocytic, or monocytic, or may show mixed differentiation (ie, both granulocytic and monocytic).

A critical differentiation in AML is between *de novo* AML and *secondary* AML.

- **De novo (primary) AML** occurs in patients with no previous history of hematologic disease. The patients tend to be younger, have a better response to therapy, and an overall better survival. Reciprocal chromosomal translocations are characteristically present.
- **Secondary AML** occurs in patients with a preceding hematologic disease such as a myelodysplastic syndrome or a chronic myeloproliferative disorder or in patients who have received chemotherapy for another malignancy. In general, secondary AML occurs in older patients and is associated with a poor response to therapy and an overall poor prognosis. Cytogenetic analysis usually shows numerical abnormalities rather than reciprocal translocations.

A second critical distinction in AML is between *acute promyelocytic leukemia (APL)* and other subtypes because there is a unique therapy for APL called all-*trans*-retinoic acid (**ATRA**). All other subtypes are treated essentially the same.

The standard classification for AML has been the **FAB classification** (Table 13–6), which defines eight subtypes based on the degree of maturation and lineage differentiation. The FAB classification is based largely on standard morphology and simple cytochemical stains and does not include cytogenetic abnormalities, the presence of dysplastic features, or a history of previous therapy for a neoplastic disease, all of which are critical prognostic factors in AML. A basic criterion for the diagnosis of AML in the FAB system is that *at least 30% of cells in the bone marrow or blood must be myeloblasts.*

There are some clinical differences between the FAB subtypes; for example, the monocytic types (AML-M4 and AML-M5) are strongly associated with tissue invasion, including gums and the CNS (leukemic meningitis). Acute promyelocytic leukemia is strongly associated with disseminated intravascular coagulation (DIC). There are also associations between some FAB subtypes and certain recurrent chromosomal translocations; however, the FAB classification has limited prognostic significance.

The **World Health Organization (WHO) classification** (Table 13–7) distinguishes those cases of AML associated with specific chromosomal translocations that have prognostic and treatment implications. It also identifies cases with myelodysplastic features, which are associated with a poorer outcome than cases without myelodysplastic features, and identifies AML associated with previous therapy for malignant disease (*therapy-related AML*), which is generally associated with a poor outcome.

⇨ An important change in the WHO classification from the FAB is that **the threshold number of myeloblasts in the marrow is reduced from 30%** (in the FAB) **to 20%** (in the WHO). In the FAB classification, cases with 20 to 30% myeloblasts in the marrow are diagnosed as a myelodysplastic syndrome: refractory anemia with excess blasts in transformation (RAEB-T). In the WHO classification, these cases are diagnosed as AML.

Epidemiology

The annual incidence of AML in the United States is approximately 2.4 per 100,000. Acute myeloid leukemia occurs at all ages but is predominantly a disease of older adults. The incidence rises progressively with age, reaching 12.6 per 100,000 in adults ≥65 years. Approximately 85% of acute leukemias in adults are AML, compared to 15% of acute leukemias in children.

Predisposing factors for AML include trisomy 21, Fanconi's anemia, ataxia-telangiectasia, and Bloom syndrome. There appears to be a familial predisposition to AML. First-degree relatives of AML patients have about a three-fold increase in risk, and there is increased concordance for AML in identical twins. (If one identical twin gets AML, the other twin has an increase in risk.) Exposure to ionizing radiation increases the risk of AML, including patients treated for diseases such as ankylosing spondylitis or rheumatoid arthritis. Benzene and its derivatives have been linked to AML.

Table 13–6
FAB Classification of AML

Category	Features	Comment
M0: Minimally differentiated AML	<3% of blasts have MPO or SBB staining, but there is expression of myeloid antigens on flow cytometry	5–10% of AML; morphologically resembles ALL; Auer rods and lymphoid antigen expression must be absent
M1: AML without maturation	>90% of myeloid cells are blasts; >3% of blasts positive for MPO or SBB	10–20% of AML
M2: AML with maturation	>10% of myeloid cells have maturation to promye-locyte or later stage; ≥30% myeloblasts	30–45% of AML; t(8;21) present in ~25% of cases
M3: Acute promyelocytic leukemia (APL): • Hypergranular variant • Microgranular variant (M3v)	• Hypergranular (75%): Predominant cell is abnormal promyelocyte with large cytoplasmic granules or numerous Auer rods • Microgranular (25%): Abnormal promyelocytes with small granules and folded nuclei	5–10% of AML; associated with rearrangements of *RARα* gene on chromosome 17 Disseminated intravascular coagulation common Both variants respond to all-*trans*-retinoic acid (ATRA)

Continued

Table 13–6
FAB Classification of AML—Continued

Category	Features	Comment
M4: Acute myelomonocytic leukemia (AMML): • Subtype: AMML with abnormal marrow eosinophils (M4Eo)	Monocytosis in blood; ≥20% of marrow cells are monocytic • M4Eo: Abnormal eosinophils with large basophilic granules present in marrow	15–25% of AML; propensity for tissue involvement, including gums and CNS • M4Eo variant associated with inv(16) or t(16;16); ~15–30% of AML-M4
M5: Acute monocytic leukemia: • M5A • M5B	• M5A: >80% of marrow cells are monoblasts • M5B: Predominance of promonocytes	• M5A: 5–8% of AML; more common in younger patients • M5B: 3–6% of AML; more common in older individuals
M6: Acute erythroleukemia	>50% of nucleated marrow cells are erythroid precursors; >30% of nonerythroid cells are myeloblasts	5% of AML; more common in older individuals
M7: Acute megakaryocytic leukemia	>50% of myeloblasts express megakaryocytic markers by flow cytometry	8–10% of AML; flow cytometry required for diagnosis; often associated with marrow fibrosis

MPO = myeloperoxidase; SBB = Sudan black B.

Table 13–7
WHO Classification of AML

AMLs with recurrent cytogenetic translocations:

AML with t(8;21); *AML1*(*CBFα*)/*ETO*. Favorable

APL (AML with t(15;17)(q22;q11-12) and variants; *PML/RARα*). Favorable

AML with abnormal marrow eosinophils (inv(16)(p13;q22) or t(16;16)(p13;q11); *CBFβ/MYH11X*). Favorable

AML with 11q23 (*MLL*) abnormalities. Unfavorable

AML with multilineage dysplasia: Generally unfavorable

With prior myelodysplastic syndrome

Without prior myelodysplastic syndrome

AML and myelodysplastic syndromes, therapy related: Generally unfavorable

Alkylating agent related

Epipodophyllotoxin related (some may be lymphoid)

Other types:

AML not otherwise categorized*

AML minimally differentiated

AML without maturation

AML with maturation

Acute myelomonocytic leukemia

Acute monocytic leukemia

Acute erythroid leukemia

Acute megakaryocytic leukemia

Acute basophilic leukemia

Acute panmyelosis with myelofibrosis

*This category could be used if cytogenetic/molecular analysis is unavailable or normal.

It appears that people who work in the leather and rubber industries, truck drivers, gas station attendants, and people who work in the petroleum industry, who are all exposed to benzene and other hydrocarbons, have an increased incidence of AML. Cancer chemotherapy drugs including alkylating agents and topoisomerase II inhibitors are also associated with AML (therapy-related AML). There is a higher incidence of AML in cigarette smokers, possibly due to benzene and other carcinogenic chemicals in cigarette smoke. However, *in most cases, no obvious predisposing factor is present.*

Clinical Features

The clinical presentation of AML symptoms resembles that of ALL. Symptoms related to bone marrow infiltration and suppression of normal hematopoiesis are common. Fever is present in 15 to 20% of patients; this should be presumed due to infection and treated as such until proven otherwise but may be due to hypermetabolism. Physical examination may show mild splenomegaly; prominent lymphadenopathy is unusual.

Tissue involvement is more common in AML than in ALL. Skin involvement occurs in approximately 10% of patients, particularly in patients with monocytic subtypes; it presents as violaceus nontender plaques or nodules. Involvement of the gums is common, and patients may present initially to the dentist, complaining of bleeding gums. Leukemic meningitis occurs in approximately 5 to 7% of patients at diagnosis and is more common with high WBC counts and monocytic subtypes.

Hyperleukocytosis with leukostasis is also more common in AML than ALL. There is a risk of leukostasis with blast counts ≥50,000/μL, and the risk increases significantly with blast counts ≥100,000/μL. **Hyperleukocytosis with leukostasis represents a medical emergency**, and prompt lowering of the blast count with leukapheresis should be performed as soon as possible.

Metabolic complications of AML may include hyperuricemia, hyper- or hypokalemia, hyperphosphatemia, and the *tumor lysis syndrome* with acute renal failure. Patients with high blast counts may have spurious hypoglycemia or hypoxemia if blood samples are not analyzed promptly, due to consumption of glucose or oxygen by the blasts. Spurious hyperkalemia may also occur.

Disseminated intravascular coagulation may occur in AML. It is most frequent in acute promyelocytic leukemia (APL) but may also occur with other types.

Laboratory

Anemia and thrombocytopenia are almost always present. The platelet count given by automated hematology analyzers may be spuriously increased due to fragments of the leukemic blasts, which are counted as platelets by the instrument. Examination of a blood smear gives a more accurate assessment of the platelet count in this circumstance. The white cell count is variable; it is elevated in more than half of patients and may exceed 100,000/μL, but may also be decreased. Blasts are usually present on blood smear but occasionally may be absent or hard to find.

Careful examination of a blood smear for circulating blasts is required. The blasts in AML tend to be larger and more variable in appearance than those in ALL, with more irregular nuclei, but may be impossible to distinguish from lymphoblasts. *The only morphologic feature that absolutely confirms myeloid lineage is the presence of **Auer rods*** (Figure 13–4).

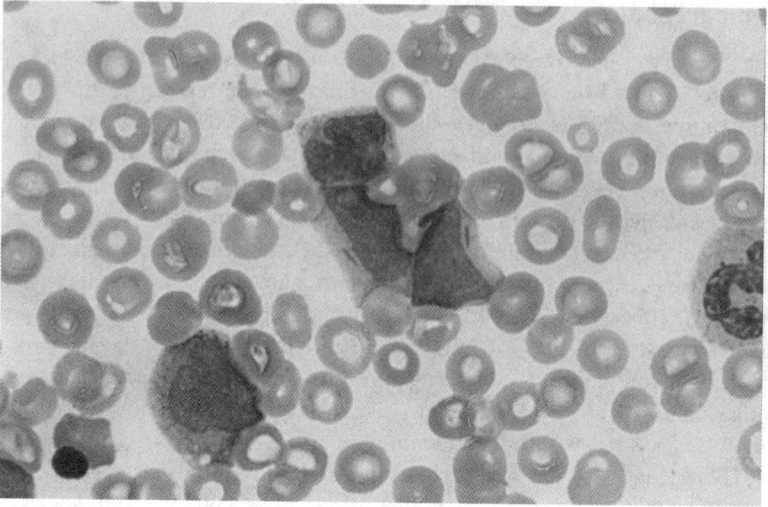

Figure 13–4 Acute myelogenous leukemia (AML) blood smear. The two cells in the center contain Auer rods.

Bone Marrow

The bone marrow is typically hypercellular, with a predominance of blasts or other immature cells (Figure 13–5). Normal hematopoietic precursors are decreased.

Cytochemical stains may be performed on peripheral blood (if there is a high circulating blast count) or on bone marrow aspirate smears. By FAB criteria, staining for myeloperoxidase and/or Sudan black B must be present in ≥3% of blasts in AML, except for the M0 subtype. Staining for the naphthol ASD chloroacetate ("specific") esterase may be seen in AML with granulocytic differentiation, and staining for the α-naphthyl butyrate ("nonspecific") esterase may be seen in AML with monocytic differentiation. Finely granular cytoplasmic staining with the PAS reaction is common in AML and must not be interpreted as ALL. Coarse "block" positivity resembling that seen in ALL may be present in erythroleukemia and in megakaryocytic leukemia.

Immunophenotype

Immunophenotyping by flow cytometry is most useful in identifying myeloid lineage and distinguishing between AML and ALL. Phenotyping can suggest specific subtypes of AML, particularly megakaryocytic leukemia, but definitive subclassification usually requires correlation with morphology and cytochemical stains.

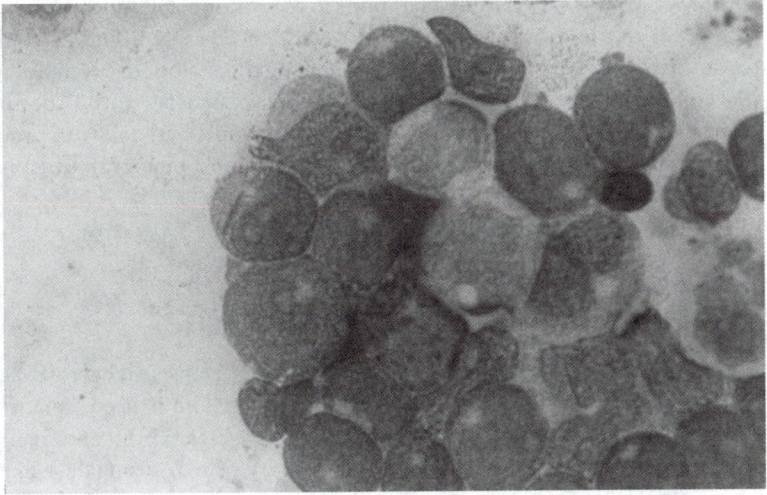

Figure 13–5 **Acute myelogenous leukemia (AML) bone marrow aspirate.** Note the prominent Auer rod in the cell on the edge of the cluster.

- Myeloid lineage–associated markers include **CD13**, **CD15**, and **CD33**. Of these, CD33 is the most sensitive. CD15 is usually seen in more differentiated granulocytic leukemias. None of these markers are totally specific for AML.
- CD7 (usually thought of as a T-cell marker) is often found on AMLs with minimal maturation (M0 and M1 in the FAB classification). Other markers usually associated with lymphoid lineage may also be seen in AML, including CD2, CD4, CD19, CD10 (cALLA), and TdT.
- Expression of HLA-DR (a Class II histocompatibility antigen) may be helpful. HLA-DR is expressed in most cases of AML, with the striking exception of acute promyelocytic leukemia (APL) which usually lacks HLA-DR.
- Expression of CD19 on AML blasts is associated with, but not specific for, the t(8;21) translocation.
- In addition to lacking HLA-DR, APL often expresses CD4. CD34 (the human progenitor cell antigen) is usually absent.
- Diagnosis of acute megakaryocytic leukemia depends on detection of platelet-associated antigens such as CD41 and CD61.

Cytogenetics

Cytogenetic analysis has become critical in the diagnosis and treatment of AML. As in ALL, recurring chromosomal abnormalities can be divided into reciprocal translocations and alterations in chromosome number. Many of the genes involved in translocations in AML encode DNA-binding transcription factors or regulatory components of transcriptional complexes. Several of the recurring translocations have been associated with specific subtypes of AML (although the correlations are imperfect) and with prognosis. Indeed, **cytogenetic results are among the most powerful prognostic factors in AML** (Table 13–8).

Differential Diagnosis

The differential diagnosis of AML includes the following:

- **Reactive leukocytosis (*leukemoid reaction*):** Reactive leukocytosis can usually be distinguished from AML by the predominance of mature cells rather than blasts. The hemoglobin and platelet count are usually normal, unless they are altered by the primary illness causing the leukemoid reaction.
- **Acute lymphoblastic leukemia (ALL):** The distinction between ALL and AML was discussed above.
- **Chronic myeloproliferative disorders:** The chronic myeloproliferative disorders such as chronic myelogenous leukemia (CML) can usually be distinguished from AML by the predominance of relatively mature granulocytes and the rarity of blasts in the blood and marrow in the chronic myeloproliferative disorders.
- **Aplastic anemia:** Aleukemic leukemia can mimic aplastic anemia. The presence of a hypocellular marrow in aplastic anemia, versus the hypercellular marrow typically seen in AML, usually makes the distinction straightforward. However, rare cases of AML are associated with a hypocellular marrow and can be more difficult to distinguish from aplastic anemia.
- **Recovery from myelosuppression of any type:** Recovery from myelosuppression from any cause (drugs, infection, chemical exposure) can be associated with a transient predominance of blasts in the marrow. This can be difficult to distinguish from AML if the preceding myelosuppression is not recognized. If this is a possibility, observing the patient for a few weeks without therapy to see if he or she recovers may be helpful.
- **Myelodysplasia:** The distinction between myelodysplasia and AML is based upon the number of myeloblasts in the marrow: if there are <20% myeloblasts, it is myelodysplasia; if there are ≥20% myeloblasts, it is AML (<30% or ≥30%, respectively, if you use the FAB criteria). Sometimes the distinction can be difficult. In such cases, the presence of a cytogenetic translocation characteristic of AML strongly favors that diagnosis. Otherwise, it might be a good idea to observe the patient for a few weeks without therapy to see if there is progression.

Table 13–8
Cytogenetic Abnormalities in AML

Trans- location	Genes	Association	Significance
t(8;21):	*AML1* (*CBFα*) on 21; *ETO* on 8	AML with differen- tiation (FAB-M2)	Favorable
inv(16) or t(16;16)	*CBF*β on 16q; *MYH11* on 16p	AML with abnormal bone marrow eosinophils (FAB-M4Eo)	Favorable
t(15;17)	*PML* on 15; *RARα* on 17	Acute promyelocytic leukemia (FAB-M3)	Favorable; responds to all-*trans*-retinoic acid (ATRA)
t(11q23;var)	*MLL* on 11q23; more than 40 translocation partners	AML in infants; AML associated with topoisomerase II inhibitors; AML with monocytic differentiation	Unfavorable

Other Cytogenetic Abnormalities	Genes	Association	Significance
Numerical chromosome abnormalities:	Unknown	AML in older adults; secondary AML; AML associated with alkylating agent chemotherapy	Unfavorable
Deletion of chromosome 7,	Unknown	AML in older adults; secondary AML; AML associated with alkylating agent chemotherapy	Unfavorable
Deletion of chromosome 5 or the long arm of chromosome 5,	Unknown	AML in older adults; secondary AML; AML associated with alkylating agent chemotherapy	Unfavorable
Chromosome 8 trisomy, others	Unknown	AML in older adults; secondary AML; AML associated with alkylating agent chemotherapy	Unfavorable

Treatment

Treatment of AML can be divided into *remission induction* and *postinduction (postremission)* phases.

- **Remission induction:** Standard induction therapy includes an anthra-cycline and cytosine arabinoside (cytarabine; ara-C). Daunorubicin has

been the standard anthracycline, but idarubicin and mitoxantrone ar
also popular. A common regimen is "3 + 7": 3 daily doses of daunoru
bicin plus 7 daily doses of cytarabine. With standard regimens, a CR ca
be achieved in approximately 70 to 80% of patients ≤60 years of age an
in ~50% of older patients. However, postinduction treatment i
required to prevent relapse.

- **Postinduction (postremission) therapy:** Postinduction regimens ca
include chemotherapy at various levels of intensity (maintenance, con
solidation, or intensification), allogeneic bone marrow transplant* o
high-dose chemotherapy with autologous bone marrow transplant. Th
choice of therapy depends on the individual patient, the prognosis a
determined by cytogenetic results on the bone marrow among othe
factors, and also whether the patient has a suitable bone marrow dono
Chemotherapy: A commonly used regimen in younger patients is high
dose cytosine arabinoside (HiDAC; 2–12 g/m2/day). Standard-dos
cytarabine plus an anthracycline is a common regimen for olde
patients.
Allogeneic bone marrow transplant: Allogeneic BMT performed dur
ing remission is the most effective therapy available for decreasin
relapse of AML. It is used predominantly in younger patients consid
ered to be at high risk of relapse. Older individuals are generally no
considered candidates for allogeneic transplant due to higher trans
plant-related mortality, but the age limit has been rising because o
improvements in supportive care.
Autologous bone marrow transplant: Hematopoietic progenitor cell
can be harvested after the patient has achieved a CR and either give
after intensive chemotherapy in first remission or saved to be used i
case of relapse. The early morbidity and mortality of autologous BM
is lower than that of allogeneic BMT, but the relapse rate is higher, giv
ing an overall survival that is approximately equivalent. Autologou
BMT can be used in patients who are too old for allogeneic BMT or wh
do not have a suitable donor.

Prognosis

The overall long-term disease-free survival of patients less than 65 years ol
with AML is approximately 40%. The prognosis is worse for older patient
and those with secondary AML. Patients with AML can be divided int

*The term bone marrow transplant includes peripheral blood progenitor cells as well a
actual bone marrow. Allogeneic means that the stem cells were obtained from another per
son; autologous means that the stem cells came from the patient; syngeneic would be from
an identical twin.

ree broad prognostic groups, predominantly on the basis of cytogenetic
·sults:

- **Favorable prognostic group:** This group includes patients <60 years
  old with the t(8;21), t(15;17), inv(16), or t(16;16) cytogenetic abnormalities, no previous hematologic disease, and AML that is not therapy
  related. This group makes up ~20% of patients <60 years. They have a
  high CR rate (>85%) and a relatively low risk of relapse (30 to 40%).
- **Unfavorable prognostic group:** This group includes patients with
  cytogenetic abnormalities involving more than two chromosomes,
  monosomies of chromosomes 5 or 7, deletion of the long arm of 5
  (del5q), or abnormalities of the long arm of chromosome 3. Patients
  with abnormalities involving chromosome 11q23 (*MLL* gene) are
  sometimes also considered to be in this group. These abnormalities are
  more often present in older individuals and patients with secondary
  AML. This group makes up ~15% of patients who are 15 to 60 years old.
  They tend to have a lower CR rate and a higher relapse rate, and survival
  at 5 years is <20%. No current treatment approach is considered satisfactory for these patients. Patients over 60 years of age generally have an
  unfavorable prognosis, with 5-year-survival rates <10%.
- **Intermediate (standard) prognostic group:** Patients in this group have
  either a normal karyotype or chromosomal abnormalities not included
  in the other groups.

pecial Types of Acute Myeloid Leukemia

everal types of AML deserve special mention:

- **Acute promyelocytic leukemia (APL; FAB-M3):** Acute promyelocytic
  leukemia with the t(15;17) is distinct because it responds to a specific
  therapy: ATRA. Acute promyelocytic leukemia most commonly occurs
  in younger individuals. The white cell count is often relatively low, and
  DIC is very common. There are two subtypes of APL: the hypergranu-
  lar variant (~75%) and the microgranular variant (M3v). The hyper-
  granular variant is characterized by cells that contain numerous Auer
  rods and prominent basophilic granules (Figures 13–6 and 13–7). The
  microgranular variant is characterized by cells with fine cytoplasmic
  granularity and folded (monocytic-appearing) nuclei. All-trans-
  retinoic acid induces differentiation of the leukemic promyelocytes; it
  is not a cytotoxic agent and does not induce bone marrow aplasia. It is
  able to induce a complete hematologic remission in the majority of APL
  patients, but relapse invariably occurs if ATRA is used as a single agent.
  Therefore, a cytotoxic agent of some type is also given, either together
  with ATRA to induce remission or as consolidation following remission

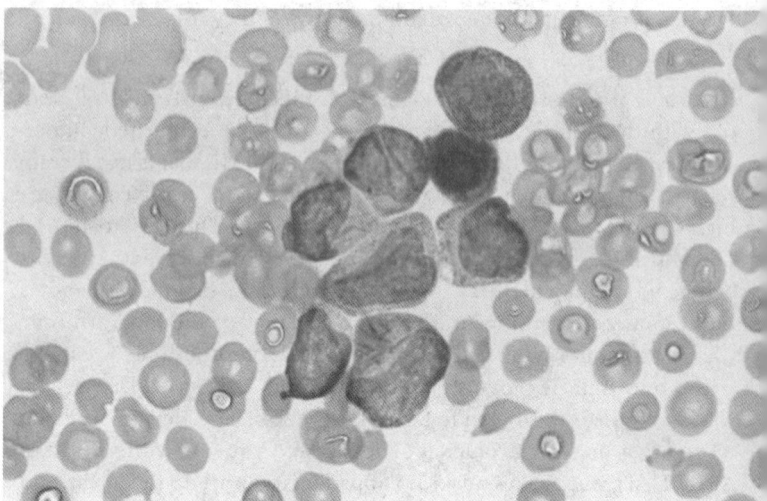

Figure 13–6 Acute promyelocytic leukemia (FAB AML-M3) blood smear. Note the cytoplasmic granules in the cell at the top and the multiple Auer rods in the cell at the bottom. The patient was in florid disseminated intravascular coagulation (note the schistocytes and the complete absence of platelets).

induction with ATRA. All-*trans*-retinoic acid also improves the coagulopathy associated with APL. All-*trans*-retinoic acid may be associated with the "retinoic acid syndrome," which includes a capillary leak syndrome with fever, respiratory failure, impaired renal function, and, in some patients, cardiac failure. **Arsenic trioxide** also appears to be effective in APL.

- **Therapy-related AML:** Therapy-related AML now represents approximately 10 to 20% of AML cases in the United States. Therapy-related AML may follow treatment for Hodgkin's or non-Hodgkin's lymphoma, ALL, or non-hematologic neoplasms. The drugs that are implicated include alkylating agents (cyclophosphamide, mechlorethamine, chlorambucil, busulfan, BCNU, and CCNU) and topoisomerase II inhibitors including epipodophyllotoxins (etoposide and tenoposide) and anthracyclines (daunorubicin and doxorubicin). Therapy-related AML is usually resistant to standard therapy, and the overall prognosis is poor. Younger patients should be considered for immediate allogeneic BMT if a suitable donor is available. Therapy-related AML is divided into two types based on the drug treatment that induced it:
  - **Related to alkylating agents:** Therapy-related AML develops in 3 to 10% of patients given alkylating agents for Hodgkin's disease, non-

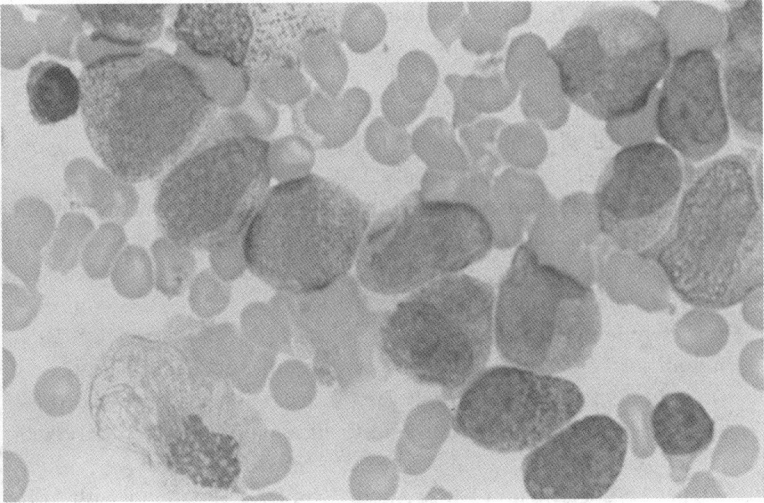

Figure 13–7 Acute promyelocytic leukemia (FAB AML-M3) bone marrow aspirate.
Note the prominent Auer rod in the center cell.

Hodgkin's lymphoma, breast carcinoma, or other malignancies. The risk of AML peaks at ~5 to 10 years after the chemotherapy. Patients often pass through a myelodysplastic phase prior to development of AML. Common chromosomal abnormalities in this group include deletions of chromosomes 5 and 7.

- **Related to topoisomerase II inhibitors:** A second type of therapy-related AML occurs in patients given topoisomerase II inhibitors, particularly epipodophyllotoxins such as etoposide (VP16). The latency period after chemotherapy is relatively short (2 to 3 years), and patients usually do not progress through a myelodysplastic phase. Chromosomal abnormalities involving 11q23 are common in this group.

- **Granulocytic sarcoma (extramedullary myeloid tumor):** Granulocytic sarcomas (sometimes called *chloromas* because they may have a green color on section due to myeloperoxidase) are tumor masses composed of myeloblasts. They may occur in subcutaneous tissue, around the orbit, in the epidural space or brain, in the testes, or in other sites. Initial transformation of a chronic myeloproliferative disorder into an acute myeloid leukemia may occur in the form of a granulocytic sarcoma. Blood and bone marrow involvement is usually present at diagnosis of the granulocytic sarcoma, but patients may present with apparently solitary granulocytic sarcomas, without blood or bone marrow involvement (*primary extramedullary myeloid tumor*).

- **Acute myeloid leukemia in infancy and early childhood:** AML in infancy and children less than 2 years of age is rare but has a less favorable prognosis than AML in older children. They tend to have high white cell counts, DIC, hepatosplenomegaly, and extramedullary disease (primarily skin and CNS). Cytogenetic analysis often shows abnormalities involving the *MLL* gene at 11q23.

- **Acute myeloid leukemia in the elderly:** AML in the elderly (over about 65 years) differs from AML in younger patients because many older patients have a previous history of myelodysplasia or have myelodysplastic features. Unfavorable cytogenetic abnormalities are common, and often there is expression of the multidrug-resistant protein *MDR1*. In addition, older patients often have significant medical problems, which limits their ability to tolerate the aggressive therapy needed for AML. Complete remission rates up to 40 to 60% have been observed, but remission durations tend to be short (median <1 year).

- **Relapsed and refractory AML:** About 40 to 80% of patients with AML relapse after achieving a remission, and 10 to 20% of patients never achieve CR despite therapy (*refractory AML*). The prognosis of patients with relapsed or refractory disease is usually poor; patients with refractory AML and patients with early relapse from CR (within 6 months) have a particularly poor outlook. In general, patients who have relapsed cannot be cured with chemotherapy alone. Allogeneic transplant should be performed for patients who have suitable donors and appear able to tolerate the procedure. Autologous BMT using cryopreserved stem cells harvested during the first remission can be used during second remission but is probably inferior to allogeneic BMT.

Additional Readings

Farhi DC, Rosenthal NS. Acute lymphoblastic leukemia. Clin Lab Med 2000;20: 17–28.

Löwenberg B, Downing JR, Burnett A. Acute myeloid leukemia. N Engl J Med 1999;341:1051–62.

Pui C-H, Evans WE. Acute lymphoblastic leukemia. N Engl J Med 1998;339: 605–29.

14

The Chronic Myeloproliferative Disorders and the Myelodysplastic/ Myeloproliferative Disorders

The chronic mycloproliferative disorders (CMPDs) are clonal hematopoietic stem cell disorders in which regulation of proliferation is impaired, but differentiation and maturation are generally maintained. Thus, they are characterized by *increased cell counts*, but the increase consists predominantly of *mature cells*. The different CMPDs each feature a predominant increase in a single cell line: granulocytes in chronic myelogenous leukemia, erythrocytes in polycythemia vera, and platelets in primary thrombocythemia. However, offspring of the neoplastic clone differentiate into all of the different myeloid cell lines and sometimes also B lymphocytes. There is overlap between the different CMPDs; therefore, the platelet count can be elevated in chronic myelogenous leukemia (CML), and the leukocyte count can be elevated in primary thrombocythemia.

Idiopathic myelofibrosis (IM; also known as *agnogenic myeloid metaplasia* and *myelofibrosis with myeloid metaplasia*) differs from the other CMPDs in that it is often characterized by cytopenias rather than increased cell counts. The major feature of IM is increased collagen production by bone marrow fibroblasts; the fibroblasts themselves are not part of the malignant clone but are driven to produce excess collagen by neoplastic megakaryocytes and monocytes.

Chronic myelogenous leukemia is the second most common adult leukemia in the United States, following chronic lymphocytic leukemia. The other chronic myeloproliferative disorders are all relatively uncommon. All of the CMPDs share a predisposition to evolve into acute leukemia; this occurs in the majority of patients with CML, but only a small proportion of patients with the other CMPDs. Survival in CML and idiopathic myelofibrosis tends to be relatively short. Polycythemia vera and primary thrombocythemia are associated with long survival.

The **myelodysplastic/myeloproliferative disorders** (**MDS/MPDs**) are characterized by both *dysplastic morphologic features* and *increased cell counts* and thus have features of both the myelodysplastic syndromes and the CMPDs. This category of disease is defined in the new World Health Organization (WHO) classification of diseases of the hematopoietic and lymphoid tissues. Three diseases are included in this group: **atypical** (*Philadelphia chromosome–negative*) **chronic myelogenous leukemia** (**aCML**), **juvenile myelomonocytic leukemia** (**JMML**), and **chronic myelomonocytic leukemia** (**CMML**).

CHRONIC MYELOGENOUS LEUKEMIA (CHRONIC GRANULOCYTIC LEUKEMIA)

Pathophysiology

Chronic myelogenous leukemia (also known as **chronic granulocytic leukemia**, or **CGL**) is caused by a reciprocal translocation between the long arm of chromosome 9 and the long arm of chromosome 22 [**t(9;22)**], known as the **Philadelphia chromosome** (**Ph¹**). The translocation results in juxtaposition of the *abl* (*Abelson leukemia virus*) gene on chromosome 9 and the *bcr* (*breakpoint cluster region*) gene on chromosome 22. The result is a fusion gene, *bcr/abl*, which codes for a fusion protein designated **p210**.

The normal *abl* gene codes for a tyrosine kinase enzyme. The BCR-ABL p210 protein produced by the *bcr/abl* fusion gene is a more potent tyrosine kinase than the normal ABL protein and acts as an oncogene.

⇨ The *bcr/abl* fusion gene in nearly all CML patients produces a protein with a molecular weight of 210,000 daltons (210 kD). The rearrangement in most cases of Philadelphia chromosome–positive acute lymphoblastic leukemia (ALL) occurs in a different place in the *bcr* gene, resulting in a fusion protein with a molecular weight of ~190 kD (**p190**). The p190 protein in ALL is an even more potent tyrosine kinase than is the p210 protein in most cases of CML. However, some cases of ALL have the same p210 protein found in CML.

Chronic myelogenous leukemia classically occurs in three phases: a *chronic phase*, an *accelerated phase*, and termination in *blast crisis*.

Epidemiology

Chronic myelogenous leukemia represents ~20% of all leukemias in the United States. Chronic myclogenous leukemia occurs at all ages, but predominantly in older adults. There is a slight male predominance (~1.5:1). Chronic myclogenous leukemia has been linked to exposure to ionizing radiation; no other predisposing factors are known.

Clinical Features

In nearly half of patients, CML is discovered as an incidental finding on a routine CBC. Symptomatic patients may have fatigue, lethargy, low-grade fever, and weight loss. There may be early satiety or left upper quadrant discomfort due to splenomegaly. Gout is occasionally the presenting feature, due to hyperuricemia. Hyperviscosity due to leukostasis may be present if the WBC count is very high.

Splenomegaly is almost always present on physical examination and can be massive. Mild hepatomegaly is common; lymphadenopathy is unusual. The characteristics of CML are summarized in Table 14–1.

Laboratory

The white blood cell count can range from ~25,000/µL to >300,000/µL. Mild anemia is common. Thrombocytosis is present in ~30 to 50% of patients, and the platelet count can exceed 1,000,000/µL.

The blood smear in CML is very characteristic (Figure 14–1). There is a marked granulocytosis including all stages of granulocytic maturation, from blasts to segmented neutrophils. There is a predominance of more mature forms, from myelocytes to segmented neutrophils. Myeloblasts are typically only 1 to 2% of WBCs and are always <10% in the chronic phase. **Basophils** are **always** *increased in number and usually in the percentage of WBC.* Eosinophils are also frequently increased, but monocytes are not. Occasional nucleated RBCs may be present. Giant platelets and megakaryocyte nuclear fragments may be present.

Serum chemistries often show an increase in lactic dehydrogenase (LDH) and uric acid. The cobalamin (vitamin B_{12}) level is often increased.

A very helpful test is the **leukocyte alkaline phosphatase (LAP) score** (sometimes called the *neutrophil alkaline phosphatase [NAP] score*). **The LAP score is characteristically *decreased* in CML**, whereas it is normal or increased in most of the other conditions in the differential diagnosis of CML. However, the LAP score in CML can increase with infections, treatment, and with progression to the accelerated phase or blast crisis.

⇨ The LAP score test is done by performing a chemical reaction on a blood smear that causes cells with the alkaline phosphatase enzyme to

Table 14–1

Characteristics of Chronic Myelogenous Leukemia (Chronic Phase)

Blood:
- Granulocytosis
- Full range of granulocyte precursors
- Predominance of myelocytes and segmented neutrophils
- Myeloblasts typically ~1–2%; always <10%
- Basophilia
- Thrombocytosis common

Bone Marrow:
- Hypercellular
- Granulocytic hyperplasia (increased M:E ratio)
- Increased megakaryocytes, particularly small megakaryocytes
- Mild fibrosis in one-third of patients

Splenomegaly

Decreased LAP score

Philadelphia chromosome [t(9;22)] and/or *bcr/abl* rearrangement

Elevated serum cobalamin (vitamin B_{12}) and uric acid

M:E = myeloid to erythroid; LAP = leukocyte alkaline phosphatase.

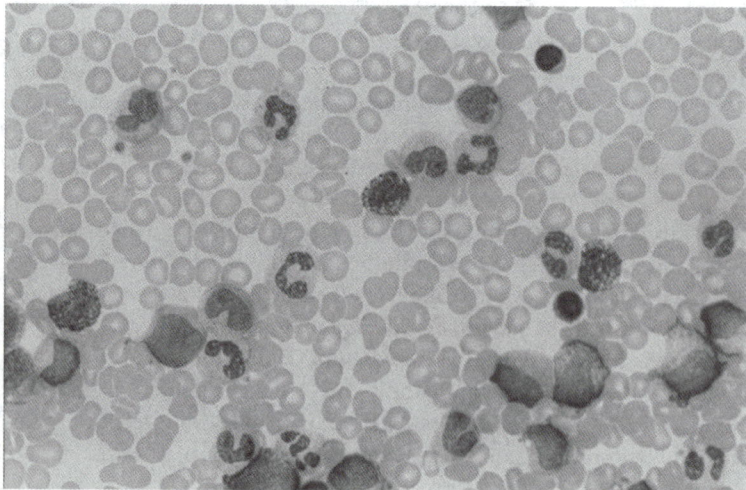

Figure 14–1 Chronic myelogenous leukemia blood smear. All stages of granulocyte maturation are present, with a predominance of mature forms; several basophils are present.

have granular colored staining. The blood smear is viewed under a microscope, and the degree of granular staining in mature neutrophils (bands and segs) is graded from 0 (no staining) to 4+ (dense granular staining). The LAP score is the sum of staining for 100 cells. The normal range is ~20 to 100. The two main conditions with a low LAP score are CML and paroxysmal nocturnal hemoglobinuria (PNH).

Bone Marrow

The bone marrow in CML is hypercellular, with an increase in the ratio of granulocytic to erythroid precursors (~10 to 30:1; normal ~2 to 4:1). Granulocyte precursors mature normally, and myeloblasts are <10% in the chronic phase. Megakaryocytes are often increased in number; a characteristic feature is numerous small megakaryocytes. There may be focal marrow fibrosis, and occasional cases have moderate to severe fibrosis.

Cytogenetics

The Philadelphia chromosome [t(9;22)(q34;q11)] is present in ~85 to 95% of cases analyzed by standard cytogenetic analysis. A variant cytogenetic abnormality is present in ~5 to 10% of cases. In occasional cases, there is no Philadelphia chromosome or other detectable abnormality by standard cytogenetics, but a t(9;22) is detected by fluorescence in situ hybridization (FISH), or a *bcr/abl* rearrangement is detected by molecular tests. The clinical presentation and biologic behavior of such cases appear to be identical to cases with the typical Philadelphia chromosome. *If there is no Philadelphia chromosome or variant by standard cytogenetics, and no evidence of a* bcr/abl *rearrangement by molecular tests, then the diagnosis is **not** CML!*

Additional cytogenetic abnormalities may be present at diagnosis. In general, it appears that these patients have the same course as patients lacking additional cytogenetic abnormalities at diagnosis. Additional cytogenetic abnormalities often appear with transformation to the accelerated phase or blast crisis. The most significant of these are an additional Philadelphia chromosome, isochrome 17q (two long arms of chromosome 17 joined together at the centromere), and trisomy of chromosome 8.

Molecular Diagnostic Tests

Fluorescence in situ hybridization can detect the t(9;22) translocation using probes to the *abl* and *bcr* loci. The *bcr/abl* rearrangement can also be detected by reverse transcription-polymerase chain reaction (RT-PCR). These tests are useful in cases that appear to be CML but lack the Philadelphia chromosome by standard cytogenetics. They can also be used to detect residual disease after bone marrow transplant or other therapy.

Differential Diagnosis

- **Leukemoid reaction:** A granulocytic leukemoid reaction can sometimes be difficult to distinguish from CML (Table 14–2). Leukemoid reactions typically show a predominance of mature cells (bands and segs), without the immature cells seen in CML. *Basophils are not usually increased in leukemoid reactions but are almost always increased in CML.* The LAP score is usually increased in leukemoid reactions and decreased in CML. Finally, cytogenetic analysis on the bone marrow or peripheral blood should be normal in a leukemoid reaction.
- **Leukoerythroblastic reaction:** A leukoerythroblastic reaction due to a space-occupying lesion in the bone marrow usually shows more nucleated RBCs, "teardrop" RBCs, and fewer myelocytes and metamyelocytes. If the distinction is not clear, a bone marrow biopsy should be done.
- **Other chronic myeloproliferative disorders:** CML can resemble any of the other myeloproliferative disorders, particularly primary thrombocythemia. Although the WBC count is usually higher and the platelet count lower in CML than primary thrombocythemia, occasionally CML can present with a striking thrombocytosis and less prominent leukocytosis. It has been recommended that cytogenetic analysis and/or molecular analysis on the marrow be done in all cases of suspected chronic myeloproliferative disorder, of any type, in order to exclude CML. If a Philadelphia chromosome or *bcr/abl* rearrangement is found, the diagnosis is CML.
- **Atypical (Philadelphia chromosome–negative) CML (a*CML*):** Atypical CML is characterized by a predominance of segmented neutrophils, with fewer myelocytes and metamyelocytes. The characteristic basophilia of

Table 14–2
Distinction of CML from a Neutrophilic Leukemoid Reaction

Characteristic	CML	Leukemoid Reaction
Known cause for leukemoid reaction	Absent	Often present
WBC count	Often >70,000/μL	Usually <70,000/μL
Leukocyte differential	Complete spectrum of granulocyte precursors	Predominance of mature neutrophils; rare immature granulocytes
Basophilia	Present	Absent
LAP score	Decreased	Normal or increased
Splenomegaly	Present	Absent

true CML is usually lacking. Dysplastic changes are usually present in aCML and lacking in true CML. *By definition,* there is *no* Philadelphia chromosome or molecular evidence of a *bcr/abl* rearrangement in aCML.

- **Chronic myelomonocytic leukemia (CMML):** Monocytosis is required for a diagnosis of CMML, rare in CML. Chronic myelomonocytic leukemia usually shows dysplastic changes, which are typically absent in CML.
- **Acute leukemias:** Acute leukemias with the Philadelphia chromosome (usually lymphoblastic, less often myeloid) can be difficult to distinguish from the rare cases of CML presenting in blast crisis. Patients should be given appropriate therapy for ALL or AML, depending on the phenotype of the blasts.

Disease Course

As noted, CML tends to occur in two or three phases: chronic phase, accelerated phase, and blast crisis. Some patients progress directly from chronic phase to blast crisis, without an intermediate accelerated phase.

- **Chronic phase:** Most patients are diagnosed in chronic phase. The chronic phase lasts a median of ~3 to 4 years but can vary from a few months to >15 years. Approximately 5% of patients transform within the first year after diagnosis, and ~20 to 25% of surviving patients transform each year thereafter.
- **Accelerated phase:** Accelerated phase can be difficult to define and diagnose. Patients may have a gradual increase in blasts in the blood or bone marrow, an increase in basophils in the blood, or an increase in fibrosis in the marrow. Increasing doses of medications may be required to control the WBC count. Finally, patients may have systemic symptoms (fever, weight loss, night sweats) that are not responsive to therapy and for which another cause cannot be found. The presence of additional cytogenetic abnormalities may be helpful in confirming transformation to an accelerated phase (Table 14–3). The accelerated phase tends to be short; patients either transform to unequivocal blast crisis within a few months or die during the accelerated phase.
- **Blast crisis:** Blast crisis is defined by the presence of **>30% blasts in the blood and/or bone marrow.** In most cases, the blasts have a myeloid phenotype, but **approximately 25 to 30% of cases have a lymphoid phenotype, usually precursor B cell.** Occasional cases express erythroid or megakaryocytic markers. Survival after development of myeloid blast crisis is ≤3 months in most cases. Patients with a lymphoid phenotype may respond to therapy for ALL, but survival is usually only slightly improved (≤4 to 6 months).

Table 14–3
Characteristics of Accelerated Phase of CML

Marked leukocytosis unresponsive to medications

5–30% peripheral blood blasts

Peripheral blood blasts + promyelocytes >30%

Marrow blasts >10% but <30%

Increasing basophilia

Systemic symptoms (fever, night sweats, weight loss) without precipitating cause

Increasing splenomegaly unresponsive to medication

Marked marrow fibrosis

Cytogenetic progression: additional Philadelphia chromosome, trisomy 8, isochromosome 17q

- Occasional patients may first demonstrate transformation to blast crisis in an extramedullary site, as a granulocytic sarcoma. Systemic dissemination usually follows within a few months.
- A small number of cases develop a "burnt out" fibrotic phase resembling end-stage idiopathic myelofibrosis (agnogenic myeloid metaplasia). This may be a short transition period in the development of blast crisis, or patients may die in the fibrotic phase without transforming to acute leukemia.

Treatment

Treatment for CML can be divided into *palliative therapy* (control of the WBC count and other disease manifestations) and *curative therapy*. At present, the only proven curative therapy is allogeneic bone marrow transplant.* Allogeneic bone marrow transplantation has become the treatment of choice for young patients with a histocompatible stem cell donor, in the hope of curing the disease. The results from allogeneic transplant are better if the transplant is performed early in the course of the disease; therefore, *consider the possibility of a bone marrow transplant as soon as the patient is diagnosed* with CML.

- **Conventional cytotoxic chemotherapy:** Hydroxyurea (Hydrea) is the drug of choice to control the WBC count and systemic symptoms. Hydroxyurea has a rapid onset of action and a low incidence of serious

---

*The term bone marrow transplant is used to designate all types of hematopoietic stem cell therapy.

side effects and does not increase the toxicity of bone marrow transplant. The starting dose is approximately 2 g/day, and the dose is subsequently titered to the WBC count.

- Busulfan used to be the most common chemotherapy drug used for CML. It has been replaced by hydroxyurea because the results of bone marrow transplants are worse in patients with previous busulfan therapy.

- **Interferon-α:** Interferon-α has become a standard therapy for patients with chronic-phase CML. It induces a complete hematologic response (normalization of the CBC) in a high proportion of patients (≥70%) and has been shown to decrease the proportion of cells in the marrow that carry the Philadelphia chromosome (cytogenetic response) in many cases. A *major cytogenetic response* (<35% of metaphases showing the Philadelphia chromosome) can be achieved in ~10 to 15% of patients and is associated with prolonged survival. A small proportion of patients achieve a complete cytogenetic response (absence of the Philadelphia chromosome by standard cytogenetics); some of these patients are maintained in complete remission for years and may be cured. Toxicity of interferon-α includes a flu-like syndrome at the start of therapy, arthralgias, myalgias, impotence, weight loss, headache, and fever. Memory loss and depression may occur, particularly in older patients. Autoimmune phenomena, including immune thrombocytopenia or hemolysis, lupus, and hypothyroidism, may occur. Overall, up to 25% of patients discontinue therapy due to toxicity. **Response to interferon-α can be quite slow.** The median time to hematologic response is ~6 to 8 months, and cytogenetic response takes longer (up to 2 years). It has been suggested that patients who respond more quickly have a better prognosis. The mechanism of action of interferon-α is unclear.

- **Allogeneic bone marrow transplant:** Allogeneic bone marrow transplant is the only proven curative therapy in CML and is the treatment of choice in young patients who have a histocompatible donor. The long-term disease-free survival rate in patients who receive a related histocompatible transplant during chronic phase is ~45 to 70%, and young patients transplanted within the first year of diagnosis have a ≥70% long-term survival rate. Relapses occur in up to 20% of patients; infusion of donor leukocytes may induce a second remission, presumably due to a "graft-versus-leukemia" effect. Unrelated transplants have higher transplant-related mortality rates, but ~35 to 45% of patients are relapse free at 2 years from transplant. Allogeneic transplant is associated with acute toxicity, and there is a significant mortality rate. Thus, the patient has to balance the chance of cure for an otherwise uniformly fatal disease against the acute toxicity and chance of early mortality in bone marrow transplant. **If transplant is a possibility, it is better to do it early**. Any delay runs the risk of progression to accelerated phase or blast crisis, and the results of transplant after progression are worse than in first chronic phase. Patients transplanted early in chronic phase appear to do better than patients transplanted after being in chronic phase for several years.

- **Autologous bone marrow transplant:** Several centers have tried autologous bone marrow transplant for CML. Studies have suggested prolonged survival, but most patients eventually relapse.

- **Tyrosine kinase inhibitors:** *Gleevec* (imatinib mesylate; STI571) is an orally administered inhibitor of the *bcr-abl* tyrosine kinase, recently approved by the FDA. The results of initial clinical trials for chronic- and accelerated-phase CML and myeloid blast crisis of CML are promising.

Treatment of Accelerated Phase and Blast Crisis

Treatment of accelerated phase and blast crisis is generally unsatisfactory. Combination chemotherapy as for AML (or ALL for patients with lymphoid blast crisis) is used. Occasional patients achieve a second chronic phase (~25 to 30% of patients in accelerated phase, <20% of patients in blast crisis), but the second chronic phases tend to be short. Allogeneic bone marrow transplant is less successful in accelerated phase or blast crisis than in first chronic phase, with ~35% survival for patients transplanted in accelerated phase and 12% for patients transplanted during blast crisis. The results are slightly better in patients who are transplanted in second chronic phase.

Chronic Neutrophilic Leukemia

Chronic neutrophilic leukemia (CNL) is a rare variant of CML that is characterized by a predominance of mature segmented neutrophils in the blood, without the immature granulocytes and basophils seen in CML. The LAP score is normal or increased rather than decreased; splenomegaly is less prominent. The disease course tends to be indolent, with long survival and a low incidence of transformation to acute leukemia. The Philadelphia chromosome can be present. Recently, it has been shown that the breakpoint in the *bcr* gene in chronic neutrophilic leukemia differs from that in CML or ALL and produces a larger protein (p230). The different BCR-ABL protein may explain the difference in clinical course of CNL.

POLYCYTHEMIA VERA

Pathophysiology

Polycythemia vera (**p. vera**; also known as *polycythemia rubra vera*) is characterized by an **increase in the red cell mass**, measured as increased hemoglobin and hematocrit. Like CML, p. vera is a clonal disorder of hematopoietic stem cells. Early erythroid precursors (BFU-E and CFU-E) are able to grow in culture in the absence of added erythropoietin (*endogenous erythroid colony growth*), suggesting that they are independent of erythropoietin.

The main complications of p. vera are thrombosis and hemorrhage. Patients may develop a "burnt out" stage characterized by bone marrow fibrosis. Occasional patients transform to acute myelogenous leukemia.

Epidemiology

Polycythemia vera is uncommon, with an estimated incidence of 0.5 to 2 per 100,000 population per year. The median age at diagnosis is about 60 years, and there is a slight male predominance. Exposure to ionizing radiation predisposes to p. vera. The incidence is also higher in people who work in petroleum refineries and chemical plants.

Clinical Features

Many patients are found to have an elevated hemoglobin as an incidental finding on screening blood counts. Symptoms of p. vera may be due to *increased blood viscosity, splenomegaly, bleeding,* and *hypermetabolism.*

- **Increased blood viscosity:** The increased red cell mass results in an increase in blood viscosity. Symptoms related to this include headache, dizziness, tinnitus, visual disturbances, syncopal episodes, numbness or tingling in the fingers, blurred vision, dyspnea on exertion, and weakness. Cerebrovascular accidents (strokes) may be a presenting feature.
- **Splenomegaly:** Splenomegaly is present in ~70% of patients and may cause left upper quadrant discomfort and early satiety due to compression of the stomach.
- **Bleeding:** Bleeding is common in patients with p. vera. The most common sites of bleeding are mucous membranes, the skin, and the gastrointestinal tract.
- **Hypermetabolism:** Hyperuricemia is common, and patients may have gouty arthritis or renal stones. Hypermetabolism may also result in systemic symptoms, such as night sweats and weight loss.
- **Other symptoms:** Other symptoms can include weight loss, pruritis, and *erythromelalgia* (reddening, swelling, and pain in the digits). *Pruritus after taking a hot shower* is a classic symptom of p. vera.

Physical Examination

The complexion is ruddy, often with red or dark blotches on the skin. Hypertension is common (~70% of patients). Splenomegaly is present in the majority of patients; moderate hepatomegaly is present in ~40%.

Laboratory

The CBC shows an increase in the hemoglobin, hematocrit, and the red cell count. The hemoglobin may range from ~18 to 24 g/dL; the hematocrit is usually >60% in men and >55% in women. The white cell count is elevated in about half of patients, predominantly due to mature granulocytes. Basophils are often slightly increased. Moderate thrombocytosis is present in ~80% of patients. Erythrocyte morphology on the blood smear is usually unremarkable, except for mild anisocytosis and sometimes microcytosis. Marked anisocytosis, numerous teardrop erythrocytes, or other striking morphologic abnormalities in RBCs suggest another diagnosis. Giant bizarre platelets or megakaryocyte fragments may be present. Serum chemistries show an increase in the uric acid and the LDH. The serum cobalamin (vitamin B_{12}) level may be increased.

Measurement of the red cell mass (dilution studies using the patient's red cells labeled with radioactive chromium) shows a marked increase. The plasma volume is normal or decreased.

- Red cell mass and plasma volume levels may not be needed if the hemoglobin is >18.5 g/dL in men or >16.5 g/dL in women, particularly if there is other evidence for p. vera such as a palpable spleen, thrombocytosis, or leukocytosis.

A useful laboratory test is a *serum erythropoietin level*, using sensitive immunoassays for erythropoietin (EPO). The serum EPO level is decreased in ~60 to 80% of cases of p. vera, whereas it is normal or increased in patients with secondary polycythemia.

Bone Marrow

The bone marrow is hypercellular. There is an increase in all cell lines, with a predominant increase in erythroid precursors, resulting in a decrease in the ratio of myeloid to erythroid cells (M:E ratio). Mild fibrosis is present in ~10 to 15% of cases. A characteristic feature is an **absence of stainable iron in the marrow**.

Cytogenetics

There is no characteristic cytogenetic abnormality in p. vera, and the results of chromosomal analysis are usually normal. The most important role for cytogenetics in polycythemia is to exclude CML.

Differential Diagnosis

Diagnostic criteria for p. vera are presented in Tables 14–4 and 14–5.

Table 14–4
Diagnostic Criteria for Polycythemia Vera

A1: Raised red cell mass: • Male ≥36 mL/kg body weight • Female ≥32 mL/kg	B1: Thrombocytosis (>400,000/μL)
A2: Normal arterial oxygen saturation (≥92%)	B2: Leukocytosis >12 × 10⁹/L without fever or infection
A3: Splenomegaly	B3: Raised LAP score or raised B$_{12}$ level

Diagnosis of p. vera is acceptable if the following combinations are present: A1 + A2 + A3 or A1 + A2 + any two from category B.
LAP = leukocyte alkaline phosphase.
Reproduced with permission from Berlin NI. Diagnosis and classification of polycythemia. Semin Hematol 1975;12:339–51.

The most important differential considerations are *relative erythrocytosis* and *secondary polycythemia*. The other CMPDs, particularly CML, must also be considered.

- **Relative erythrocytosis:** Relative erythrocytosis is excluded by finding a normal red cell mass and a decreased plasma volume. The serum EPO level is normal.
- **Secondary polycythemia:** Secondary polycythemia is an increase in red cell mass due to some other condition, such as chronic lung disease with hypoxemia or right-to-left shunt. Causes of secondary polycythemia were discussed in Chapter 9.
- **Other chronic myeloproliferative disorders:** The most important disorder to consider is CML, and chromosomal analysis should be performed on the marrow. Idiopathic myelofibrosis and primary thrombocythemia can also overlap with p. vera. Marked fibrosis in the marrow and a prominent leukoerythroblastic reaction in the blood would favor idiopathic myelofibrosis, whereas marked thrombocytosis would favor primary thrombocythemia.

Disease Course

Most patients with p. vera have a prolonged course. The median survival is >10 years. Major complications can include the following:

- **Thrombosis:** *Thrombosis is the most frequent cause of death in patients with p. vera* (~30 to 40% of patients). Patients may develop deep venous thromboses in the lower extremities, pulmonary emboli, cerebrovascular accidents (strokes), or coronary artery or peripheral arterial occlusions. Thrombosis at unusual sites may occur, including the splenic vein, hepatic vein (*Budd-Chiari syndrome*), and portal and mesenteric

Table 14–5

Proposed Modified Criteria for the Diagnosis of Polycythemia Vera

A1:	Raised red cell mass (>25% above mean normal predicted value)	B1:	Thrombocytosis (> 400 × 10^9/L)
A2:	Absence of cause of secondary erythrocytosis	B2:	Neutrophilic leukocytosis (neutrophil count >10 × 10^9/L)
A3:	Palpable splenomegaly	B3:	Splenomegaly demonstrated on examination or imaging studies
A4:	Clonality marker or acquired abnormal marrow karyotype	B4:	Characteristic BFU-E growth or reduced serum erythropoietin

A1 + A2 + A3 or A1 + A2 + A4 establishes p. vera
A1 + A2 + two of B criteria establish p. vera
Adapted from Messinezy M, Pearson TC. The classification and diagnostic criteria of the erythrocytoses (polycythaemias). Clin Lab Haematol 1999;21:309–16.

veins. Older patients (particularly >70 years) and those with previous thromboses are at particularly high risk. Control of the hematocrit decreases the thrombotic tendency.

- **Progressive myelofibrosis:** Progression to a "spent" or "burnt out" phase with myelofibrosis, resembling idiopathic myelofibrosis, occurs in ~25% of patients (*post-polycythemic myeloid metaplasia*). This occurs on average ~10 years after diagnosis.

- **Transformation to AML:** The risk of transformation to AML is <5% in patients treated with phlebotomy alone. It is dramatically increased in patients who receive alkylating agent chemotherapy (such as chlorambucil) or radioactive phosphorous. Patients may pass through a fibrotic phase prior to transformation, or transformation may be abrupt.

Treatment

- **Phlebotomy:** *Phlebotomy is the primary treatment for p. vera* and may be the only treatment needed. It controls the hematocrit by inducing a state of iron deficiency. Approximately 250 to 500 mL of blood can be removed every 2 to 3 days (less frequently for older patients and patients with cardiovascular disease) until the hematocrit is ≤42 to 45%. Thereafter, one unit is removed as needed to maintain the hematocrit at that level.

- **Hydroxyurea:** Hydroxyurea is usually the first choice in addition to phlebotomy to control the hematocrit, elevated WBC count, and platelet count in patients who are refractory to phlebotomy alone.

- **Interferon-α:** Interferon-α can be used to control the hematocrit and WBC and platelet counts in patients who are not controlled by phlebotomy with or without hydroxyurea.
- **Low-dose aspirin:** Low-dose aspirin (~50 mg per day) is often given to prevent thromboses. Higher doses are associated with a high risk of hemorrhage and should be avoided.
- **Radioactive phosphorous:** In older patients, radioactive phosphorous (^{32}P) given orally can be very useful to control the hematocrit in older patients who are intolerant of or refractory to phlebotomy. It increases the risk of transformation to AML; however, the risk of AML does not increase for ~5 to 7 years. It is generally avoided in younger patients.
- **Anagrelide:** Anagrelide (Agrylin) selectively decreases the platelet count and may be useful in patients with marked thrombocytosis. It is discussed further in the section on primary thrombocythemia below.

PRIMARY THROMBOCYTHEMIA

Pathophysiology

Primary thrombocythemia (also known as *essential thrombocythemia*) is a clonal hematopoietic stem cell disorder that manifests primarily as a marked increase in the platelet count. The *major clinical consequences* of primary thrombocythemia are *thrombosis and hemorrhage*. Transformation to AML occurs but is rare. The occurrence of thrombosis or hemorrhage appears to be related to qualitative platelet abnormalities since patients with reactive thrombocytosis are not prone to such complications despite having similar platelet counts. The occurrence of thrombosis or hemorrhage does not correlate well with either the platelet count or platelet function abnormalities. However, lowering of the platelet count appears to decrease the incidence of complications.

Epidemiology

The estimated incidence of primary thrombocythemia is ~1 to 2 per 100,000 per year. It occurs predominantly in older people, with an average age at diagnosis of ~50 to 60 years, but there is a significant incidence in young patients (20 to 50 years). There appears to be a higher incidence in women, particularly in the younger group.

Clinical Features

Most patients are asymptomatic at diagnosis, and thrombocytosis is discovered as an incidental finding on a routine CBC. Common clinical symptoms include the following:

- **Microvascular occlusions:** Microvascular occlusions usually invol\
the digits and can cause pain, acrocyanosis, necrosis, and gangrene (
the fingertips or toes. *Erythromelalgia* (redness and burning pain in th\
digits which is relieved by aspirin) is a common symptom.
- **Large vessel thromboses:** Large vessel thromboses usually involve th\
arteries to the lower extremities but can involve the coronary, rena\
mesenteric, subclavian, or carotid arteries. Thrombosis of the hepati\
veins (Budd-Chiari syndrome), splenic veins, and veins of the lowe\
extremities may occur.
- **Bleeding:** Gastrointestinal bleeding is common. Other sites of bleedin\
include the urinary tract, skin, eyes, gums, joints, and brain. *Most bleed\
ing episodes are minor; major hemorrhage is unusual.*
- **Neurologic events:** Headaches, paresthesias, transient ischemic attacks\
visual disturbances, and seizures can occur.

Physical Examination

The physical examination in primary thrombocythemia is generally unre\
markable. There may be discoloration or gangrene of the toes or fingertips\
Mild splenomegaly may be present; marked splenomegaly suggests anothe\
disease.

Laboratory

By definition, the platelet count is >600,000/μL, and is >1,000,000/μL in\
the majority of patients. The hemoglobin is usually normal, but mild ane\
mia is not uncommon. Mild leukocytosis (<20,000/μL) is often present.\
The leukocyte differential shows a mild left shift, and mild eosinophilia and\
basophilia are often present. **Giant platelets, other bizarre platelet shapes,**\
and **megakaryocyte nuclear fragments** are often present on the blood\
smear (Figure 14–2). There should not be numerous nucleated RBCs,\
teardrop RBCs, or immature granulocyte precursors.

Serum chemistries may show a mild increase in LDH and uric acid.

Bone Marrow

The bone marrow is hypercellular, with a marked increase in megakary\
ocytes. **Clustering of megakaryocytes is characteristic** (Figure 14–3). There\
is often granulocytic and erythroid hyperplasia. Mild fibrosis may be pres\
ent, but marked fibrosis (>one-third the biopsy area) *must* be absent. Stain\
able iron must be present for a diagnosis of primary thrombocythemia.

Cytogenetics

Cytogenetic abnormalities are found in less than 25% of patients, and no\
characteristic abnormality has been described. The Philadelphia chromo-

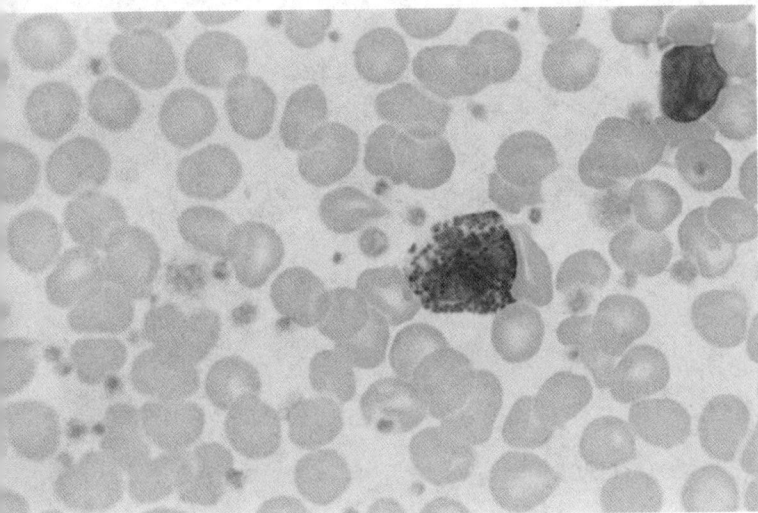

Figure 14–2 Primary thrombocythemia blood smear. Platelets are markedly increased; a basophils is present in the center. The cell in the top right is a megakaryocyte nuclear fragment.

some must be absent. The diagnostic criteria for primary thrombocythemia are summarized in Table 14–6.

Differential Diagnosis

The most important differential diagnostic considerations are reactive thrombocytosis, CML, and idiopathic myelofibrosis.

- **Reactive thrombocytosis:** The distinction between reactive thrombocytosis and primary thrombocythemia is discussed in Chapter 11. Features that favor primary thrombocythemia include numerous giant or bizarre platelets on blood smear, marked clustering of megakaryocytes in the bone marrow, and thrombosis or hemorrhage without an apparent cause.
- **Chronic myelogenous leukemia:** The WBC count is usually higher and the platelet count lower in CML than primary thrombocythemia, but there is overlap. The presence of a low LAP score and significant splenomegaly would favor CML. The presence of a Philadelphia chromosome or *bcr/abl* rearrangement would make a definitive diagnosis of CML.
- **Idiopathic myelofibrosis (*agnogenic myeloid metaplasia*):** Idiopathic myelofibrosis can usually be distinguished from primary thrombocythemia by a marked leukoerythroblastic reaction in the blood, marked splenomegaly, and the presence of marked fibrosis in the marrow (≥one-third the area of the biopsy).

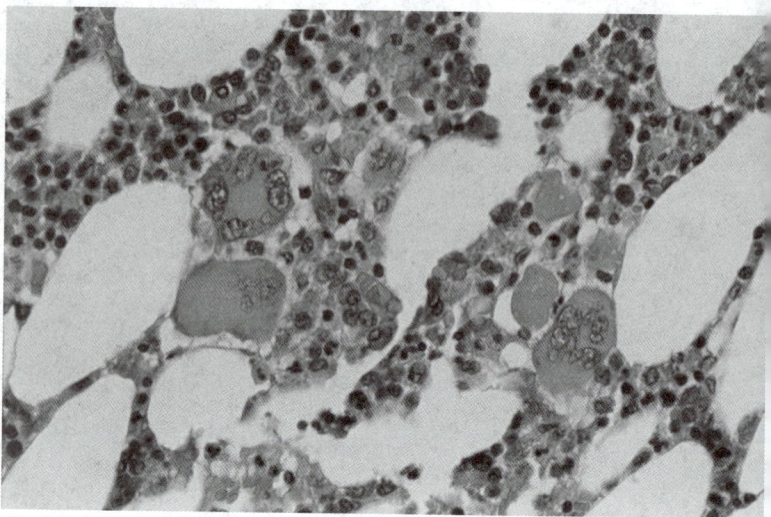

Figure 14–3 Primary thrombocythemia bone marrow biopsy. A cluster of megakaryocytes is present.

Disease Course

Primary thrombocythemia is generally associated with the longest survival of any of the chronic myeloproliferative disorders. Progression to end-stage myelofibrosis or transformation to acute leukemia occur, but both are rare (<5% of patients). The major threat to life is thromboembolic events. The primary risk factors for thrombosis and hemorrhage are older age (>60 years) and a previous history of thrombosis.

Table 14–6
Diagnostic Criteria for Primary Thrombocythemia

Platelet count >600,000/μL

Normal red cell mass

Stainable iron in marrow or failure of iron trial (<1 g/dL increase in hemoglobin after 1 month of iron therapy)

No Philadelphia chromosome [t(9;22)] or *bcr/abl* rearrangement

Marrow fibrosis absent or < one-third biopsy area

No known cause for reactive thrombocytosis

Treatment

Asymptomatic patients may not require treatment. Symptomatic patients and those at high risk of thrombosis require therapy. Several agents can be used:

- **Low-dose aspirin:** Low doses of aspirin (75 to 100 mg/day) help control vasomotor symptoms and decrease the risk of thrombosis. Antiplatelet agents should be used with caution in patients with hemorrhagic manifestations.
- **Hydroxyurea:** Hydroxyurea lowers the platelet count within 2 to 6 weeks. The main side effect is leukopenia, which is reversible upon discontinuing or lowering the dose of hydroxyurea.
- **Anagrelide:** Anagrelide (Agrylin) selectively lowers the platelet count, probably by interfering with megakaryocyte maturation. The starting dose is 0.5 mg three to four times daily by mouth; after 1 week, the dose is adjusted to maintain a platelet count <600,000/μL. It is generally well tolerated, and most side effects are mild and decrease with time. Major side effects are due to vasodilation, including headache, tachycardia, cardiac arrhythmias, angina, fluid retention, and dizziness. Myocardial infarcts and congestive heart failure have been reported. Other complications may include diarrhea, abdominal pain, nausea and vomiting, and skin rashes. It is contraindicated during pregnancy.
- **Plateletpheresis:** Plateletpheresis rapidly lowers the platelet count and is useful in patients with extreme thrombocytosis and acute complications. The effect is transient; therefore, it must be used in combination with other measures.
- **Interferon-α:** Interferon-α can be used in high-risk women of childbearing age. The initial dose is 3 to 5 million units subcutaneously, three to five times weekly, adjusted to keep the platelet count at the desired level.

IDIOPATHIC MYELOFIBROSIS (AGNOGENIC MYELOID METAPLASIA)

Pathophysiology

Idiopathic myelofibrosis (**IM**; also known as *agnogenic myeloid metaplasia* [**AMM**] and *myelofibrosis with myeloid metaplasia* [**MMM**]) is characterized by a **leukoerythroblastic reaction in the blood** (nucleated RBCs and immature granulocytes), **splenomegaly**, and **fibrosis in the marrow** (Table 14–7).

Like the other chronic myeloproliferative diseases, IM is a clonal disease of hematopoietic stem cells. The excess collagen in the marrow is produced by marrow fibroblasts, which are polyclonal and not part of the neoplastic

Table 14–7
Characteristics of Idiopathic Myelofibrosis

Leukoerythroblastic reaction: nucleated RBCs and immature granulocytes in blood

Extramedullary hematopoiesis, predominantly in the spleen

Splenomegaly, often marked

Marrow fibrosis

clone. They are driven to produce the excess collagen by megakaryocyte and monocytes, which do belong to the malignant clone. The cytokines that are involved include *transforming growth factor-β* (**TGF-β**), *platelet derived growth factor* (**PDGF**), and others. There is extramedullary hematopoiesis in the spleen, causing splenomegaly.

Epidemiology

Idiopathic myelofibrosis is an uncommon disease; the estimated incidence is ~0.5 to 1.5 per 100,000 per year. It predominantly occurs in older individuals, with a median age of ~65 years at diagnosis, but there is a wide age range. Idiopathic myelofibrosis has been linked to exposure to benzene and other hydrocarbons and also to ionizing radiation.

Some authors designate myelofibrosis developing out of another chronic myeloproliferative disease (p. vera or primary thrombocythemia) as *secondary myelofibrosis* and would then designate IM as *primary myelofibrosis*. Approximately 10% of cases of myelofibrosis develop out of a preceding myeloproliferative disorder.

Clinical Features

Symptoms may include fatigue, cachexia, weight loss, low-grade fever, and night sweats. Marked splenomegaly may cause early satiety, left upper quadrant pain, and diarrhea. Up to 25% of patients are asymptomatic at diagnosis and are diagnosed as a result of a routine CBC or detection of splenomegaly on a routine physical.

Physical Examination

Splenomegaly is the most striking finding of examination; the spleen is firm and may extend across the midline and down to the pelvic brim. Hepatomegaly is present in approximately half of patients but tends to be less striking. Petechiae, purpura, and signs of portal hypertension may be present.

aboratory

nemia is present in most patients at diagnosis. The WBC count is creased in about half of patients due to granulocytosis but may be ecreased. Eosinophilia and basophilia may be present. The platelet count increased in half of patients at diagnosis.

The most striking laboratory findings appear on the blood smear, which lows numerous teardrop RBCs, nucleated erythrocytes, immature granu-cyte precursors, and giant platelets (Figure 14–4).

Serum levels of uric acid, LDH, alkaline phosphatase, and vitamin B_{12} e often increased.

one Marrow

he bone marrow usually cannot be aspirated ("dry tap"). The biopsy can ary in appearance from hypercellular with relatively inapparent fibrosis to ear-total replacement by collagen to osteosclerosis with replacement of the marrow space by bone (Figure 14–5). Megakaryocytes are typically icreased in number and morphologically abnormal. A characteristic fea-are is groups of immature hematopoietic cells within dilated marrow nuses.

The initial type of collagen produced is **reticulin**, which is demon-rated by a silver (reticulin) stain. Later, mature collagen may be present nd is detected by the trichrome stain. Cases with only subtle fibrosis, which

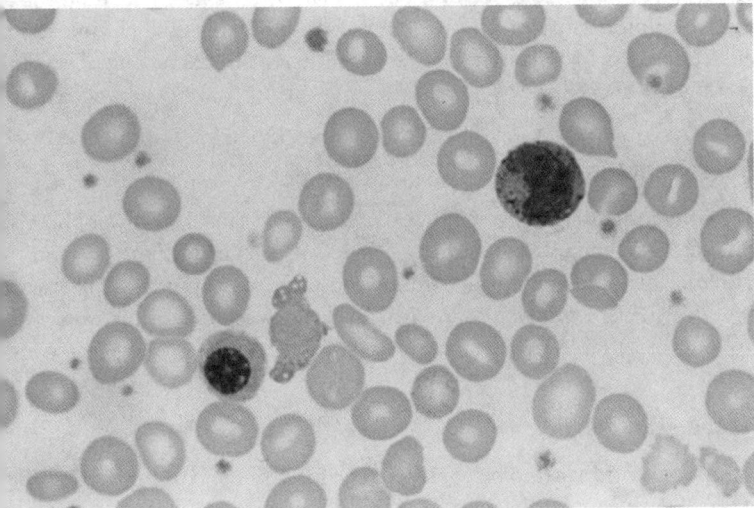

igure 14–4 Idiopathic myelofibrosis blood smear. Nucleated erythrocyte, bizarre latelet, and basophil are seen.

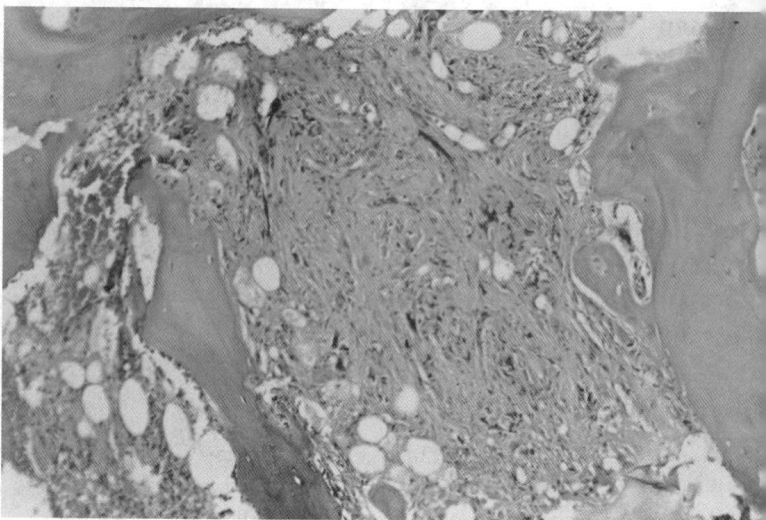

Figure 14–5 Idiopathic myelofibrosis bone marrow biopsy (hematoxylin and eosin stain). The solid pink area represents dense fibrosis.

are likely to be missed unless a reticulin stain is done, have been designated the "cellular phase" of IM.

Cytogenetics

Cytogenetic results are abnormal in about half of patients. There is no characteristic abnormality in IM. By definition, the Philadelphia chromosome must be absent. Molecular tests may be useful in excluding a *bcr/abl* rearrangement.

Differential Diagnosis

The differential diagnosis of IM includes benign causes of myelofibrosis, hairy cell leukemia, CML and the other CMPDs (including "post-polycythemic myeloid metaplasia" following p. vera), acute leukemia with myelofibrosis, myelodysplasia with myelofibrosis, and other causes of myelofibrosis (Table 14–8).

Disease Course

The course in IM used to be considered grim, with median survival of 3 to 5 years. Recently, it has been recognized that younger patients and patients without anemia may have a more indolent course. The median survival of

Table 14–8
Causes of Bone Marrow Fibrosis

Neoplastic Causes	Non-neoplastic Causes
Chronic myeloproliferative disorders: • Idiopathic myelofibrosis (IM) • Chronic myelogenous leukemia (CML) • Polycythemia vera (p. vera)	Granulomatous diseases: • Mycobacterial infections • Fungal infections • Sarcoidosis
Acute megakaryoblastic leukemia (FAB-M7)	Paget's disease of bone
Myelodysplasia with myelofibrosis	Hypoparathyroidism
Hairy cell leukemia	Hyperparathyroidism
Acute lymphoblastic leukemia	Renal osteodystrophy
Multiple myeloma	Osteoporosis
Metastatic carcinoma	Vitamin D deficiency
Systemic mastocytosis	Autoimmune diseases: • Systemic lupus erythematosus (SLE) • Systemic sclerosis

Adapted from Lee RG, Foerster J, Lukons J, et al, editors. Wintrobes's clinical hematology, 10th ed. Baltimore: Williams & Wilkins, 1999. p. 2391.

patients ≤55 years may exceed 10 years, and younger patients without anemia may survive up to 15 years. The major causes of death are **hemorrhage**, **infection**, **heart failure**, and **leukemic transformation**. Leukemic transformation occurs in up to 20% of patients within the first 10 years. The marked splenomegaly may cause portal hypertension, and patients may develop hematemesis from gastroesophageal varices.

An unusual complication of IM is the development of extramedullary hematopoietic foci. These may occur in lymph nodes, skin, the pleural or peritoneal cavities, the central nervous system, and other organs. Complications can include compression of the spinal cord or other nerves and pleural or peritoneal effusions.

Treatment

Treatment for IM is largely palliative. The only possible curative therapy is bone marrow transplantation; however, most patients are too old at diagnosis to consider BMT. Treatment options include the following:

• **Transfusions:** Red cell transfusions are used for symptomatic anemia.
• **Corticosteroids and androgens:** Corticosteroids and androgens (nandrolone or oxymetholone) may improve anemia. Corticosteroids can

decrease hemolysis if present; androgens stimulate erythropoiesis. Only a minority of patients respond, and responses tend to be partial and temporary.

- **Hydroxyurea:** Hydroxyurea is considered the drug of choice to control leukocytosis and thrombocytosis in IM; it may also decrease the spleen size.
- **Splenectomy:** Splenectomy is indicated to decompress the portal vein in patients with portal hypertension. Splenectomy also decreases abdominal discomfort due to massive splenomegaly and may increase cell counts by eliminating splenic sequestration. Unfortunately, there are significant operative mortality and morbidity rates (~9% and 38% respectively).
- **Splenic irradiation:** Splenic irradiation can be used as an alternative to splenectomy in patients who are poor candidates for operation. The effect is often temporary, and some patients may develop pancytopenia.
- **Interferon-α:** Interferon-α has been used, with occasional benefit.
- **Bone marrow transplantation:** Allogeneic bone marrow transplant has been used in some younger patients, with hematologic response in up to 70% of patients and regression of fibrosis in up to 40%. It is usually reserved for younger patients with poor prognostic factors.

THE MYELODYSPLASTIC/MYELOPROLIFERATIVE DISORDERS

The category of myelodysplastic/myeloproliferative disorders (MDS/MPDs) was created in the new WHO classification system to include cases with *both* proliferative *and* myelodysplastic features. The three diseases included in this category are **atypical** (*Philadelphia chromosome–negative*) **chronic myelogenous leukemia (aCML)**, **juvenile myelomonocytic leukemia (JMML)**, and **chronic myelomonocytic leukemia (CMML)**. These are all rare and will be discussed only briefly.

Atypical Chronic Myelogenous Leukemia

Approximately 5% of cases that are initially considered CML lack both the Philadelphia chromosome and *bcr/abl* rearrangement and are then designated aCML. The blood smear shows leukocytosis consisting predominantly of segmented neutrophils, without the metamyelocytes, myelocytes, and basophils characteristic of Philadelphia chromosome–positive CML. Monocytosis and dysplastic changes are more prominent than in typical CML. Anemia and thrombocytopenia are more common, and splenomegaly is less prominent. It occurs in an older population (median age in the sixties), with a slight male predominance. Overall survival tends to be worse than typical CML, with a median survival slightly over 1 year (Table 14–9).

Table 14–9

Characteristics of Atypical Chronic Myelogenous Leukemia

Median age: 60s

Slight male predominance

Monocytosis: 3–10% of WBC

Dysplastic changes

No basophilia

Anemia and thrombocytopenia common

Splenomegaly mild or absent

No Philadelphia chromosome or *bcr/abl* rearrangement

Short survival

Juvenile Myelomonocytic Leukemia

Juvenile myelomonocytic leukemia (previously called juvenile CML and juvenile CMML) is a rare condition usually occurring in children below the age of 4 years (40% occur within the first year and 60% within the first 2 years). There is a slight male predominance. Clinical signs include fever, bleeding, hepatosplenomegaly, lymphadenopathy, and skin involvement. The WBC count is usually ~20,000 to 30,000/μL; monocytosis is frequent (often >5,000/μL); blasts are usually <3%. Anemia and thrombocytopenia are common. A characteristic finding is an *increase in the fetal hemoglobin* (Hb F) *level in erythrocytes* (Table 14–10). The clinical course is variable with about one-third having a relatively indolent course, one-third having an aggressive course, and the remainder having an intermediate course. Children below 1 year of age at diagnosis tend to have longer survival. Allogeneic bone marrow transplant is considered the treatment of choice for patients with aggressive disease.

Table 14–10

Characteristics of Juvenile Myelomonocytic Leukemia

Age below 4 years

Slight male predominance

Fever

Hepatosplenomegaly and lymphadenopathy

Skin rashes

Leukocytosis 20,000–30,000/μL with monocytosis >1,000/μL

Anemia and thrombocytopenia

Fetal erythropoiesis: increased Hb F, decreased Hb A_2

Associated with neurofibromatosis type 1

Table 14–11
Characteristics of Chronic Myelomonocytic Leukemia

Older age group (median ~60–70 years)

Males > females

Monocytosis >1,000/μL in blood; >5% monocytes in bone marrow

Myelodysplastic changes

Variable WBC count: decreased to increased

Hepatosplenomegaly in ~25%

Variable clinical course

Transformation to AML in ~15%

Chronic Myelomonocytic Leukemia

Chronic myelomonocytic leukemia is classified as a myelodysplastic syndrome in the FAB classification of myelodysplasias. It occurs predominantly in older individuals (median age 60 to 70 years), with a male predominance. Required features include monocytosis (>1,000/μL) in the blood, increased monocytes in the bone marrow (>5%), and dysplastic changes. Chronic myelomonocytic leukemia is heterogeneous. Some cases are characterized by a low or normal neutrophil count, multilineage marrow dysplasia, no organomegaly, and blood and marrow monocytosis (*myelodysplastic picture*). Other cases have neutrophilia, monocytosis, and splenomegaly (*myeloproliferative picture*). Survival is variable; some patients have an indolent course with prolonged survival, whereas others have a more aggressive course with survival of only a few months. About 15% of patients transform to AML and others die of bone marrow failure (Table 14–11). No therapy has been shown to have substantial benefit.

Additional Readings

Aricò M, Biondi A, Pui H-H. Juvenile myelomonocytic leukemia. Blood 1997; 90:479–88.
Barosi G. Myelofibrosis with myeloid metaplasia: diagnostic definition and prognostic classification for clinical studies and treatment guidelines. J Clin Oncol 1999;17:2954–70.
Sawyers CL. Chronic myeloid leukemia. N Engl J Med 1999;340:1330–40.
Tefferi A. Myelofibrosis with myeloid metaplasia. N Engl J Med 2000;342: 1255–65.
Tefferi A, Solberg LA, Silverstein MN. A clinical update in polycythemia vera and essential thrombocythemia. Am J Med 2000;109:141–9.

15

The Myelodysplastic Syndromes

The myelodysplastic syndromes (MDS) are a heterogeneous group of diseases with highly variable clinical and morphologic features. Like the acute leukemias and the chronic myeloproliferative disorders, they are clonal proliferations of hematopoietic stem cells. Unlike the acute leukemias, there is at least partial preservation of maturation and differentiation; however, in the myelodysplastic syndromes, these are disordered and inefficient. Many cells die in the marrow (*ineffective hematopoiesis*). Thus, the myelodysplastic syndromes are characterized by cytopenias, abnormal morphologic appearances, and sometimes impaired function of the cells that are produced (Table 15–1).

⇨ In summary, the myelodysplastic syndromes are characterized by a *decreased number* of *morphologically abnormal cells* that often *do not function properly.*

Table 15–1
Characteristics of the Myelodysplastic Syndromes

Predominantly older age group

More common in men than women

Decreased blood cell counts

Abnormal cellular appearance (dysplasia)

Defective cell function

Transformation into AML (~25% of patients)

Majority of patients die of bone marrow failure

Patients with myelodysplasia may transform into acute myeloid leukemia (AML), and therefore the myelodysplastic syndromes have also been called *preleukemias* and *smoldering acute leukemias*. However, only a minority of patients with MDS transform into AML (~25% overall), and some subtypes have a very low incidence of leukemic transformation. The majority of patients with MDS die of bone marrow failure.

The myelodysplastic syndromes vary in behavior from indolent diseases with fairly long survival to aggressive diseases with survival of only months. At the aggressive end, the myelodysplastic syndromes form a morphologic and clinical continuum with AML. Distinction between MDS and AML is sometimes arbitrary and can be difficult.

⇨ **Myelodysplastic changes are *not* specific for the myelodysplastic syndromes**. Similar morphologic changes can be seen in a wide variety of conditions, some of which are reversible. *The term myelodysplastic syndromes should be restricted to cases that are idiopathic and/or not due to a reversible cause.*

CLASSIFICATION OF THE MYELODYSPLASTIC SYNDROMES

The standard classification of MDS has been the **French-American-British** (**FAB**) **classification**, which designates five subtypes of MDS (Table 15–2). Classification in the FAB system is based predominantly on the number of myeloblasts in the blood and bone marrow. The FAB system has some abil-

Table 15–2
FAB Classification of the Myelodysplastic Syndromes

Subtype	Features
Refractory anemia (RA)	Dysplastic changes in blood and bone marrow <1% myeloblasts in blood <5% myeloblasts in marrow
Refractory anemia with ringed sideroblasts (RARS)	>15% of nucleated erythroid precursors are pathologic ringed sideroblasts <1% myeloblasts in blood <5% myeloblasts in marrow
Refractory anemia with excess blasts (RAEB)	1–5% myeloblasts in blood 5–20% myeloblasts in marrow
Refractory anemia with excess blasts in transformation (RAEB-t)	20–30% myeloblasts in marrow *or* Auer rods present
Chronic myelomonocytic leukemia (CMML)	>1,000 monocytes/µL in blood Monocytosis in marrow

ity to predict survival and probability of leukemic transformation; however, it does not take critical prognostic factors into account, such as cytogenetic alterations or a history of previous therapy for malignant disease, and its prognostic ability is therefore limited. The new World Health Organization (**WHO**) classification of hematopoietic and lymphoid neoplasms includes a new classification system for myelodysplasias (Table 15–3), which will probably replace the FAB classification in the future.

The primary differences between the two systems are as follows:

- **Refractory anemia (RA)** and **refractory anemia with ringed sideroblasts (RARS)**, in the WHO system, are limited to cases with *dysplastic changes restricted to the erythroid series* (ie, not present in granulocytes or megakaryocytes). These patients generally have long survival, with low risk of leukemic transformation. R**efractory anemia with ringed sideroblasts** is diagnosed when >15% of nucleated erythroid precursors in the marrow are ringed sideroblasts on iron stain.
- The category **refractory cytopenia with multilineage dysplasia (RCMD)** was created in the WHO system to contain cases with <5% myeloblasts in the marrow but with dysplastic changes in two or more cell lines. These patients have shorter survival than patients with dys-

Table 15–3

WHO Classification of the Myelodysplastic Syndromes

Subtype	Features
Refractory anemia (RA)	Dysplastic changes in erythroid series only <5% myeloblasts in marrow
Refractory anemia with ringed sideroblasts (RARS)	Dysplastic changes in erythroid series only >15% of nucleated erythroid precursors are ringed sideroblasts <5% myeloblasts in marrow
Refractory cytopenia with multilineage dysplasia (RCMD)	Dysplasia in two or more cell lines <5% myeloblasts in marrow
Refractory anemia with excess blasts (RAEB): • Subtypes RAEB-1 and RAEB-2	RAEB-1: 5–10% myeloblasts in marrow RAEB-2: 10–20% myeloblasts in marrow *or* Auer rods present
5q-syndrome	Refractory macrocytic anemia Normal or increased platelet count Monolobated megakaryocytes in marrow Deletion of long arm of chromosome 5 (5q-) No other cytogenetic abnormalities
Myelodysplasia, not further classified	Cases that do not fit into the other defined categories

plastic changes restricted to the erythroid line. Ringed sideroblasts may be present.

- **Refractory anemia with excess blasts** (**RAEB**) is subdivided into two categories in the WHO system: **RAEB-1** and **RAEB-2**, depending on the myeloblast count and the presence or absence of Auer rods. There is usually dysplasia in multiple cell lines. Patients with RAEB tend to have shorter survival than patients with RA, RARS, or RCMD.

- The FAB category **refractory anemia with excess blasts in transformation** (**RAEB-t**) is eliminated in the WHO system. Cases that fit this category in the FAB system are now classified as AML. **The threshold marrow myeloblast count for the diagnosis of AML is reduced from 30 to 20%.**

- Myelodysplasia arising in patients who previously received chemotherapy for a malignant disease is now classified with the acute myeloid leukemias. This group was sometimes designated *therapy-related myelodysplasia* (t-MDS). These patients usually progress to overt AML over a relatively short time and have poor survival.

- Patients with one of the characteristic recurring translocations in AML [t(8;21), t(15;17) or inversion (16)] are classified as AML, even if the blast count is low. Previously, these patients were often classified as MDS if the blast count was <30%.

- The category **5q- syndrome** was created in the WHO system. This category recognizes a subset of patients with a deletion of the long arm of chromosome 5 (5q-) and relatively long survival.

- The category **chronic myelomonocytic leukemia** (**CMML**) was moved to a new disease category: the **myelodysplastic/myeloproliferative syndromes** (discussed in Chapter 14).

- The category **myelodysplastic syndrome, unclassifiable** was created to include cases of myelodysplasia that do not fit into any of the defined categories.

EPIDEMIOLOGY

Myelodysplasia appears to be about twice as common as AML, and the incidence appears to be increasing. The myelodysplastic syndromes are predominantly diseases of older adults, with a median age of ~65 years at diagnosis. Myelodysplasia does occur in younger individuals, including rare cases in childhood. However, *the diagnosis of myelodysplasia should always be questioned in a younger patient* (below ~50 years) *and reversible causes aggressively excluded.*

Most series show a higher incidence in men than women.

The cause of most cases of myelodysplasia is unknown. Exposure to mutagenic agents appears to increase the risk of myelodysplasia, such as onizing radiation and alkylating agent chemotherapy. Exposure to benzene, other organic solvents, petrochemicals, and insecticides has also been linked to myelodysplasia.

CLINICAL FEATURES

At present, about half the cases are detected as incidental findings on routine blood counts. Symptoms are usually related to cytopenias; fatigue due to anemia is the most common symptom. Approximately 30% of patients have a history of multiple infections. Despite the relatively high incidence of thrombocytopenia, bleeding is not a common major complaint (<10% of patients).

The physical examination in MDS is generally unremarkable. Patients may have evidence of infection, petechiae, purpura, or other signs of bleeding. Mild splenomegaly may be present, but marked splenomegaly suggests a chronic myeloproliferative disorder or some other disease rather than MDS.

LABORATORY

The diagnosis of MDS depends on finding both *quantitative* and *qualitative* abnormalities in blood and bone marrow cells. Nearly all patients with MDS are anemic; the mean corpuscular volume is normal or slightly increased. Leukopenia is present in ~50 to 60% of patients at diagnosis, and thrombocytopenia is present in ~40 to 60%. Up to half of patients are pancytopenic. Rare patients may have isolated decreases in the WBC count or platelet count as the initial manifestation of MDS.

The blood smear often shows macrocytosis, ovalocytosis, and anisocytosis of erythrocytes. Neutrophils may be hypogranular or have abnormal nuclear segmentation. A common appearance of neutrophils is the pseudo-Pelger-Huët anomaly: bilobed nuclei resembling "pince-nez" eyeglasses with abnormally condensed nuclear chromatin (Figure 15–1). Giant and hypogranular platelets may be present.

Neutrophils may show decreased myeloperoxidase activity or may show aberrant staining for both myeloperoxidase and α-naphthyl-butyrate (monocytic) esterase.

BONE MARROW

The bone marrow is usually hypercellular. Erythroid precursors are often enlarged and show delayed nuclear maturation relative to the cytoplasm (megaloblastoid change). Nuclei may appear bi- or multilobated or have budding; they may appear karyorrhexic; multinucleated cells may be present (Figure 15–2). The cytoplasm may appear vacuolated or have irregular

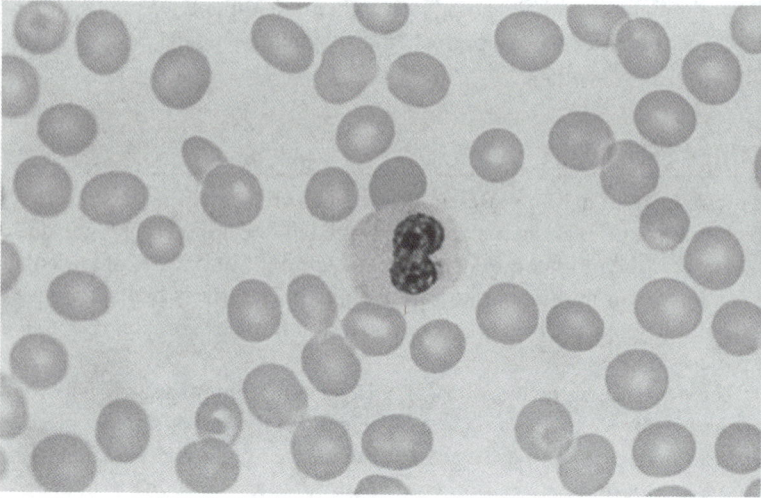

Figure 15–1 Myelodysplasia blood smear. Pseudo-Pelger-Huët phenomenon (hyposeg-mented neutrophil). The neutrophil is also hypogranular. Platelets are greatly decreased.

hemoglobinization. Granulocyte precursors may have nuclear-cytoplasmic asynchrony or hypogranularity (Figure 15–3). Giant metamyelocytes and bands may be present. Myeloblasts may be increased. Megakaryocytes may be small, multinucleated, or have hypolobated or hyperlobated nuclei.

Ringed sideroblasts are nucleated erythroid precursors containing ≥5 granules adjacent to the nucleus and covering ≥one-third the diameter of the nucleus on Prussian blue (iron) stain. **Refractory anemia with ringed sideroblasts is defined by >15% of nucleated erythroid precursors being ringed sideroblasts.** However, if there are dysplastic changes in two or more cell lines, the proper diagnosis is RCMD. If ≥5% of cells are myeloblasts, the proper diagnosis is RAEB.

The bone marrow biopsy may show disarray of the normal architecture, with cells present in abnormal locations. For example, megakaryocytes or erythroid precursors may be located next to bone trabecula (they are nor-mally located *away* from bone). Clusters of immature myeloid precursors located away from bone trabecula, designated *abnormal localization of imma-ture precursors* (**ALIP**), have been considered an adverse prognostic indicator in MDS. Mild fibrosis may be present, but marked fibrosis is uncommon.

CYTOGENETICS

Cytogenetic analysis has become a crucial part of diagnosis and prognosis in myelodysplasia. Clonal cytogenetic abnormalities are found in ~30 to 50%

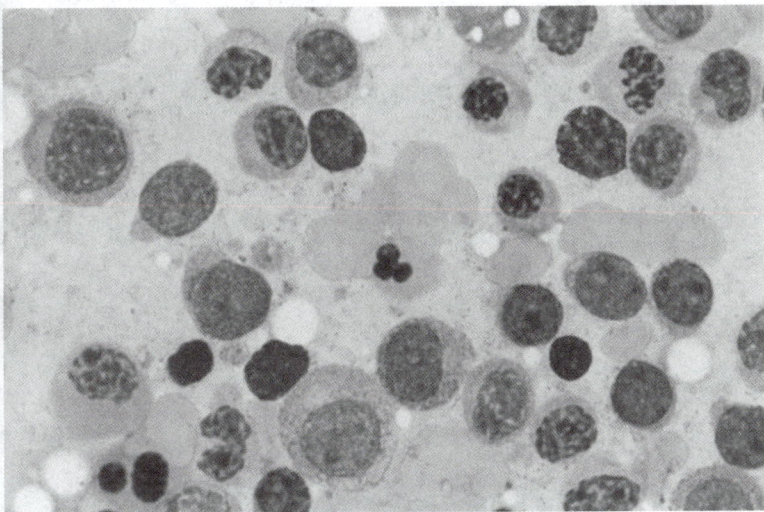

Figure 15–2 Myelodysplasia bone marrow aspirate. Abnormal erythroid precursor with multilobated nucleus.

of cases in de novo MDS and in >80% of cases of therapy-related MDS. The most common abnormalities are partial or complete chromosome deletions. The most frequently involved chromosomes are 5, 7, 8, 20, X, and Y. Balanced reciprocal translocations, as seen in AML, are rare in MDS. The presence of cytogenetic abnormalities and the specific abnormalities present are critical prognostic factors in MDS (Table 15–4).

DIFFERENTIAL DIAGNOSIS

Myelodysplasia is a diagnosis of exclusion (Table 15–5). Cytopenias with myelodysplastic changes can be seen in a variety of conditions, some of which

Table 15–4
Cytogenetic Abnormalities in Myelodysplastic Syndromes

Favorable Prognosis	Unfavorable Prognosis	Intermediate Prognosis
Normal	Complex abnormalities involving ≥3 chromosomes	All others
-Y		
5q- (sole abnormality)	Abnormalities of chromosome 7	
20q- (sole abnormality)		

-Y = deletion of Y chromosome.
5q- = deletion of long arm of chromosome 5.

Table 15–5
Differential Diagnosis of Myelodysplastic Syndromes

Nutritional deficiency: cobalamin, folate, copper, severe cachexia

Alcohol abuse

Zinc excess (causes copper malabsorption)

Myelosuppressive drugs or medications: immunosuppressive medications such as methotrexate or azathioprine; chloramphenicol; anti-HIV medications

Occupational or hobby exposure to toxic chemicals: benzene, organic solvents, pesticides, fertilizers

HIV infection

Other infections: parvovirus B19

Acute myeloid leukemia

Chronic myeloproliferative disorders

Aplastic anemia

are reversible. *It is critical to exclude these reversible causes before giving a patient the diagnosis of myelodysplasia or starting treatment for MDS.* A summary of the evaluation for possible myelodysplasia is given in Table 15–6.

- **Nutritional deficiency** can mimic MDS, including deficiencies of folate, cobalamin (vitamin B_{12}) and copper. Chronic alcoholism can also mimic MDS.

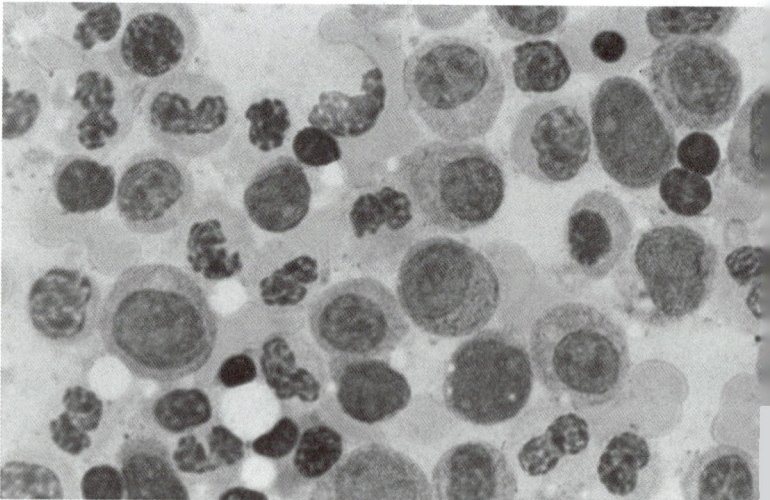

Figure 15–3 Myelodysplasia bone marrow aspirate. Hypogranular hyposegmented neutrophils.

Table 15–6
Evaluation of Possible Myelodysplasia

Past medical history, particularly treatment for malignancy

Occupational and hobby history: chemical or radiation exposure

Review medications, current and previous, including over-the-counter medications and dietary supplements

Careful review of blood smear

Cobalamin, folate, and ferritin or iron/iron-binding capacity levels

HIV serologies (if any risk factors for HIV)

Bone marrow examination

Cytogenetic analysis of bone marrow

Immunophenotyping by flow cytometry*

*In general, immunophenotyping by flow cytometry has limited usefulness in the diagnosis of MDS. Some flow cytometry laboratories use altered expression of myeloid antigens, or aberrant expression of antigens associated with other cell lines, as indicating myelodysplasia. This requires a lot of experience and is not available at most hospitals.

- **Cobalamin**, **folate,** and **ferritin or iron/iron-binding capacity** levels should be checked.
- **Medications:** A complete **drug history**, including previous as well as current medications, must be taken, including "over-the-counter" medications and dietary supplements.
- *Stop all nonessential medications* and *substitute less myelosuppressive ones* for any essential medications that may be myelosuppressive.
- **Current and past medical illnesses** must be considered. Of particular interest would be any history of blood diseases or treatment for malignancy.
- **Family history of hematologic diseases:** A family history of blood disease would favor an inherited blood disorder, such as an inherited sideroblastic anemia or a congenital dyserythropoietic anemia.
- **Chemical, toxin, or radiation exposure:** A complete **occupational history**, with particular attention to chemical and radiation exposure, is required. Hobbies and other activities should also be questioned.
- **Human immunodeficiency virus:** HIV can cause striking dysplastic changes in the marrow. Human immunodeficiency virus serologies should be checked in any young person with a possible diagnosis of myelodysplasia or anyone with risk factors for HIV infection in whom the diagnosis of myelodysplasia is being considered.
- **Parvovirus B19:** Parvovirus B19 is usually associated with aplastic crises in patients with hemolytic anemia, such as sickle cell disease. However, it can cause a chronic red cell aplasia (and occasionally

cytopenia of other cell lines) in immunosuppressed patients. It is associated with giant proerythroblasts on bone marrow aspirate and intranuclear inclusions on the biopsy.

- **Acute myeloid leukemia:** The distinction between AML and MDS depends primarily on the number of myeloblasts in the marrow: <20% = MDS, ≥20% = AML (<30% or ≥30% in the FAB system). The distinction is arbitrary and can be difficult: for example, it is not clear that a patient with 19% myeloblasts has a different disease than a patient with 21% myeloblasts. For treatment purposes, it probably does not matter much in such cases. Sometimes it is a good idea to observe the patient for a little while to see if the disease declares itself; AML will usually become more obvious with time.

- **Erythroleukemia:** Distinction between erythroleukemia (M6 in the FAB classification) and MDS can be particularly difficult. In the FAB system, **if >50% of nucleated marrow cells are erythroid precursors, the myeloblast percent should be calculated in terms of** *nonerythroid cells*. If >50% of cells are erythroid precursors, and myeloblasts are >30% of *nonerythroid* cells, the diagnosis is erythroleukemia. If myeloblasts are <30% of nonerythroid cells, the diagnosis is MDS.

  - Example: A patient is found to have 70% erythroid precursors in the marrow, and myeloblasts are 15% of *total* cells. Calculated as a percentage of nonerythroid cells (100% – 70% erythroid precursors = 30% nonerythroid cells), myeloblasts are 50% of *nonerythroid cells,* and the diagnosis is erythroleukemia [15% myeloblasts ÷ 30% nonerythroid cells = 50%].

  - Example: A patient has 70% erythroid precursors in the marrow, and myeloblasts are 5% of *total* cells. Myeloblasts are 17% of *nonerythroid cells* and the diagnosis is MDS: RAEB [5% myeloblasts ÷ 30% nonerythroid cells = 16.67%].

- **Chronic myeloproliferative disorders:** The chronic myeloproliferative disorders are usually characterized by increased (rather than decreased) cell counts, and dysplastic changes are usually absent.

- **Aplastic anemia:** Aplastic anemia is easily distinguished from MDS in most cases by the presence of a hypocellular marrow instead of the normocellular or hypercellular marrow characteristic of MDS. However, rare cases of MDS are associated with a hypocellular marrow, but the presence of striking dysplastic changes or a characteristic MDS cytogenetic abnormality would indicate MDS rather than aplastic anemia.

⇨ *Avoid giving a diagnosis of myelodysplasia to anyone who has severe acute medical problems or multiple chronic medical problems and anyone who has been in the hospital for more than a few days.* In the latter circumstance, see what the CBC was on admission: if the CBC on admission was normal, MDS is unlikely. A careful inspection of the medication list is often beneficial.

⇨ Cytogenetic analysis may be very helpful in confirming or excluding a diagnosis of MDS. If you are trying to decide between MDS and a benign condition, the presence of a clonal cytogenetic abnormality (particularly one of the common ones in MDS) would strongly favor MDS. If you are trying to decide between MDS and AML, the presence of one of the characteristic AML translocations [t(8;21), t(15;17) or inv(16)] would strongly favor AML. Numerical abnormalities or partial deletions of chromosomes 5, 7, or 20 would not be helpful since they can be seen in both MDS and AML. The presence of a Philadelphia chromosome [t(9;22)] would indicate chronic myelogenous leukemia, not MDS.

DISEASE COURSE

The disease course in MDS is highly variable. In general, RA and RARS are considered the low-grade variants of MDS, with prolonged survival and a low rate of transformation to AML. Refractory anemia with excess blasts and RAEB-t (in the FAB) are considered high-grade variants (Table 15–7). Refractory cytopenia with multilineage dysplasia (in the WHO) probably falls in between. The most common causes of death are infection, hemorrhage, and leukemic transformation. The most important prognostic factors are age, percent myeloblasts in the bone marrow, number of cell lines with cytopenia, and cytogenetic results.

An international workshop on prognosis in myelodysplasia has formulated a prognostic scoring system for myelodysplasia[1] (Tables 15–8 and 15–9). Patients are divided into four groups based on percent myeloblasts, karyotype, and number of cytopenias. As the risk score increases, patients have a shorter survival, higher risk of transformation to AML, and shorter time to leukemic transformation. Patients with a low score tend to die of

Table 15–7
Survival and Transformation to AML

	FAB Subgroups				
	RA	RARS	RAEB	RAEB-t	CMML
Median survival (months)	43	73	12	5	20
Transformation to AML (%)	15	5	40	50	35
% Patients	25	15	35	15	10

Reproduced with permission from Hoffman R, Benz EJ, Shattil SJ, et al, editors. Hematology: basic principles and practice. 3rd ed. New York, Churchill Livingstone, 2000. p. 1118.

Table 15–8
International Prognostic Scoring System (IPSS) for MDS

	Score Value				
Prognostic Variable	**0**	**0.5**	**1.0**	**1.5**	**2.0**
BM blasts (%)	<5	5–10	—	11–20	21–30
Karyotype*	Good	Intermediate	Poor	—	—
Cytopenias†	0/1	2	3	—	—

Reproduced with permission from Greenberg P, Cox C, LeBeau M, et al. International scoring system for evaluating prognosis in myelodysplastic syndromes. Blood 1997;89:2079–88.
Score: low = 0; INT-1 = 0.5–1.0; INT-2 = 1.5–2.0; high = ≥2.5
*Karyotype: Good = normal, -Y, del(5q) alone, or del (20q) alone; Poor = complex (≥3 abnormalities) or chromosome 7 abnormalities; Intermediate = other abnormalities.
†Hemoglobin <10 g/dL, absolute neutrophil count <1,500/µL, or platelet count <100,000/µL each count as one cytopenia.

bone marrow failure; patients with a high score usually die from acute leukemia. This prognostic index predicted survival better than the FAB classification and was able to define groups with different prognoses within single FAB categories.* Age was not included in the IPSS score. Patients >60 years had a worse prognosis at every risk level.

TREATMENT

Treatment for myelodysplasia has to be highly individualized. Most patients with MDS are older and have comorbid illnesses, and therefore are less able to tolerate aggressive therapy than younger or healthier patients. Some patients with MDS may have prolonged survival; older patients with low-grade myelodysplasia may be more likely to die of illnesses other than MDS. Therefore, possible benefit from therapy has to be carefully balanced against the risks or complications. *In many patients, control of symptoms is the primary goal of therapy.* In younger or healthier patients, aggressive therapy in an attempt to achieve cure might be warranted, even at the risk of significant toxicity or even death. At present, the only therapy that can be considered potentially curative is allogeneic bone marrow transplant.

---

*Only patients with de novo MDS were included in the analysis; patients with therapy-related or other secondary MDS were excluded. Patients with "proliferative type" CMMI (WBC >12,000/mL) were also excluded. Patients were classified according to the FAB system; some patients in the study (those with >20% marrow myeloblasts) would be classified as AML rather than MDS in the WHO classification.

Table 15–9
IPSS: Survival and Transformation to AML

Risk Group	Low	INT-1	INT-2	High
Median survival (years)	5.7	3.5	1.2	0.4
Time to 25% transformation to AML (years)	9.4	3.3	1.1	0.2

Data from Greenberg P, Cox C, LeBeau M, et al. International scoring system for evaluating prognosis in myelodysplastic syndromes. Blood 1997;89:2079–88.

⇨ **A major goal is to identify, treat, or exclude any reversible causes.**

Options for therapy include the following:

- **Supportive care:** Supportive care includes red cell transfusions for anemia, antibiotics for infections, and platelet transfusions for thrombocytopenia with hemorrhage.
- **Pyridoxine:** Pyridoxine supplementation may be beneficial in a proportion of patients with RARS but is of no benefit for patients in any other category.
- **Hematopoietic growth factors:** Hematopoietic growth factors (erythropoietin, granulocyte colony–stimulating factor [G-CSF], granulocyte-macrophage colony–stimulating factor [GM-CSF]) have a limited role in treatment of myelodysplasia. Erythropoietin increases the hemoglobin level in approximately 15 to 25% of patients; patients with low transfusion requirements, low serum erythropoietin levels, and RA are most likely to respond. Both G-CSF and GM-CSF increase the neutrophil count in a majority of patients and may decrease the infection rate or improve the patient's response to infection. However, the effects are transient. Overall, use of growth factors can help some patients, but the high cost plus the requirement for continuous use and parenteral administration have limited their use in MDS.
- **Chemotherapy:** Combination chemotherapy as used in AML has been tried in some patients with MDS, with generally disappointing results. Compared to patients with de novo AML, patients with MDS have lower response rates (~40 to 60% versus 70 to 80% in AML), higher relapse rates (~90% versus 65–80%), and shorter remission durations. The use of combination chemotherapy is also limited by the older age of the MDS population; many patients are not candidates for aggressive chemotherapy regimens.
- **Allogeneic bone marrow transplant:** Allogeneic bone marrow transplant (BMT) remains the only real potentially curative therapy for MDS. Unfortunately, the use of allogeneic BMT for MDS is limited by the older age of most patients and the fact that only a minority of

patients have histocompatible bone marrow donors. However, the use of allogeneic BMT is being extended to older patients, and the existence of a national bone marrow donor registry has allowed matched unrelated transplants. Several trials of allogeneic BMT in MDS have been performed; overall, ~40% of patients in these trials have long-term disease-free survival and may be cured. The results are better in patients with RA and RARS, those with low-risk cytogenetics, and patients transplanted early in the course of disease. Patients with high-grade MDS (RAEB and RAEB-t) have higher relapse rates and overall poor results. Patients with MDS have high transplant-related mortality rates (~30 to 35%). Infection, graft-versus-host disease and single- or multi-organ failure are the most common causes of death. Related histocompatible transplants achieve better results than unrelated transplants in most series. The results in patients with therapy-related MDS have generally been poor.

- **Autologous bone marrow transplant:** Cytogenetically normal stem cells can be demonstrated in some patients after combination chemotherapy. Therefore, attempts have been made to do autologous stem cell transplants in MDS patients using cells harvested after the induction of remission with chemotherapy. Some patients have done well, but many patients in these trials have not made it to the transplant stage because of severe and prolonged myelosuppression following induction chemotherapy or because of an inability to collect sufficient stem cells for transplantation.

- **Immunosuppressive agents:** Immunosuppressive agents were found to be beneficial in patients with hypocellular MDS and are now being tried in patients with other MDS variants. Patients with features of paroxysmal nocturnal hemoglobinuria (in addition to MDS) also appear to respond to immunosuppressive agents.

- **Experimental agents:** A variety of other agents are undergoing clinical trials. Among them are amifostine (a cytoprotective agent), 5-azacytidine, thalidomide, and monoclonal antibodies directed against the CD33 myeloid-associated antigen.

MYELODYSPLASIA VARIANTS

A few distinct variants of MDS deserve mention:

- **The 5q- syndrome:** The 5q- syndrome is characterized by refractory macrocytic anemia, normal or increased platelet counts, increased numbers of monolobated megakaryocytes in the bone marrow, and deletion of the long arm of chromosome 5 (5q-) as the sole cytogenetic abnormality. Survival is relatively long, with a low rate of leukemic

transformation. The majority of patients are older women. Iron overload from transfusion can become a significant problem in these
patients, and iron chelation therapy may be required.

↪ *Not all patients with 5q- have the 5q- syndrome* or the favorable prognosis associated with it. Patients who have other cytogenetic abnormalities, in addition to 5q-, have a less favorable prognosis.

- **Therapy-related myelodysplasia:** Therapy-related myelodysplasia
  (t-MDS) currently accounts for ~10 to 15% of MDS cases.[†] There is a
  high incidence of adverse cytogenetic abnormalities, particularly abnormalities involving chromosomes 5 and 7. Hypocellular myelodysplasia
  and myelodysplasia with myelofibrosis are more common in patients
  with t-MDS. Most patients have a relatively brief myelodysplastic phase
  and progress to overt leukemia within a few months.
- **Hypocellular myelodysplasia:** Approximately 10 to 15% of patients
  with myelodysplasia have a hypocellular marrow rather than the typical normocellular or hypercellular marrow. These patients may be difficult to distinguish from aplastic anemia; the key to proper diagnosis is
  to note the presence of striking myelodysplastic changes. A trial of
  immunosuppression may be warranted.

Reference

1. Greenberg P, Cox C, LeBeau M, et al. International scoring system for evaluating prognosis in myelodysplastic syndromes. Blood 1997;89:2079–88.

[†]In the WHO classification, therapy-related MDS is classified with therapy-related AML
rather than myelodysplasia.

16

The Chronic Lymphocytic Leukemias

*T*he chronic lymphocytic leukemias are a heterogeneous group of conditions characterized by an *increased number of small, mature-appearing lymphocytes in the blood*. By far the most common is a proliferation of small B cells that express the T cell–associated antigen CD5; the term chronic lymphocytic leukemia (**CLL**) refers to this entity unless specified otherwise. This type of CLL is closely related to B-cell *diffuse small lymphocytic lymphoma* (**SLL**). Less common B-cell CLLs include *hairy cell leukemia* (**HCL**) and B-cell *prolymphocytic leukemia* (**B-PLL**). Patients with non-Hodgkin's lymphomas may develop lymphocytosis, and occasionally lymphocytosis is the presenting feature of the lymphoma.

Mature T-cell lymphoproliferations occur, but these are rare. They include *T-prolymphocytic leukemia* (**T-PLL**) and *large granular lymphocytic leukemia* (*T-γ lymphocytosis*). A form of T-cell proliferation designated *adult T-cell leukemia/lymphoma* (**ATL/L**) has been linked to the human T-cell lymphocytotrophic virus I (HTLV-I). It is common in parts of the Far East, but rare in the United States. *Sézary syndrome* (SS) is a proliferation of T helper cells, related to a cutaneous T-cell lymphoma (mycosis fungoides).

- The **chronic lymphocytic leukemias** differ from **acute lymphoblastic leukemia** (**ALL**) in that the *cells appear mature* and have a *mature phenotype*. Acute lymphoblastic leukemia is a proliferation of immature cells (blasts).
- The distinction between **chronic lymphocytic leukemia** and **non-Hodgkin's lymphoma** (NHL) primarily depends on the *presence or absence of peripheral blood involvement*; however, the distinction is sometimes arbitrary and often clinically insignificant. The new World

Health Organization (WHO) classification of hematopoietic and lymphoid neoplasms de-emphasizes the difference between lymphocytic leukemia and lymphoma of the *same cell type*.

B-CELL CHRONIC LYMPHOCYTIC LEUKEMIA/SMALL LYMPHOCYTIC LYMPHOMA

Epidemiology

B-cell chronic lymphocytic leukemia/small lymphocytic lymphoma (**CLL** for short) is the most common adult leukemia in the United States and western Europe (~30% of adult leukemias). Chronic lymphocytic leukemia is uncommon in the Far East and other parts of the world. Chronic lymphocytic leukemia is predominantly a disease of older ages; the median age at diagnosis is ~55 to 65 years. It is uncommon below the age of 40 years; however, onset in the early thirties is not unheard of. Chronic lymphocytic leukemia is 1.5 to 2 times more common in men than women.

The cause of CLL is unknown. Some studies have shown a higher incidence of CLL in people who work in agriculture and in the asbestos industry, suggesting an occupational link; however, other studies have not confirmed this association. Chronic lymphocytic leukemia does not seem to be related to alkylating agents or exposure to ionizing radiation.

Pathophysiology

Chronic lymphocytic leukemia is characterized by a *slow but relentless accumulation of small lymphocytes*. The cells in CLL are arrested at a functionally immature level.

Chronic lymphocytic leukemia cannot be distinguished from B-cell SLL on examination of lymph nodes or bone marrow biopsy. Chronic lymphocytic leukemia is diagnosed if there is lymphocytosis in the blood (>5,000 lymphocytes/μL), SLL if there is no lymphocytosis. Many people now group the two together.

The **major complications of CLL** can be considered in relation to four factors:

- **Immunosuppression**
- **Autoimmune phenomena:** Patients with CLL are prone to autoimmune phenomena, usually involving blood cells (autoimmune hemolytic anemia and autoimmune thrombocytopenia)
- **Mass effects:** The neoplastic lymphocytes invade and colonize lymph nodes, the spleen, the bone marrow, and eventually virtually every organ in the body. The enlarged lymph nodes may compress other organs and compromise organ function
- **Transformation to large cell lymphoma**

The immunologic deficiency in CLL is complex. Hypogammaglobulinemia is common; therefore, patients are predisposed to infections with encapsulated organisms such as *Streptococcus pneumoniae*. There are also abnormalities in T-cell numbers and function, including a decreased ratio of T helper to T suppressor (CD4/CD8) cells and impaired cell-mediated immunity. Therapy for CLL may increase the immunosuppression.

Clinical Features

Many patients with CLL are asymptomatic at diagnosis; lymphocytosis is detected as an incidental finding on a routine CBC. Symptoms, when present, are usually due to anemia and include fatigue, dizziness, or dyspnea on exertion. Patients may have nonspecific systemic symptoms such as fever, night sweats, and weight loss.

The physical examination in CLL may be completely normal. The most common abnormality is lymphadenopathy, which may be localized or generalized. The lymph nodes are usually slightly to moderately enlarged, firm or rubbery, nontender, and freely movable. Mild or moderate hepatosplenomegaly may be present.

Laboratories

By definition, there must be **>5,000 lymphocytes/μL** in the blood. The neutrophil count is decreased as a percentage of white cells, but the absolute neutrophil number may be normal, increased, or decreased. Mild anemia and/or thrombocytopenia are common at diagnosis, but significant decreases (hemoglobin <11 g/dL, platelets <100,000/μL) are less common (≤15%).

The blood smear in CLL is very characteristic (Figures 16–1 and 16–2). There is an increased number of small mature-appearing lymphocytes. The cells usually look monotonous; however, some cases have a variable lymphocyte appearance. The nuclear chromatin appears condensed, giving the impression of dense chunks of chromatin surrounded by white spaces (aptly described as a "soccer ball" nucleus). Characteristically, there are many disintegrated cells on the smear ("smudge" or "basket" cells). *The combination of many "soccer ball" lymphocytes with numerous "smudge" cells in the background is almost diagnostic for CLL.* There may be occasional prolymphocytes (larger cells, with less condensed nuclear chromatin and prominent central nucleoli); by definition, these must be ≤10% of lymphocytes. Erythrocytes usually look unremarkable. Other white cells and platelets are normal in appearance but may be decreased in number.

Other routine laboratories are usually unremarkable, although, occasionally, the lactic dehydrogenase (LDH) or serum calcium is elevated.

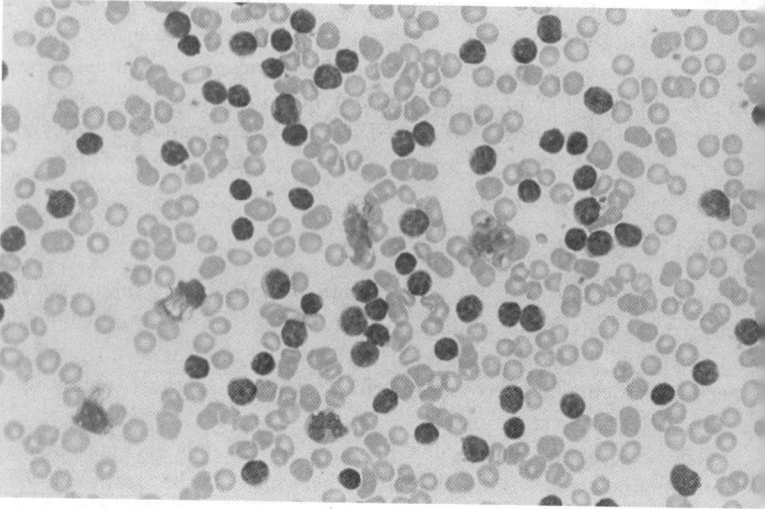

Figure 16–1 B-cell chronic lymphocytic leukemia, low power. Lymphocytosis of small mature-appearing lymphocytes. Numerous "smudge" cells are present.

A positive direct antiglobulin (Coombs') test is uncommon at diagnosis (~1% of patients) but becomes common (up to 35%) as the disease progresses.

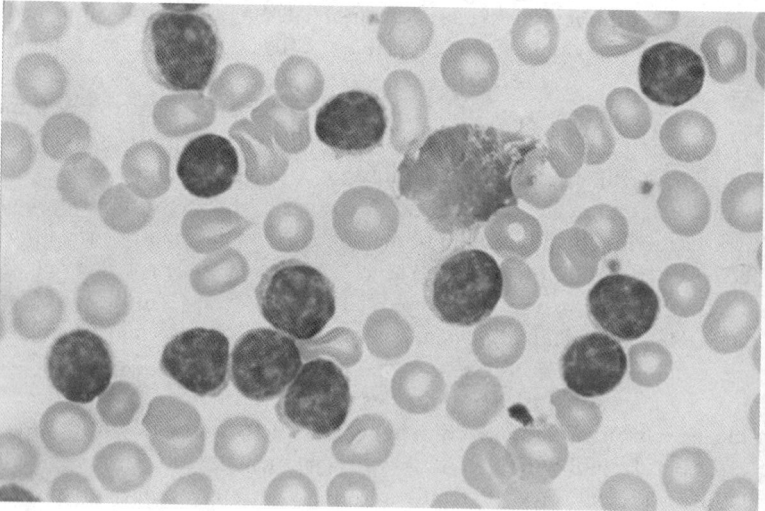

Figure 16–2 B-cell chronic lymphocytic leukemia, high power. Condensed "soccer ball" nuclear chromatin; one "smudge cell" is present.

Hypogammaglobulinemia is present in up to 60% of patients at diagnosis. A small monoclonal protein (usually IgM type) is found in ~5 to 10% of patients on routine serum protein electrophoresis, more frequently when sensitive methods are used.

Bone Marrow

The bone marrow aspirate usually shows ≥30% small lymphocytes. The marrow biopsy may show three patterns of involvement: (1) *nodular* (discrete aggregates of small lymphocytes), (2) *interstitial* (the lymphocytes infiltrate around the fat cells and normal hematopoietic cells), and (3) *diffuse* (total marrow replacement by the leukemic cells). The presence of a diffuse pattern of infiltration is an adverse prognostic feature.

The features of B-cell CLL/SLL are listed in Table 16–1.

Immunophenotype

Chronic lymphocytic leukemia has a **highly characteristic immunophenotype**: (1) expression of B-cell markers (CD19, CD20, CD23), (2) coexpression of **CD5** (usually considered a T-cell marker), and (3) weak surface immunoglobulin with light chain restriction (a marked imbalance in the expression of kappa and lambda light chains instead of the normal 2:1 ratio of light chain expression). Expression of CD5 is found on a small proportion of normal B cells in the blood and on mantle zone B cells in lymph

Table 16–1
Features of B-Cell CLL/SLL

Predominantly older age group

Moderate lymphadenopathy and splenomegaly

Lymphocytosis (>5,000/μL):
- Small mature-appearing lymphocytes
- Condensed ("soccer ball") nuclear chromatin
- Numerous "smudge cells"

Immunophenotype:
- CD5 coexpression
- Immunoglobulin light chain restriction
- Dim surface immunoglobulin and CD20
- Expression of CD23; absence of FMC-7

Predisposition to infection

Autoimmune phenomena, particularly autoimmune hemolytic anemia

Transformation to large cell lymphoma (Richter's syndrome)

nodes; however, expression of CD5 on a *predominant* B-cell population strongly suggests malignancy. Expression of CD5 is typical of only two B-cell neoplasms: Chronic lymphocytic leukemia/SLL and mantle cell lymphoma. CLL/SLL can usually be distinguished from mantle cell lymphoma by the weak (dim) expression of surface immunoglobulin and CD20, presence of CD23, and absence of FMC-7. Mantle cell lymphoma has *moderate to bright* surface immunoglobulin and CD20, expression of FMC-7, and absence of CD23 (Table 16–2).

Cytogenetics

Standard cytogenetic analysis is difficult to do in CLL because of the low mitotic rate of the cells and is not part of routine CLL evaluation in most centers. Overall, cytogenetic abnormalities are found in ~50% of cases by standard chromosome analysis. The most common abnormality found is trisomy 12, in ~20% of cases. The next most common abnormalities are structural deletions of the long arms of chromosomes 13 and 14.

Chromosomal abnormalities are found more often by fluorescence in situ hybridization (FISH) than by standard cytogenetics, with abnormalities present in ≥80% of cases. Deletions of l3q are the most common abnormality found by FISH.

Differential Diagnosis

The differential diagnosis of CLL primarily includes reactive lymphocytosis, other types of CLLs, leukemic phase of non-Hodgkin's lymphomas, and

Table 16–2
Immunophenotype of Small B-Cell Neoplasms

Marker	CLL/ SLL	Mantle Cell Lymphoma	Follicular Lymphoma	Hairy Cell Leukemia	Marginal Zone Lymphoma
CD5	+	+	−	−	−
CD10 (cALLA)	−	−	+	−	−
CD20	Dim	+	+	+	+
CD23	+	−	+/−	+/−	−
FMC-7	−	+	+	+/−	+
Surface Ig*	Dim	Moderate or bright	+	+	+
Other				CD11c, CD25, and CD103	

+ = positive; − = negative; +/− = variable.
*Surface immunoglobulin.

acute leukemias (Table 16–3). Reactive (benign) lymphocytosis is the most important differential.

- **Reactive lymphocytosis:** Reactive lymphocytosis is more common in younger individuals; however, the age range can overlap with CLL. In most cases of reactive lymphocytosis, the lymphocytes are more variable and may have an "atypical" appearance (more abundant cytoplasm, larger nuclei with more prominent nucleoli, and characteristic "hugging" of erythrocytes). The primary condition causing the lymphocytosis may be evident.
- **Leukemic phase of non-Hodgkin's lymphoma:**
  - *Small lymphocytic lymphoma* (**SLL**): The distinction between CLL and SLL is arbitrary and largely meaningless: >5,000 lymphocytes/μL = CLL, ≤5,000/μL = SLL.
  - *Mantle cell lymphoma* (**MCL**): Up to ~20% of cases of mantle cell lymphoma can be leukemic at diagnosis, and lymphocytosis can be the initial presenting feature of MCL. The lymphocytes in MCL tend to have more granular nuclear chromatin, and the characteristic "smudge cells" seen in CLL are usually not present in MCL. Immunophenotyping by flow cytometry is usually able to make the distinction. As noted above, MCL is the other CD5-positive B-cell malignancy but differs in intensity of surface immunoglobulin and CD20 expression, absence of CD23, and presence of FMC-7.

Table 16–3
Differential Diagnosis of Chronic Lymphocytic Leukemia

Reactive Lymphocytosis:
- Viral infections, particularly EBV, CMV, viral hepatitis
- *Bordetella pertussis* (whooping cough)
- Toxoplasmosis
- Brucellosis
- Acute infectious lymphocytosis
- Tertiary or congenital syphilis
- Drug hypersensitivity reactions
- Endocrine disorders: thyrotoxicosis, Addison's disease, hypopituitarism
- Persistent polyclonal B-cell lymphocytosis

Malignant Lymphoproliferative Disorders:
- Leukemic phase of non-Hodgkin's lymphomas (mantle cell, follicular, marginal zone, splenic lymphoma with villous lymphocytes)
- Hairy cell leukemia
- Prolymphocytic leukemia (B cell and T cell)
- Acute lymphoblastic leukemia; acute myeloid leukemia (FAB-M0 and M1)

EBV = Epstein-Barr virus; CMV = cytomegalovirus.

- *Follicular lymphomas*: Leukemic presentation of follicular lymphomas is uncommon but does occur. The lymphocytes in follicular lymphomas have prominent nuclear folds or clefts, and it is often possible to make the distinction based on the blood smear. The immunophenotype of follicular lymphomas differs from that of CLL.
- Other lymphomas can occasionally present with leukemic involvement of the blood, including marginal zone lymphomas, splenic lymphoma with villous lymphocytes, and large cell lymphomas. The appearance on blood smear and/or immunophenotyping will usually allow distinction.
- **Hairy cell leukemia:** Hairy cell leukemia is discussed below.
- **Prolymphocytic leukemias:** Prolymphocytic leukemias are uncommon. They can be distinguished from CLL by larger cell size, less condensed nuclear chromatin, and prominent central nucleoli. The immunophenotype is also different (usually CD5 negative).
- **Acute leukemias:** Acute leukemia is easily distinguished from CLL in most cases by the predominance of immature cells rather than mature lymphocytes.

Staging

Two staging systems are used for CLL: the **Rai** or **modified Rai** (Table 16–4) and the **Binet** system (Table 16–5). The modified Rai system is commonly

Table 16–4

Rai and Modified Rai Staging Systems for CLL

	Rai Staging	Modified Rai Staging*	
Stage 0:	Lymphocytosis only (blood and marrow)	Low risk	Rai stage 0
Stage I:	Lymphocytosis plus enlarged nodes	Intermediate risk	Stages I and II
Stage II:	Lymphocytosis plus enlarged spleen and/or liver, ± nodes		
Stage III:	Lymphocytosis plus anemia (Hgb <11 g/dL), ± above	High risk	Stages III and IV
Stage IV:	Lymphocytosis plus thrombocytopenia (<100 × 10⁹/L) ± above		

*Currently, the modified Rai system is used more often.
± = with or without.

Table 16–5
Binet Staging System for CLL

Stage	≥3 Lymphoid Sites	Hemoglobin <10 g/dL +/or Platelets <100,000/μL
A	—	—
B	+	—
C	+/−	+

A = lowest stage; B = intermediate; C = highest.
+ = present; − = absent; +/− = present or absent.

used in the United States; the Binet system is used more in Europe. The stage in both systems depends on the presence of lymphadenopathy and bone marrow compromise, with the presence of bone marrow compromise indicating advanced stage. Both systems correlate with survival; patients with more advanced disease have shorter survival.

A proportion of patients with low-stage disease at diagnosis have rapid progression of disease and short survival, but neither system is able to identify these patients. Other factors that can help predict disease course include the following:

- **Lymphocyte doubling time:** Observing the patient for a time without treatment allows calculation of the time it would take for the lymphocyte count to double. A doubling time of <**12 months** suggests **aggressive disease**; doubling time >**12 months** suggests **indolent disease**.
- **Abnormal chromosome analysis:** The presence of cytogenetic abnormalities by standard metaphase analysis suggests more aggressive disease. Deletions of 17p and trisomy 12 are associated with shorter survival. Deletions of 13q appear to be associated with indolent disease and long survival.
- **Diffuse pattern of bone marrow infiltration:** A diffuse pattern of bone marrow infiltration suggests more aggressive disease, whereas nodular or interstitial patterns suggest more indolent disease.

Elevated serum levels of β_2-microglobulin and soluble CD23 have also been reported to predict aggressive disease, as has the presence of abnormalities involving the p53 tumor suppressor gene. Expression of CD38 on ≥30% of lymphocytes by flow cytometry has also been reported to indicate more aggressive disease.

Disease Course

The majority of patients with CLL have indolent disease, with long survival. A small number of patients follow a relatively aggressive course, with survival of only a few years. Overall, the median survival in CLL is ~6 to 10 years. Most patients have a gradual increase in the lymphocyte count, with eventual development of lymphadenopathy and splenomegaly. The disease can usually be controlled for some years but eventually becomes resistant to therapy.

Many patients, especially older patients, have few problems related to CLL and die of unrelated illnesses. The life expectancy of asymptomatic patients ≥70 years with stage 0 CLL is essentially identical to the age-matched population without CLL. On the other hand, symptomatic or advance-stage CLL results in significant shortening of life expectancy, even in older patients.

Complications of CLL include the following:

- **Infections:** Infections are the number one cause of death in CLL patients. Bacterial infections are most common in untreated CLL patients. The organisms include *S. pneumoniae, Staphylococcus aureus, Haemophilus influenzae,* and gram-negative enteric organisms such as *Escherichia coli, Klebsiella pneumoniae,* and *Pseudomonas aeruginosa.* The most common type of infection is pneumonitis; others include sinusitis, urinary tract infections, skin and soft tissue infections, and septicemia. Opportunistic infections (*Pneumocystis carinii, Listeria, Nocardia,* mycobacteria, and herpes viruses) may occur in patients treated with nucleoside analogues such as fludarabine.
- **Autoimmune phenomena:** Patients with CLL are predisposed to autoimmune phenomena, usually antibodies against blood cells. The most common is autoimmune hemolytic anemia, which has been described in ~10 to 35% of patients. Pure red cell aplasia and immune thrombocytopenia also occur but are much less common.
  - *Autoimmune hemolytic anemia* in CLL is usually the warm-reacting type and closely resembles idiopathic warm autoimmune hemolytic anemia. The antibodies are produced by residual normal B cells, not the neoplastic CLL cells. They are the IgG type, polyclonal, and usually directed against an antigen in the Rh blood group that is present on the red cells of nearly all people. In most cases, autoimmune hemolytic anemia occurs in patients with long-standing CLL. Treatment for immune hemolytic anemia in CLL is similar to treatment of idiopathic immune hemolytic anemia. Prednisone is the cornerstone of therapy.
  - *Pure red cell aplasia* (**PRCA**) in CLL is uncommon, but CLL is the most common cause of PRCA. The diagnosis is made by the com-

bination of severe anemia with decreased reticulocyte count and an absence of erythroid precursors in the marrow. Prednisone is the primary therapy; cyclosporine has also shown effectiveness.

- *Immune thrombocytopenia* occurs in ~1 to 3% of CLL patients. Unlike immune hemolytic anemia, it may occur early in the course of the disease. Treatment is similar to idiopathic immune thrombocytopenic purpura.
- *Evans's syndrome* is simultaneous autoimmune hemolytic anemia and autoimmune thrombocytopenia occurring in CLL.

- **Progression to large cell lymphoma (Richter's syndrome):** The development of large cell non-Hodgkin's lymphoma in patients with CLL has been termed *Richter's syndrome*. The quoted incidence of Richter's syndrome is ~10 to 15%, but the actual incidence is probably 3 to 5%. Richter's syndrome is characterized by systemic symptoms (fever, night sweats, weight loss) and rapidly progressive lymphadenopathy. The lymphoma is usually a large cell histologic type. In most cases, the large cell lymphoma appears to represent a transformation of the original CLL clone. In some cases, however, it appears to be an unrelated second malignancy. The lymphoma is characteristically unresponsive to therapy, and survival after Richter's transformation is usually only a few months.
- **Transformation to other malignancies:** Transformation of CLL to other types of hematologic malignancy has been described. The most common of these is prolymphocytic transformation, which occurs in ~5 to 10% of CLL patients. This is defined as >55% of prolymphocytes in the blood (larger cells with more abundant cytoplasm, larger nuclei with less condensed chromatin, and single central nucleoli). Prolymphocytic transformation tends to be resistant to therapy and is associated with short survival. Transformation to ALL or multiple myeloma has been described but is extremely rare.

Treatment

Chronic lymphocytic leukemia is incurable with conventional therapy. Therefore, *the primary goal of therapy for most patients is control of symptoms and maximizing quality of life.* Since many patients have indolent disease, with long survival and few complications, treatment for CLL may not be required at initial diagnosis. *Lymphocytosis per se is **not** usually an indication for treatment.*

   Indications for treatment in CLL include the following:

- Progressive systemic symptoms (fever, night sweats, weight loss)
- Progressively worsening anemia or thrombocytopenia
- Autoimmune hemolytic anemia or thrombocytopenia
- Bulky lymphadenopathy that is compressing vital structures or is cosmetically unacceptable

- Massive splenomegaly
- Marked lymphocytosis (>150,000 to 200,000/μL)

    Treatment modalities for CLL can include the following:

- **Alkylating agents:** Alkylating agents (chlorambucil or cyclophosphamide) have been the standard chemotherapy for CLL, used alone or in combination with prednisone. Chlorambucil can be given either as a daily dose or as an intermittent bolus therapy every 3 to 4 weeks.
- **Prednisone or other corticosteroids**: Glucocorticoids are often used in combination with chlorambucil or cyclophosphamide. Prednisone (~40 to 80 mg/day, given 5 to 7 days per month) is the most common corticosteroid used. Prednisone is the standard therapy for CLL-related autoimmune hemolytic anemia and immune thrombocytopenia.
- **Purine analogues (fludarabine):** The purine analogue fludarabine (Fludara) has become the first choice of many hematologists for treating CLL. It is administered as a 30-minute intravenous infusion at a dose of ~25 mg/m^2/day for 5 days, at 4-week intervals. Compared to chlorambucil, fludarabine results in higher overall response rates and longer progression-free survival. A significant number of patients achieve apparent complete responses. Fludarabine may be effective in patients who are resistant to chlorambucil. Initial studies suggested that fludarabine increased overall survival in CLL; however, other studies have not shown a survival advantage for fludarabine. Toxicities of fludarabine include myelosuppression and immunosuppression. Patients on fludarabine may be subject to opportunistic infections, including *P. carinii, Listeria, Nocardia*, mycobacteria, and herpes viruses. Autoimmune hemolytic anemia has also been linked to fludarabine.
- **Combination chemotherapy:** Combination chemotherapy as used for aggressive non-Hodgkin's lymphomas has been tried in CLL. These regimens may have a higher complete response rate than chlorambucil with or without prednisone but have higher toxicity rates and have generally not shown improvements in survival.
- **Monoclonal antibody therapy (rituximab):** Monoclonal antibodies against lymphocyte-associated cell surface antigens are now being used in CLL. **Rituximab** (also called Rituxan) is a monoclonal antibody directed against the CD20 B-cell antigen. Patients with high lymphocyte counts can have severe infusion-related reactions to rituximab, including fever, rigors, hypotension, dyspnea, and bronchospasm. Starting therapy at a lower dose appears to decrease the incidence of infusion-related reactions. Antibodies against other B-cell antigens are being developed.

- **Bone marrow transplantation (BMT):** Bone marrow transplants* have been used in a relatively small number of CLL patients. Allogeneic transplants may add an immunologic "graft-versus-leukemia" effect to the therapeutic effects of chemotherapy and may have the potential to cure patients with CLL. Autologous transplants, using fludarabine to induce a complete response before harvesting the stem cells, have also been tried. A barrier to the use of allogeneic BMT in CLL is the older age of the majority of patients. In addition, the risk of early death due to transplant-related toxicity is a significant concern in patients with CLL, who might otherwise live for years with their disease. Transplantation would be a better option for younger patients at high risk for early disease progression and death.

Chronic Lymphocytic Leukemia in Younger Patients

Approximately 10 to 15% of patients are <50 years old at diagnosis of CLL, and diagnosis in the thirties is not that uncommon. Studies indicate that the clinical presentation and overall disease course are largely the same in younger as in older patients. However, although CLL might have little impact on overall survival in an older population, diagnosis of CLL in a younger person often indicates a significant shortening of life expectancy. A proportion of young patients will have indolent disease, with no evidence of progression over many years. Treatment of such individuals is unnecessary and may be harmful, but the remaining patients deserve an attempt to prolong survival.

The clinical prognostic factors used to predict survival in older patients also apply to young patients: advanced Rai or Binet stage, lymphocyte doubling time <12 months, and diffuse bone marrow involvement predict short survival.

Younger patients with advanced stage or a rapid lymphocyte doubling time should be considered for BMT or other clinical trials of new therapies for CLL. Patients with more indolent disease can be observed without therapy, and treatment started when disease progression is detected.

HAIRY CELL LEUKEMIA

Epidemiology

Hairy cell leukemia (HCL) is uncommon (1 to 2% of leukemias in the United States). It occurs predominantly in middle-aged and older adults;

---

*The term bone marrow transplant is used to include all forms of hematopoietic stem cell therapy.

the median age at diagnosis is ~55 years. The disease is 3 to 5 times more common in men than women. No specific etiology has been established.

Pathophysiology

Hairy cell leukemia is a clonal proliferation of mature activated B cells. The cells infiltrate into the bone marrow where they elicit fibrosis; neutropenia, anemia, thrombocytopenia, and pancytopenia are common. The neoplastic lymphocytes also infiltrate the spleen, causing splenomegaly.

Clinical Features

The most common symptoms are fatigue, weakness, and recurrent pyogenic infections. Splenomegaly may cause abdominal discomfort or early satiety due to compression of the stomach.

Splenomegaly is present on physical examination in ~80% of patients and can be massive. Hepatomegaly is common, although usually less impressive.

Laboratories

The CBC shows anemia in up to 75% of patients. Leukopenia is present in ≥50%; ~10 to 20% have lymphocytosis. *Neutropenia is common and may be severe; monocytopenia is characteristic.* Thrombocytopenia may be present in up to 80% of patients. Up to half of patients have pancytopenia.

The blood smear shows lymphocytes with filamentous cytoplasmic projections ("hairs") (Figure 16–3). The nuclei are eccentric in the cell; the nuclear chromatin is finely granular or reticular. The characteristic hairy cells may be uncommon and sometimes may require diligent searching or preparation of buffy coat smears.

- *The presence of "hairy" lymphocytes is **not** diagnostic of HCL; occasional hairy cells may be present on smears from normal people.* However, in the appropriate clinical setting, the presence of hairy cells makes the diagnosis of HCL highly likely.
- A positive reaction with the **tartrate-resistant acid phosphatase (TRAP)** stain is another very characteristic feature of HCL (Figure 16–4). T lymphocytes normally have an acid phosphatase enzyme, but the isoenzyme present in T cells is inhibited by preincubation with tartaric acid. The variant of the enzyme present in hairy cells is not inhibited by tartaric acid (ie, is *tartrate resistant*).

Bone Marrow and Spleen

It is frequently not possible to obtain a bone marrow aspirate due to fibrosis. The biopsy shows infiltration by lymphocytes with round or oval nuclei,

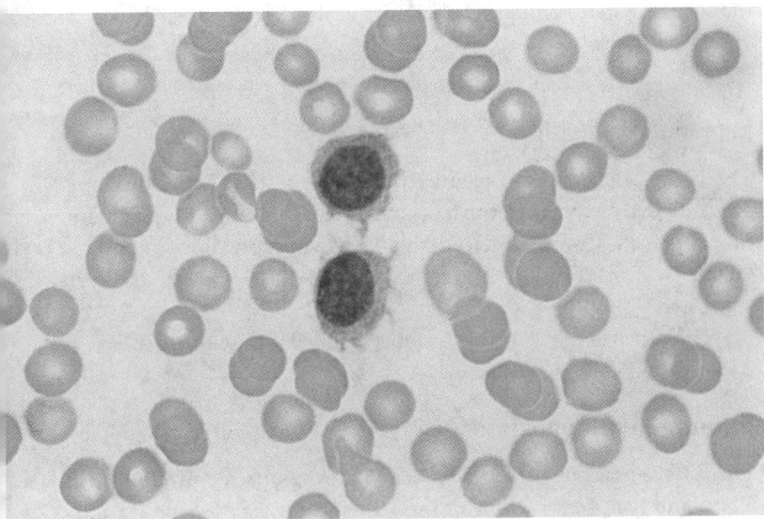

Figure 16–3 Hairy cell leukemia. Lymphocytes with filamentous cytoplasmic projections.

often surrounded by a clear space. This gives the cells a "fried egg" appearance. A reticulin stain shows an increase in reticulin fibers.

The lymphocytes infiltrate into the red pulp of the spleen, causing atrophy or replacement of the white pulp. A characteristic feature is dilated

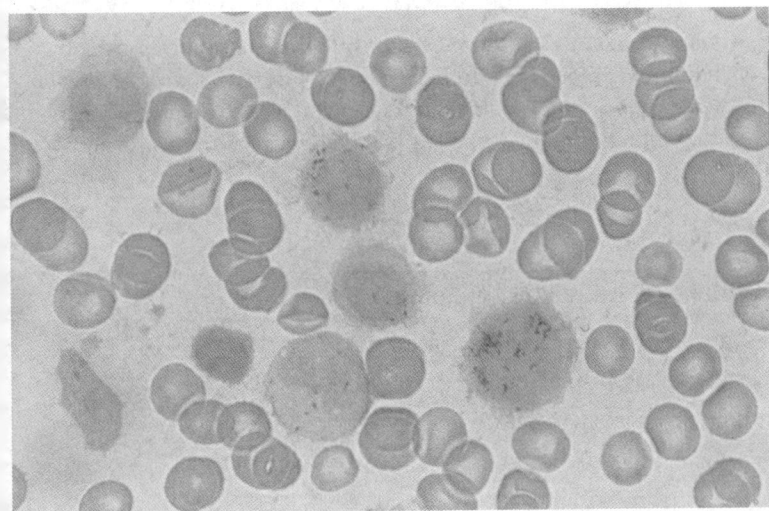

Figure 16–4 Hairy cell leukemia, TRAP stain. Acid phosphatase reaction after incubation with tartaric acid. Granular staining is seen in the lymphocytes.

blood-filled spaces lined by the hairy cells, described as "blood lakes" c "pseudosinuses."

Immunophenotype

The hairy cells express B-cell markers such as CD19 and CD20; CD22 i often strongly expressed. Surface immunoglobulin with light chain restric tion is present (λ more often than κ), CD5 coexpression is absent. **CD11c CD25** (the interleukin-2 receptor), and **CD103** are characteristicall expressed.

The features of HCL are summarized in Table 16–6.

Differential Diagnosis

The differential diagnosis of HCL includes idiopathic myelofibrosis, othe CLLs, and lymphomas with prominent splenomegaly.

- **Idiopathic myelofibrosis (agnogenic myeloid metaplasia):** Idiopathi myelofibrosis is associated with cytopenias, fibrosis in the marrow, anc splenomegaly. The characteristic circulating hairy cells are absent, anc the bone marrow lacks the lymphocytic infiltrate ("fried eggs") seen ir HCL.
- **Other chronic lymphocytic leukemias:** Other CLLs lack the typica hairy cells of CLL. The immunophenotype of HCL differs from tha of typical B-cell CLL/SLL, prolymphocytic leukemias, and T-cel leukemias.
- **Non-Hodgkin's lymphomas with splenomegaly:** The non-Hodgkin': lymphoma most likely to be confused with HCL is *splenic lymphomc with villous lymphocytes* (SLVL) since it features splenomegaly anc circulating lymphocytes with cytoplasmic projections. Lymphocytes

Table 16–6
Features of Hairy Cell Leukemia

Circulating lymphocytes with filamentous cytoplasmic projections (hairy cells)
Splenomegaly with or without hepatomegaly
Neutropenia and monocytopenia
Positive tartrate-resistant acid phosphatase (**TRAP**) stain
Expression of CD11c, CD25, and CD103; absence of CD5

of SLVL tend to have shorter projections, which may cluster at one end of the cell. The TRAP stain is usually negative, and CD25 and CD103 are absent.

Disease Course

The course of HCL is variable. Many patients have indolent disease and may survive for years with few or no complications. Before the mid-1980s, patients with symptomatic HCL had a survival of only a few years. With newer agents, particularly nucleoside analogues like 2-chlorodeoxyadenosine (cladribine), most patients have long survival with few or no problems related to HCL.

Complications of HCL can include the following:

- **Infections:** Patients with HCL are subject to recurrent bacterial infections, both gram-positive and gram-negative bacteria. Cutaneous infections are particularly common. They are also at risk of infections with opportunistic organisms such as *Listeria* and atypical mycobacteria.
- **Systemic autoimmune diseases:** An increased incidence of autoimmune diseases has been described in patients with HCL, including scleroderma, polymyositis, and polyarteritis nodosa.

Treatment

Treatment should be based on the presence or absence of symptoms. Asymptomatic patients do not necessarily require treatment. Treatment options include the following:

- **Purine nucleoside analogues (pentostatin, cladribine):** The purine nucleoside analogues 2'-deoxycoformycin (dCF; Pentostatin) and 2-chlorodeoxyadenosine (CdA; cladribine) are remarkably effective against HCL. Both have overall response rates >90%, with complete response rates of ~75 to 90%. Complete responses often last for years, and patients who relapse often have a second response to the same agent that induced the first response.
  - Cladribine is probably the most frequently used treatment for HCL. It is given as a single continuous intravenous infusion for 7 days. The primary toxicity is dose-related marrow suppression. Cladribine causes prolonged lymphopenia due to a decrease in CD4$^+$ T cells, but infections related to this are uncommon.
  - Pentostatin is given every other week for approximately 6 months or until there is maximum bone marrow response followed by two additional doses. Side effects include neutropenia, nausea and vom-

iting, fever, and fatigue. Pentostatin also induces prolonged lym
phopenia.

- **Interferon-α:** Interferon-α was the first agent shown to have rea
  effectiveness in HCL, but it has largely been replaced by cladribine an
  pentostatin.
- **Splenectomy:** Splenectomy was the only therapy that offered any ben
  efit prior to the introduction of interferon-α, but the benefit was mod
  est. With newer therapies, splenectomy is now rarely performed fo
  HCL. However, it may be useful in occasional patients with massiv
  splenomegaly who do not have a complete response to cladribine o
  pentostatin.

Hairy Cell Variant

Hairy cell variant (HCL-v) is uncommon. It resembles HCL morphologi
cally, except the cells tend to have shorter, less prominent cytoplasmic pro
jections. The WBC count is usually higher than typical HCL (ofter
>50,000/μL), and splenomegaly is usually present. The TRAP stain is vari
able in HCL-v, and expression of CD25 is usually absent. The response t
cladribine or pentostatin appears less predictable than typical HCL, anc
interferon-α appears ineffective.

UNCOMMON CHRONIC LYMPHOCYTIC LEUKEMIAS

There are a variety of uncommon lymphocytic leukemias, which will b
mentioned only briefly.

Prolymphocytic Leukemia

Prolymphocytic leukemia (PLL) can be of either B-cell or T-cell lineage
with B cell being more common. Prolymphocytes have more abundan
cytoplasm than CLL lymphocytes, larger nuclei with less condensed chro
matin, and prominent central nucleoli (Figure 16–5). B-cell prolympho
cytic leukemia (B-PLL) can arise de novo or by transformation from CLL
The de novo type is more common.

De novo B-PLL is characterized by marked lymphocytosis (ofter
>100,000/μL), with >55% prolymphocytes. Hepatosplenomegaly is com
mon; lymphadenopathy is usually minimal or absent. Phenotyping by flov
cytometry usually shows expression of B-cell markers, *absence* of CD5, anc
relatively bright surface immunoglobulin with light chain restriction. The
disease tends to be poorly responsive to therapy and survival tends to b
short (≤1 year), although some patients have more indolent disease with
longer survival.

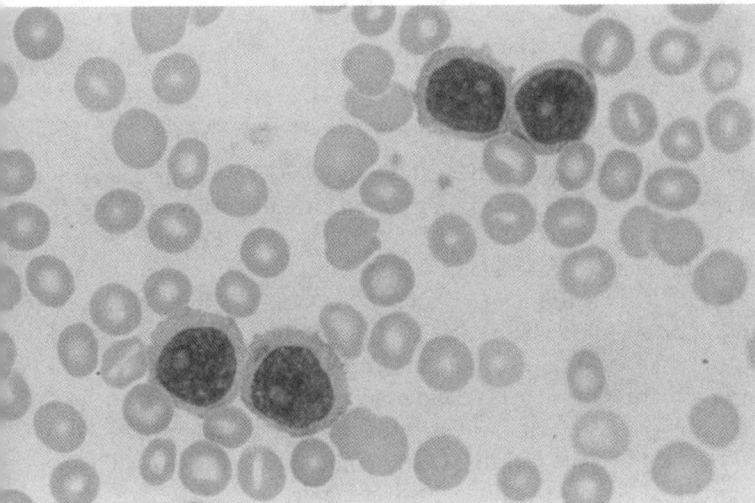

Figure 16–5 **Prolymphocytic leukemia.**

B-cell PLL can also arise in transformation from CLL. The prolymphocytes may retain the CD5 coexpression characteristic of CLL or have variable loss of CD5 expression. Like de novo PLL, PLL arising in transformation from CLL tends to respond poorly to therapy, with short survival.

Large Granular Lymphocytic Leukemia (T-γ Lymphocytosis)

Large granular lymphocytic leukemia, also known as T-γ lymphocytosis, is characterized by the presence of large lymphocytes with prominent azurophilic (reddish-purple) granules. Two different types occur. The most common type in the United States is an indolent proliferation of natural killer–like T cells associated with neutropenia, rheumatoid arthritis, and a variety of autoantibodies. The second type, which is common in the Far East but rare in the United States, is an aggressive leukemia of true NK cells. The diagnosis is suspected by finding the characteristic large granular lymphocytes on the blood smear and confirmed by flow cytometry. The common type in the United States usually expresses CD3, CD8, CD16, and CD57. The Far Eastern variant has a true NK cell phenotype (CD16 and CD56 are present; CD3, CD4, and CD8 are absent). Complications of the US variant are predominantly related to neutropenia. Treatment includes low-dose methotrexate, cyclosporine, or corticosteroids. The course is indolent, with ≥80% surviving at 10 years. The true NK cell variant seen in the

Far East is associated with Epstein-Barr virus (EBV). Clinically, it is much more aggressive, and survival is short.

Adult T-Cell Leukemia/Lymphoma

Adult T-cell leukemia/lymphoma is an aggressive lymphoproliferative disorder that is common in parts of the Far East, particularly southern Japan. It also occurs in West Africa and the Caribbean. Occasional cases occur in the United States, predominantly in the southeast.

Adult T-cell leukemia/lymphoma is associated with the **human T-cell lymphocytotrophic virus I** (**HTLV-I**), which is a retrovirus endemic in parts of the Far East, Africa, and the Caribbean. Human T-cell lymphocytotrophic virus I causes ATL/L and *tropical spastic paraparesis*, a neurologic disease. It has many similarities to the human immunodeficiency virus (HIV), including the fact that it infects the same cells (CD4$^+$ T lymphocytes), but it belongs to a different virus family.

In the United States, ATL/L predominantly occurs in young African American males. The age range is broader in Japan. Manifestations of the disease include lymphadenopathy, hepatosplenomegaly, skin lesions, and sometimes bone lesions. Patients may present with lymphadenopathy without lymphocytosis (lymphomatous form), lymphocytosis without lymphadenopathy (leukemic form), or lymphadenopathy *and* lymphocytosis (mixed). Lymphocytosis eventually develops in most cases.

Anemia and thrombocytopenia are common but usually mild. The degree of lymphocytosis is variable, from none to $\geq$500,000/μL. The lymphocytes characteristically have very convoluted nuclei (described as "florette" nuclei). Hypercalcemia is common. Serology for HTLV-I is positive.

The diagnosis is made by finding lymphocytes with the characteristic convoluted nuclei in the peripheral blood, combined with flow cytometry showing expression of CD4 and CD25 on the malignant cells. The diagnosis is confirmed by positive serologic assay for HTLV-I.

The course in the United States is aggressive, with median survival $\leq$6 months. Smoldering and chronic forms are described in Japan but are rare in the United States. No form of therapy has proven effective.

Sézary Syndrome

Sézary syndrome is a T-cell lymphocytosis related to *mycosis fungoides* (MF), a cutaneous T-cell lymphoma. In MF, the malignant lymphocytes cause cutaneous patches, plaques, or nodules. Sézary syndrome is characterized by generalized erythroderma and large numbers of atypical T cells with highly convoluted (cerebriform) nuclei in the blood (**Sézary cells**) (Figure 16–6). Sézary cells can be seen in the blood of patients with MF but usually in low numbers.

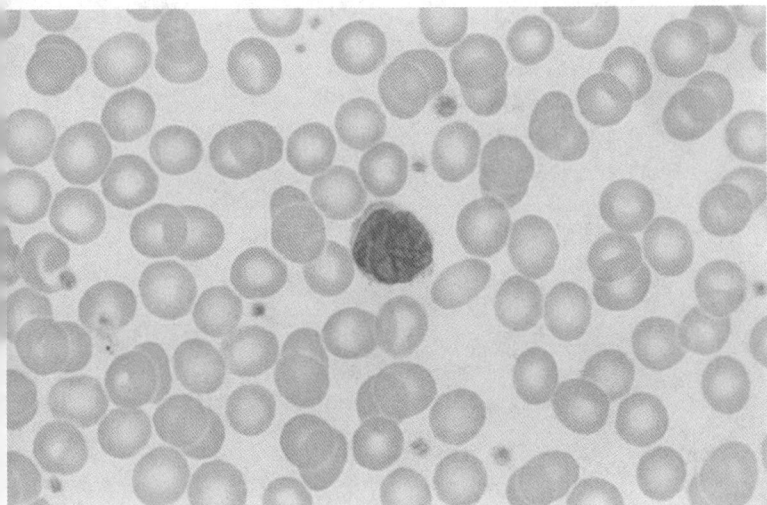

Figure 16–6 Sézary cell. Note the prominent nuclear grooves.

Both MF and SS occur predominantly at older ages, in men slightly more often than women. Mycosis fungoides is characteristically indolent, with median survival ≥10 years. Eventually, the disease becomes refractory, with progressive skin disease and visceral dissemination; survival thereafter is short. Sézary syndrome usually develops de novo, as the initial manifestation of the disease, rather than as transformation from, or terminal phase of, MF. Sézary syndrome tends to be more aggressive than MF, with a shorter survival. However, the disease may respond to a variety of therapies, and a complete response may be followed by long-term disease-free survival.

The diagnosis of SS is established by the finding of numerous lymphocytes with cerebriform nuclei in the blood of patients with generalized erythema. Flow cytometry shows cells expressing the CD4 T helper subset marker. CD25 is usually absent. The absence of CD25, as well as negative serologic assay for HTLV-I, helps differentiate SS from ATL/L.

17

Malignant Lymphomas: Non-Hodgkin's Lymphomas and Hodgkin's Disease

The category of malignant lymphomas includes two main diseases: the **non-Hodgkin's lymphomas** (**NHLs**) and **Hodgkin's disease** (**HD**; also called **Hodgkin's lymphoma**). Hodgkin's disease was described first, but the NHLs are far more common. There are important clinical differences between NHL and HD (Table 17–1), and treatment is different.

Since the NHLs are more common, they will be described first.

Table 17–1
Hodgkin's Disease versus the Non-Hodgkin's Lymphomas

Hodgkin's Disease	Non-Hodgkin's Lymphomas
Orderly contiguous spread	Noncontiguous, widely disseminated spread
Predominant central and axial lymph node involvement; rare peripheral node involvement	Frequent involvement of both central and axial and peripheral lymph nodes
Mesenteric nodes and Waldeyer's ring involved seldom or late	Frequent involvement of mesenteric nodes and Waldeyer's ring
Extranodal presentation rare	Extranodal presentation not uncommon

NON-HODGKIN'S LYMPHOMAS

- Non-Hodgkin's lymphomas are **neoplastic clonal proliferations of lymphocytes**.
- They may involve **lymph nodes, extranodal tissues, or both**. The majority involve lymph nodes, with or without involvement of the liver, spleen, and bone marrow.
- They are usually **systemic, widely disseminated diseases**. A minority are localized at diagnosis.
- Some lymphomas may exhibit **selective sites of involvement**:
  - Lymph nodes versus extranodal sites
  - Involvement of specific sites: skin, gastrointestinal tract, spleen
- They may be **tumors of B lymphocytes or T lymphocytes**. In any individual tumor, the malignant clone will be *either* B cells *or* T cells but not both.
  - In the United States, the majority of lymphomas are derived from B cells (~80 to 85%).

Epidemiology

Non-Hodgkin's lymphomas are currently the fifth leading cause of cancer death in the United States, and the incidence has nearly doubled since 1973. The reasons for the increasing incidence of NHL are not entirely clear; some of the increase is due to human immunodeficiency virus (HIV)-related lymphomas, but this does not account for the entire increase.

- Non-Hodgkin's lymphomas are more common in men than women and more common in Caucasians than African Americans.
- Non-Hodgkin's lymphomas occur at all ages but are predominantly diseases of older adults. The peak age of onset in the United States is in the sixties to seventies.
- Non-Hodgkin's lymphomas in children tend to be aggressive histologic types. Non-Hodgkin's lymphomas in adults are a mix of indolent and aggressive types.

Etiology

The etiology of NHL is, for the most part, unknown. Certain predisposing factors and possible causes have been identified:

- **Genetic predisposition:** There is an increased incidence of NHL in patients with inherited immunodeficiency disorders such as ataxia-telangiectasia, Wiskott-Aldrich syndrome, and common variable immunodeficiency.
- **Pesticides, herbicides, and other chemicals** have been linked to NHL in some studies; however, other studies have not confirmed a correlation.

- **Viruses** of several types have been linked to NHL, especially the **Epstein-Barr virus** (**EBV**). Other implicated viruses include the human T-cell lymphocytotrophic virus I (HTLV-I) and the hepatitis C virus.
  - Epstein-Barr virus infects and immortalizes B cells and stimulates B-cell replication. It appears to be very important in Burkitt's lymphomas, acquired immune deficiency syndrome (AIDS)-related lymphomas, and post-transplant lymphoproliferative disorders.
- Other infections: gastric lymphomas have been linked to *Helicobacter pylori.*
- Some autoimmune diseases increase the risk of lymphomas, including Hashimoto's thyroiditis (linked to thyroid lymphomas) and Sjögren's syndrome.
- **Immunosuppression** predisposes to lymphomas, including HIV, the inherited immunodeficiencies, and immunosuppression for organ transplants.

Cytogenetics and Molecular Biology

As part of the normal process of development, the genes for the lymphocyte antigen receptors (immunoglobulins for B cells, the T-cell receptor [TCR] for T cells) go through a process of genetic recombination, in which portions of the genes are spliced together and other parts of the genes are deleted. This process of rearrangement of the antigen receptor genes allows for the incredible diversity of the immune response but also raises the possibility of genetic accidents, which can predispose to malignancy. It has been shown that chromosomal abnormalities, predominantly reciprocal translocations, are nearly universal in NHL. Not surprisingly, these translocations often involve the lymphocyte antigen receptor genes and genes that are involved in cell proliferation or cell death (*proto-oncogenes*). In the process, the proto-oncogene is brought under the influence of the promoter for the antigen receptor gene and is overexpressed. Consequences of this process can include increased cell proliferation, characteristic of aggressive lymphomas, or resistance to apoptosis (programmed cell death), characteristic of indolent lymphomas.

There are associations between specific chromosomal translocations and specific histologic types of lymphomas (Table 17–2).

Classification of Non-Hodgkin's Lymphomas

Classification of NHL has historically been a problem. Until recently, the most widely used classification system in the United States was the **Working Formulation for the Classification of Lymphomas** (known as the *Working Formulation*), which is based on a combination of histology and

Table 17–2
Chromosomal Translocations in NHL

Translocation	Genes Involved	Lymphoma Type
t(8;14)	Immunoglobulin heavy chain gene; c-*MYC* oncogene	Burkitt's lymphoma (~85% of cases)
t(2;8); t(8;22)	Immunoglobulin light chain genes (κ and λ); c-*MYC*	Burkitt's lymphoma (~15%)
t(14;18)	Immunoglobulin heavy chain gene; *BCL-2*	Follicular lymphomas
t(11;14)	*BCL-1* (*Cyclin D1*); Immunoglobulin heavy chain gene	Mantle cell lymphoma
t(2;5)	*NPM*; *ALK*	Anaplastic large cell lymphomas

survival. The most widely used classification system in Europe was the **updated Kiel classification**, which is based upon putative cell of origin (B cell versus T cell; specific site within the lymph node). In 1994, a group of expert lymphoma pathologists from around the world proposed the **Revised European American Lymphoma Classification** (the *REAL Classification*), which has gradually been gaining acceptance in both the United States and Europe. The REAL Classification incorporated all available information about lymphomas, including standard histology, immunophenotyping, cytogenetic and molecular features, and clinical features. More recently, a group under the auspices of the World Health Organization (WHO) has put together a new Classification, based largely on the REAL classification. The new **WHO classification** will probably become the standard classification system used worldwide. Unfortunately, many older articles and textbooks use the Working Formulation system.

The **Working Formulation** divides lymphomas into three broad grades based on survival: **low grade** (survival ≥5 years), **intermediate grade** (survival ~1.5 to 3 years), and **high grade** (survival <1.5 years). The histologic features in the Working Formulation are **architecture** (*follicular* versus *diffuse*) and **cell size** (predominantly *small* versus *mixed* versus predominantly *large*) (Table 17–3).

- In general, **follicular architecture** or **small cell size** indicate **low-grade disease**.
- **Diffuse architecture** or **large cell size** indicates **aggressive** (intermediate or high-grade) **disease**.

Table 17–3

The Working Formulation for the Classification of Lymphomas

Low Grade

A. Small Lymphocytic (SLL)

B. Follicular, Predominantly Small Cleaved Cell (FSC)

C. Follicular, Mixed Small Cleaved and Large Cell (FM)

Intermediate Grade

D. Follicular, Predominantly Large Cell (FLC)

E. Diffuse, Small Cleaved Cell (DSC)

F. Diffuse, Mixed Small Cleaved and Large Cell (DM)

G. Diffuse, Large Cell (DLC)

High Grade

H. Large Cell, Immunoblastic (LCI)

I. Lymphoblastic (LBL)

J. Small Noncleaved Cell* (SNC)

Miscellaneous

*Includes Burkitt's and non-Burkitt's.

The **WHO classification** is more complex than the Working Formulation (Table 17–4). Like the REAL Classification, the WHO classification includes all types of available information about lymphoid neoplasms.

Principles of the WHO Classification

- The WHO classification divides lymphoid neoplasms into three main categories: **B-cell neoplasms**, **T-cell neoplasms**, and **Hodgkin's lymphoma**.
  - Both lymphocytic leukemias and lymphomas are included.
  - Plasma cell neoplasms (multiple myeloma) are included in the B-cell neoplasms.
- B-cell and T-cell neoplasms are subdivided into
  - **Precursor** (*immature*) types, which predominantly include the acute lymphoblastic leukemias and lymphoblastic lymphomas.
  - **Peripheral** (*mature*) types, which include chronic lymphocytic leukemias and most NHLs.
- The B-cell and T-cell types are listed according to histologic grade, and entities that resemble each other are grouped together.
- The WHO Classification does not group lymphoid neoplasms into broad clinical grades, as in the Working Formulation.
- The WHO classification includes >20 different types of lymphoid neoplasms. Fortunately, the majority of cases fall into a relatively small

Table 17–4
WHO Classification of Lymphoid Neoplasms*

B-Cell Neoplasms

Precursor B-cell neoplasms:
Precursor B-lymphoblastic leukemia/lymphoma (precursor B-cell ALL)

Mature (peripheral) B-cell neoplasms:†
B-cell chronic lymphocytic leukemia/small lymphocytic lymphoma
B-cell prolymphocytic leukemia
Lymphoplasmacytic lymphoma
Splenic marginal zone B-cell lymphoma (+/– villous lymphocytes)
Hairy cell leukemia
Plasma cell myeloma/plasmacytoma
Extranodal marginal zone B-cell lymphoma of MALT type
Nodal marginal zone lymphoma (+/- monocytoid B cells)
Follicular lymphoma
Mantle cell lymphoma
Diffuse large B-cell lymphoma
   Mediastinal large B-cell lymphoma
   Primary effusion lymphoma

Burkitt's lymphoma/Burkitt cell leukemia

T-cell and NK-cell Neoplasms

Precursor T-cell neoplasms:
Precursor T-lymphoblastic lymphoma/leukemia (precursor T-cell ALL)

Mature (peripheral) T-cell neoplasms:†
T-cell prolymphocytic leukemia
T-cell granular lymphocytic leukemia
Aggressive NK-cell leukemia
Adult T-cell lymphoma/leukemia (HTLV1+)
Extranodal NK/T-cell lymphoma, nasal type
Enteropathy-type T-cell lymphoma
Hepatosplenic γ-δ T-cell lymphoma
Subcutaneous panniculitis-like T-cell lymphoma
Mycosis fungoides/Sézary syndrome
Anaplastic large cell lymphoma, T/null cell, primary cutaneous type
Peripheral T-cell lymphoma, not otherwise characterized
Angioimmunoblastic T-cell lymphoma
Anaplastic large cell lymphoma, T/null cell, primary systemic type

Hodgkin's lymphoma (Hodgkin's disease)
Nodular lymphocyte-predominant Hodgkin's (NLPHD)
Classic Hodgkin's:
Nodular sclerosis Hodgkin's (Grades 1 and 2)
Lymphocyte-rich classic Hodgkin's
Mixed cellularity Hodgkin's
Lymphocyte depletion Hodgkin's

---

*Common entities listed in **bold**.
†Peripheral B-cell and T/NK-cell neoplasms grouped according to clinical presentation.
Reproduced with permission from Harris NL, Jaff ES, Diebold J, et al. J Clin Oncol 1999;
17:3835–49.

number of types. The remaining lymphomas are relatively uncommon and will not be described in detail. The two most common are

- Diffuse large B-cell lymphomas: ~30% of lymphomas in the United States
- Follicular lymphomas: ~20% of lymphomas in the United States

Staging of Non-Hodgkin's Lymphomas

The staging system for NHL is the **Ann Arbor staging system** (Table 17–5). The stage is determined by the anatomic spread of disease and also includes the presence or absence of systemic symptoms. In general, *localized-stage* disease (I–II) is better than *advanced-stage* disease (III–IV). The presence of systemic symptoms is a significant adverse prognostic factor.

Staging procedures

Typical staging procedures are summarized in Table 17–6 and include the following:

- History and physical examination, with particular attention to the presence of lymphadenopathy and hepatosplenomegaly
- Complete blood count and routine blood chemistries, including liver profile (lactic dehydrogenase, alkaline phosphatase, alanine aminotransferase [ALT], and aspartate aminotransferase [AST])

Table 17–5
The Ann Arbor Staging System for NHL

Stage	Features
I	Single lymph node or site; may be extranodal (designated stage IE)
II	More than one lymph node or site on the *same side of the diaphragm* (either above or below, but not both)
III	Disease on *both sides of the diaphragm*
IV	Involvement of *liver and/or bone marrow*

Systemic Symptoms Associated with NHL

Fever >38°C without infection or other cause

Severe drenching night sweats

Loss of >10% of body weight within the 6 months prior to diagnosis, not explained by dieting

Presence or absence of symptoms is designated with a suffix (A or B)

A	Systemic symptoms absent
B	Systemic symptoms present

Stage III without symptoms = IIIA; Stage III with symptoms = IIIB

- Chest and abdominal computed tomography (CT) scans
- Bone marrow aspirate and biopsies (sometimes bilateral biopsies)

Table 17–6
Routine Staging Procedures for NHL

History and physical examination
CBC and serum chemistries (liver profile, BUN and creatinine, albumin, lactic dehydrogenase)
CT scans of chest and abdomen
Bone marrow aspirate and biopsy

Indolent versus Aggressive Non-Hodgkin's Lymphomas

In a very basic way, NHLs can broadly be divided into two main types: (1) **indolent lymphomas**, predominantly those lymphomas designated low grade in the Working Formulation, and (2) **aggressive lymphomas**, which include the intermediate-grade and some of the high-grade lymphomas in the Working Formulation. There are important behavioral and treatment distinctions between the indolent and aggressive lymphomas (Table 17–7). The most important difference is that *indolent lymphomas are considered largely incurable* and are therefore usually treated for palliation; *aggressive lymphomas are considered curable* and are therefore treated with curative intent.

Indolent lymphomas may demonstrate a phenomenon known as **histologic transformation**. After a period of months or years, the histologic appearance of the lymphoma may change from an indolent to an aggressive appearance. This occurs most often in patients with follicular lymphomas but can also occur with the other indolent lymphomas. The transformed disease tends to be very aggressive and resistant to therapy, and survival after transformation is usually short.

Prognostic Factors in Non-Hodgkin's Lymphomas

Prognostic factors in NHL can be divided into pathologic factors, such as the histologic classification, and clinical prognostic factors. The **clinical prognostic factors** include the following:

- **Age:** In general, older patients do worse.
- **Stage:** *Localized disease* (stages I and II) is better than *advanced disease* (stages III and IV).

Table 17–7

Indolent versus Aggressive Lymphomas

Indolent*	Aggressive†
Predominantly older population	Occur at all ages
Majority disseminated at diagnosis	Significant proportion localized at presentation
Predominantly lymph node disease ± liver, spleen, and bone marrow; other extranodal sites involved less often or late in disease course	Extranodal disease at presentation not uncommon
Long median survival	Short median survival if untreated
Relentless relapse	Long disease-free survival possible with aggressive therapy
Majority considered incurable with conventional therapy	Significant proportion curable with conventional therapy
Treatment: controversial (conservative versus aggressive chemotherapy)	Treatment: aggressive combination chemotherapy with intent to cure
May not be treated initially if asymptomatic	Always treated immediately

*Includes histologic types categorized as low grade in the Working Formulation for the Classification of Lymphomas.
†Includes intermediate- and high-grade histologic types according to the Working Formulation.

- **Lactic dehydrogenase:** The serum lactic dehydrogenase (LD or LDH) generally reflects tumor bulk and/or aggressiveness. Elevated LDH is worse.
- **Performance status (PS):** Performance status is a measure of the physical condition of the patient. A patient who is fully ambulatory has good performance status (designated 0 to 1). A patient who is not ambulatory has poor performance status (2 to 4).
- **Extranodal disease sites:** The presence of few (≤1) extranodal sites is better than multiple (≥2) extranodal sites.

The above factors were combined into a prognostic index, known as the **International NHL Prognostic Index.** A higher risk score is associated with a decreased complete response rate to therapy, an increased probability of relapsing from complete response, and decreased overall survival (Table 17–8).

Table 17–8
The International NHL Prognostic Index

Risk Factor	Definition of Risk Factor	
Age	≤60 years	versus >60 years
Ann Arbor stage	Localized (I–II)	versus Advanced (III–IV)
Performance status	Good (0–1)	versus Poor (2–4)
Lactic dehydrogenase	≤1 × upper normal limit	versus >1 × upper normal limit
Extranodal sites	≤1	versus >1

The number of adverse risk factors (0 to 5) are added together to define a risk category.

Risk Category	Number of Risk Factors
Low	0–1
Low Intermediate	2
High Intermediate	3
High	4–5

A similar index was created for patients ≤60 years of age, omitting the age variable (the **Age Adjusted International Index**).
Adapted from Shipp MA, Harrington DP, Anderson JR, et al. N Engl J Med 1993;329:987–94.

Diagnosis of Lymphomas

Close coordination and communication between the clinician, the surgeon who does the biopsy, and the pathologist who interprets the specimen is required. A variety of special tests may be required in some cases. Important tests include the following:

- **Histology:** Routine histology is always important and, in some cases, may be all that is needed to make the correct diagnosis.
- **Immunophenotyping:** Detection of lineage-associated markers on the surface of cells can be very helpful. Immunophenotyping can be done by flow cytometry (which requires fresh tissue) or by immunohisto-chemistry on routine sections. Detection of immunoglobulin light chain restriction (ie, marked imbalance in the expression of kappa and lambda light chains on lymphocytes, rather than the normal 2:1 ratio of kappa to lambda) suggests a clonal B-cell population, which is a strong indication of B-cell malignancy.
- **Cytogenetics:** Cytogenetic analysis, either by standard karyotyping or by molecular tests, can be very helpful in subclassifying some cases of

lymphoma that are difficult to subclassify based on histology or phenotyping alone.

- **Antigen receptor gene rearrangement studies:** It is possible to detect a clonal rearrangement of the immunoglobulin or T-cell receptor genes. The presence of such a clonal rearrangement is strong evidence for lymphoid malignancy.

Specific Lymphoma Types

Certain types of lymphomas are worth mentioning, either because they are common or because they have unique clinical and pathologic features.

Diffuse Large B-Cell Lymphomas (Figures 17–1 and 17–2)

- These are the most common type of lymphoma in the United States (~30% of all NHLs).
- They are the prototypic aggressive lymphoma. Median survival is ≤1.5 years if untreated.
- A significant proportion (~30 to 50%) can be cured with aggressive combination chemotherapy.
- They are heterogeneous, with variable histologic appearances and probably diverse molecular mechanisms.

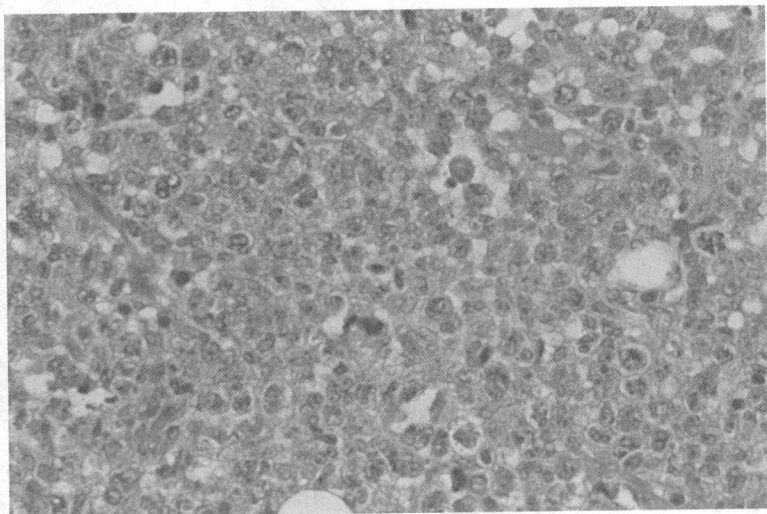

Figure 17–1 Diffuse large B-cell lymphoma, medium power.

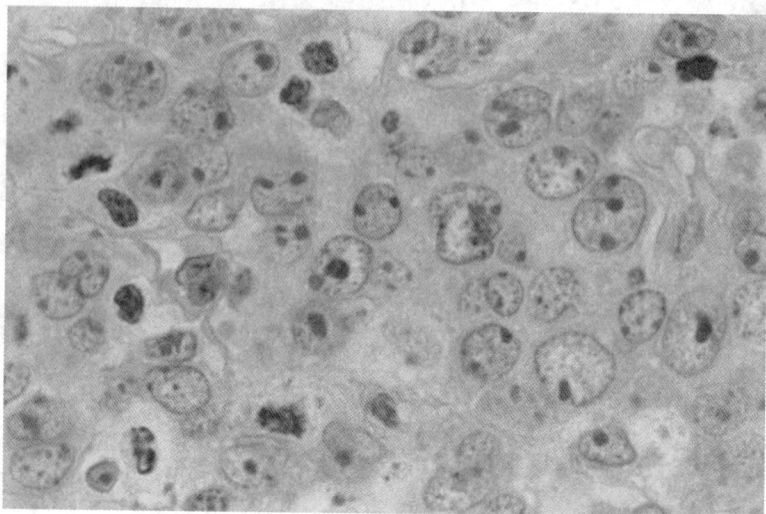

Figure 17–2 Diffuse large B-cell lymphoma, high power.

Follicular Lymphomas (Follicle Center Cell Lymphomas) (Figure 17–3)

- Follicular lymphomas together are the second most common lymphoma type in the United States (~20% of total).
- Follicular small cleaved cell lymphomas are the prototypic and most common indolent lymphoma.

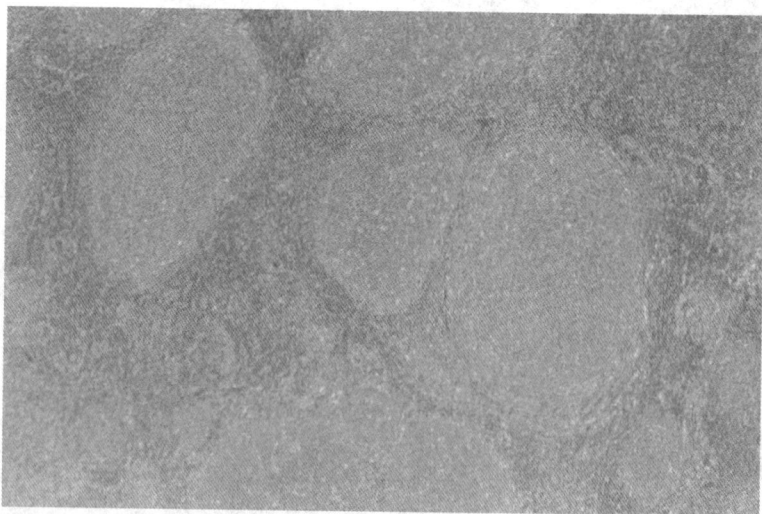

Figure 17–3 Follicular lymphoma.

- The majority of cases are advanced stage at diagnosis, with a high incidence of bone marrow and liver involvement.
- They are subdivided into three histologic grades:
  - Follicular, predominantly small cleaved cell (follicular lymphoma grade I in the WHO classification)
  - Follicular, mixed small cleaved and large cell (follicular lymphoma grade II)
  - Follicular, predominantly large cell (follicular lymphoma grade III)
- Follicular, predominantly small cleaved cell (grade I) and follicular mixed lymphomas (grade II) behave similarly: relatively indolent, with long survival but relentless relapse. Treatment is essentially similar.
- Follicular, predominantly large cell (grade III) lymphomas behave differently. They have a shorter time to relapse but with treatment may have a similar overall survival. A proportion may be curable. Treatment of follicular large cell lymphomas should include an anthracycline drug such as doxorubicin.

Small Lymphocytic Lymphoma (Figure 17–4)

- Small lymphocytic lymphoma (SLL) is the tissue-based equivalent of chronic lymphocytic leukemia (**CLL**). The distinction is based on whether or not there is lymphocytosis in the peripheral blood ($\geq 5,000$ lymphocytes/μL for CLL, $<5,000$ lymphocytes/μL for SLL). They are grouped together in the WHO classification as **B-cell CLL/SLL**.
- B-cell CLL/SLL generally behaves as a low-grade lymphoma.

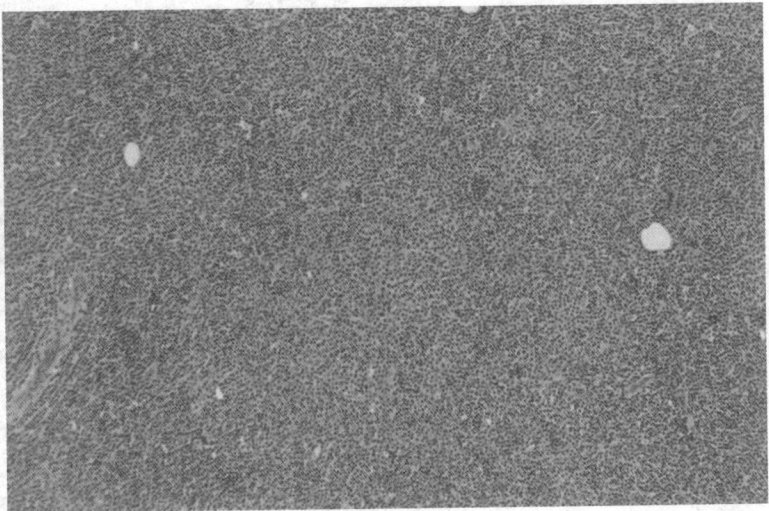

Figure 17–4 Small lymphocytic lymphoma.

- B-cell CLL/SLL has a relatively unique phenotype. The cells express an antigen designated **CD5**, which is usually considered a T-cell marker. The only other B-cell lymphoma that expresses CD5 is mantle cell lymphoma (MCL).

Lymphoma of Mucosa-Associated Lymphoid Tissue (MALT Lymphoma; Extranodal Marginal Zone Lymphoma in the WHO Classification) (Figure 17–5)

- MALT lymphomas are the most common type of extranodal lymphoma.
- The most common site is the stomach. They also occur elsewhere in the gastrointestinal (GI) tract and other mucosal sites, the salivary glands, the breasts, and the thyroid.
- They are characteristically indolent B-cell lymphomas.
- They are frequently localized at diagnosis (stage IE or IIE). Systemic dissemination occurs late, if at all.
- They may be curable with localized therapy (surgery and/or radiation therapy).
- Relapse after therapy frequently occurs at other MALT sites.
- Gastric MALT lymphomas appear to be related to chronic gastritis caused by *Helicobactor pylori*. Early stages of gastric MALT lymphoma may respond to eradication of *Helicobacter* with antibiotics.
- **It is important to note that not all lymphomas occurring in MALT sites are true MALT lymphomas**. Mantle cell lymphomas and other lym-

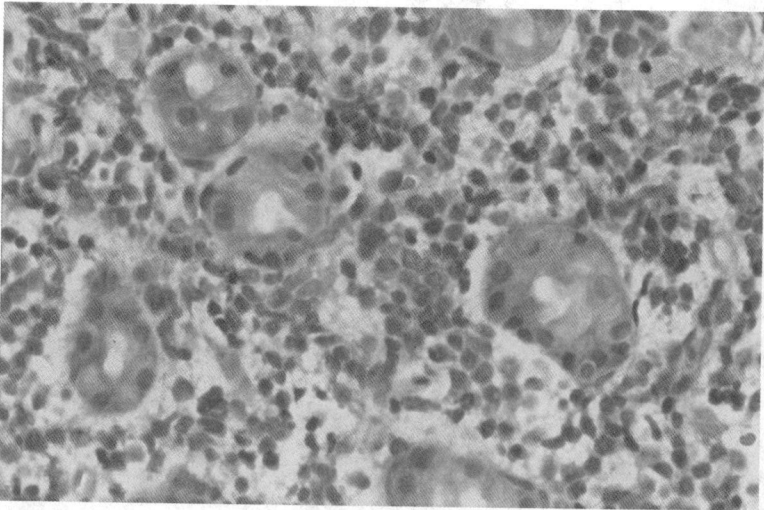

Figure 17–5 Lymphoma of mucosa-associated lymphoid tissue (MALT lymphoma) of the stomach.

phoma types can also involve the GI tract. Lymphomas composed primarily of large cells will not demonstrate the indolent behavior of typical MALT lymphomas and need to be treated as aggressive lymphomas.

Mantle Cell Lymphoma

- Approximately 5 to 10% of lymphoma cases in the United States are MCL, occurring predominantly in older individuals, with a significant male predominance.
- The majority of cases are advanced stage at diagnosis, with a high incidence of bone marrow involvement.
- Mantle cell lymphoma is characterized by generally small cells, with moderate nuclear irregularity (rounder than the cleaved cells of follicular lymphomas, more irregular than the round nuclei of small lymphocytic lymphoma). The histologic appearance can vary.
- There is a strong association with a translocation between chromosomes 11 and 14 [**t(11;14)**]. The gene on chromosome 14 is the immunoglobulin heavy chain gene. The locus on chromosome 11 was originally described as *BCL-1*, but the relevant gene is now known to be the **cyclin D1 gene** (*CCND1*). The translocation results in overexpression of cyclin D1, which is involved in passage through the cell cycle.
- Approximately 20% of patients present with leukemic blood involvement. Mantle cell lymphoma may involve the GI tract, and involvement of the central nervous system (lymphomatous meningitis) also occurs.
- Mantle cell lymphoma is considered by some people to be the worst of all lymphoma types. It has relatively short survival (median 3 to 5 years), like the aggressive lymphomas; however, it is incurable with conventional therapy, like the indolent lymphomas.
- **Mantle cell lymphoma has a characteristic immunophenotype.** Like B-cell CLL/SLL, it coexpresses B-cell markers and **CD5**, usually considered a T-cell marker.

Burkitt's Lymphoma (Working Formulation: Diffuse Small Noncleaved Cell) (Figure 17–6)

- Burkitt's lymphoma is a very high-grade NHL. It is very common in parts of Africa (*endemic Burkitt's*) but also occurs less commonly in the United States (*sporadic Burkitt's*). It characteristically occurs in children and young adults.
- *Burkitt-cell leukemia* (designated **ALL-L3** in the French-American-British classification of acute leukemia) is the leukemic equivalent of Burkitt's lymphoma. The biologic behavior and treatment are identical.
- In Africa, there is a very strong (≥95%) association with **EBV** and a high prevalence in areas of endemic **malaria**. Epstein-Barr virus and malaria

appear to be cofactors in the development of Burkitt's lymphoma. In th United States, there is less association with EBV (~25%).

- There is a universal association between Burkitt's lymphoma an translocation of the **c-MYC proto-oncogene** to one of the **immuno globulin genes** (heavy or light chain).
  - More than 80% have **t(8;14)**: *c-MYC* on chromosome 8 is translo cated to the immunoglobulin heavy chain gene (IgH) on chromo some 14. The remainder involve *c-MYC* and either the kappa ligh chain gene on chromosome 2 or the lambda light chain gene on 22
  - The *c-MYC* gene is involved with passaging cells through the cel cycle, and overexpression results in an extremely high proliferativ rate. Burkitt's lymphoma is probably the fastest growing tumor ir humans.
- The classic presentation of African Burkitt's is a huge rapidly growing jaw mass in a young child. There may be involvement of abdomina organs (particularly ovaries), and breast involvement is common ir pregnant or nursing women.
- In the United States, the majority of patients present with intra-abdom inal disease, usually involving the gastrointestinal tract. Jaw tumors are uncommon.
- Burkitt's lymphoma formerly had a dismal prognosis. Now, with very intensive chemotherapy, the prognosis in children has improved signif icantly; however, the prognosis in adults remains poor.

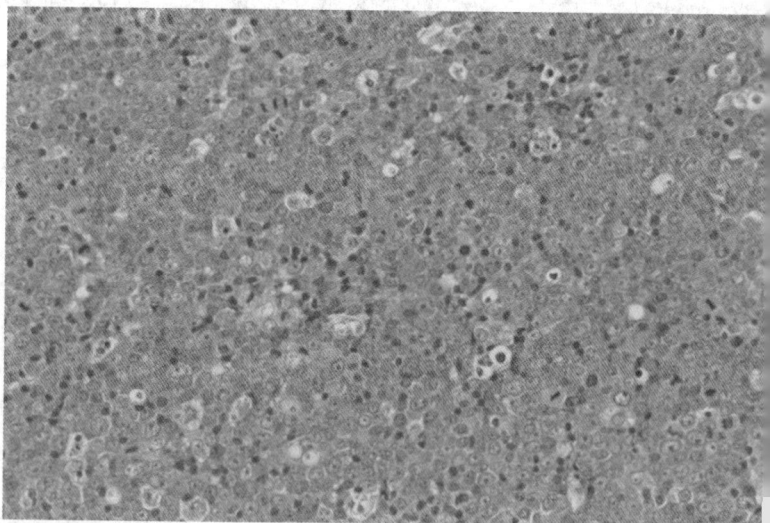

Figure 17–6 Burkitt's lymphoma. Rapidly growing jaw tumor in an 8-year-old American child. The histologic pattern is described as a "starry sky" appearance.

- Chemotherapy may result in a tumor lysis syndrome in patients with a high tumor bulk. Hydration, alkalinization of the urine, and allopurinol are usually used to prevent acute renal failure.

T-Cell Lymphomas

- T-cell lymphomas are relatively uncommon in the United States, approximately 15% of all lymphomas. T-cell lymphomas are far more common in the Far East.
- T-cell lymphomas are highly heterogeneous. The majority fall into a category designated *peripheral* (ie, post-thymic or mature) *T-cell lymphomas* (**PTCLs**). There are a variety of specific subtypes of T-cell lymphomas, most of which are rare.
- Compared to B-cell lymphomas, T-cell lymphomas tend to have a *higher incidence of extranodal disease*, are more often *advanced stage at diagnosis*, and are frequently associated with *systemic* ("B") *symptoms*. The overall prognosis appears to be worse in patients with T-cell lymphomas.

Mycosis Fungoides/Sézary Syndrome

- *Mycosis fungoides* (MF) is a cutaneous T-cell lymphoma, with a T helper (CD4$^+$) phenotype.
- It presents as patches, plaques, or tumors on the skin.
- It generally follows an indolent course, with long survival. The disease is limited to the skin for a prolonged period. Systemic/visceral spread eventually occurs after a period of years.
- *Sézary syndrome* is a related condition, in which patients present with generalized erythema (rather than plaques or nodules) and circulating atypical or "cerebriform" lymphocytes (known as Sézary cells) in the blood. Sézary syndrome tends to follow a more aggressive course than MF, with relatively short survival.

Lymphoblastic Lymphoma

- Lymphoblastic lymphoma is an uncommon high-grade lymphoma composed of **immature** (*precursor*) **lymphocytes**.
- The majority of cases (~80%) are composed of *precursor T cells*. A small number are precursor B cells.
- Lymphoblastic lymphoma is distinguished from acute lymphoblastic leukemia (ALL) by the presence or absence of bone marrow involvement. If >25% of cells in the marrow are lymphoblasts, then the diagnosis is ALL; if <25% of cells in the marrow are lymphoblasts, the diagnosis is lymphoblastic lymphoma.

- The peak age of occurrence is in adolescents to young adults (most <20 years), with a significant male predominance.
- Patients often have a large mediastinal mass, possibly related to origin in the thymus. Respiratory failure due to compression of the airways may be a lethal complication.
- Lymphoblastic lymphoma is treated similarly to ALL. The prognosis in young patients is favorable.
- As in ALL, central nervous system (CNS) relapse (*lymphomatous meningitis*) may occur if CNS prophylaxis is not given.

Anaplastic Large Cell (Ki-1⁺) Lymphoma

- Anaplastic large cell lymphoma has a distinctive morphology (characteristic large anaplastic cells with wreath-like or multiple nuclei) and often expresses the CD30 (Ki-1) phenotypic marker.
- Two clinical forms exist:
  - A cutaneous form with an indolent course, more common in adults
  - A systemic form that generally behaves like other large cell NHL, which is fairly common in children and young adults
- The majority are T-cell lineage.
- There is an association between the characteristic anaplastic large cell appearance, Ki-1 expression, and a specific chromosomal translocation: **t(2,5)(p23;q35)**.
  - The translocation involves the gene for a nucleolar phosphoprotein (nucleophosmin; **NPM**) and a putative oncogene (**ALK**), which is a protein tyrosine kinase. The result is a fusion protein designated *NPM-ALK*.
- The prognosis for the systemic variant is relatively favorable; patients have a good chance of cure with chemotherapy. The cutaneous variant tends to have a very indolent course, with long survival; systemic dissemination can occur but usually not until many years after diagnosis.

Human Immunodeficiency Virus–Related Lymphomas

- The risk of NHL is increased by ~100 to 300 times in patients with HIV infection. Non-Hodgkin's lymphoma is the AIDS-defining illness in about 3% of AIDS cases. It is the cause of death in up to 16% of HIV-infected individuals.
- Currently, ~10% of newly diagnosed lymphomas in the United States are HIV related.
- Non-Hodgkin's lymphoma occurs in all HIV risk groups. The incidence increases with duration of HIV infection and with decreasing CD4 count.
- Human immunodeficiency virus appears to play an indirect role in the development of NHL. T-cell suppression of B-cell proliferation is

removed, and B cells are stimulated to proliferate, setting the stage for genetic accidents. Epstein-Barr virus appears to be related to AIDS lymphoma; approximately half of tumors contain the EBV genome. The *c-MYC* oncogene is frequently involved.

- Nearly all cases are aggressive histologic types: ~one-third are small non-cleaved cell (Burkitt's or Burkitt-like), ~one-third are large cell immunoblastic, and most of the remainder are diffuse large cell types. The great majority have a B-cell phenotype.

- Characteristics of HIV-related lymphoma include *advanced stage at diagnosis* ($\geq 80\%$ stage IV), *frequent systemic symptoms* ($\geq 90\%$), and a *high incidence of extranodal disease*. The most common sites of involvement are the **GI tract** (~25%), **bone marrow** (20%), **liver** (10 to 25%), and **central nervous system**. The lymphoma can involve very unusual sites.

- **Primary central nervous system** lymphoma is common. In contrast, CNS lymphomas are unusual in immunocompetent people ($\leq 2\%$).

  - Up to 20% of patients with systemic (ie, not primary CNS) HIV-related lymphomas have involvement of the cerebrospinal fluid. Therefore, examination of the spinal fluid is required at diagnosis in all patients with HIV-related lymphomas, even in the absence of neurologic symptoms.

- An unusual type of lymphoma occurring in AIDS is the *primary body cavity lymphoma*, which involves the pleural or peritoneal spaces rather than lymph nodes or tissues. This appears to be related to human herpesvirus 8 (also known as the Kaposi's sarcoma–related virus) and EBV.

- Treatment of AIDS-related NHL includes systemic combination chemotherapy; the doses used are reduced compared to patients without HIV. Up to ~40% of patients have complete responses.

- The overall outlook of patients with HIV-related lymphoma is poor. Median survival after diagnosis is 8 to 12 months; however, patients with complete response to chemotherapy may have prolonged survival.

- Poor prognostic factors include age >35 years, history of intravenous drug abuse, diagnosis of AIDS prior to the diagnosis of lymphoma, CD4 count <100/μL, poor performance status, stage III or IV disease, and increased LDH.

- Human immunodeficiency virus–related primary CNS lymphoma has the worst prognosis. Median survival is ≤ 3 to 4 months in most series.

Post-Transplantation Lymphoproliferative Disorders

- Patients who are immunosuppressed to prevent organ transplant rejection are subject to a spectrum of lymphoproliferative disorders, from polyclonal and polymorphic (presumed not truly malignant) to mon oclonal, monomorphic, and high grade (highly malignant).

- The incidence varies with different organ transplants, probably relate to the intensity of immunosuppression required (greater immunosup pression leads to higher incidence):
  - Heart-lung (~4%) > heart or liver (~2%) > renal (~1%)
- There are many similarities to HIV-related lymphomas, including high incidence of extranodal disease (including the GI tract and CNS frequent advanced stage at diagnosis, and a marked excess of B-ce phenotype.
- Epstein-Barr virus appears to be important in the pathogenesis of trans plant lymphomas. The EBV genome can be found in tumor cells i nearly all cases.
- Treatment and survival depend on the phase of the disease. Patient with polymorphic B-cell hyperplasia may respond to decrease immunosuppression and acyclovir. Patients with overt malignant lym phoma have a poor response to chemotherapy and generally poo survival.

Treatment of Non-Hodgkin's Lymphomas

Treatment of NHLs will vary depending on whether the lymphoma is a indolent or an aggressive histologic type and whether it is localized (stage I–II) or advanced (stages III–IV). Therapy for certain specific types ma also vary (ie, antibiotic therapy for low-grade gastric MALT lymphoma associated with *Helicobacter*).

Indolent Lymphomas

Treatment of indolent lymphomas is somewhat controversial. At present there is little evidence that treatment at the time of initial diagnosis o *asymptomatic* patients with indolent lymphomas improves overall survival Some experts have advocated a "watchful waiting" approach: observe the patient without treatment and institute treatment when the patient has sig nificant symptoms or problems related to the lymphoma. *Symptomatic* patients, on the other hand, require immediate therapy. There are a variety of treatment options, including the following:

- **Systemic chemotherapy:** A variety of regimens have been used, includ ing chlorambucil or chlorambucil plus prednisone. Combination chemotherapy regimens include: COP (cyclophosphamide, vincristine [Oncovin], and prednisone) and COPP (cyclophosphamide, vin cristine, prednisone, and procarbazine). More aggressive regimens such as cyclophosphamide, doxorubicin (hydroxydaunorubicin; Adriamycin), vincristine, and prednisone (CHOP) have been tried but have not proven superior to the less aggressive regimens.

- **Radiation therapy:** Radiation therapy may be useful in indolent lymphomas. In particular, the rare patients with localized indolent lymphomas (stages I–II) may have prolonged disease-free survival (possibly cure) with extended field or total lymphoid irradiation.
- **Interferon:** Several trials have shown that interferon used with chemotherapy or as maintenance after chemotherapy may lead to prolonged disease-free survival. However, toxicity limits its use.
- **Fludarabine:** Fludarabine has become widely used, particularly for relapsed or refractory cases.
- **Immunologic agents:** A variety of immune-based therapies have been tried in indolent lymphomas. **Rituximab** (Rituxan), a chimeric (part mouse, part human) antibody directed against the CD20 B-cell antigen, has become widely used in indolent lymphomas. Antibodies against other lymphoid antigens are expected to become available in the future. Other immunologic therapies, such as tumor vaccines, are in clinical trials.
- **Hematopoietic stem cell transplant:** High-dose chemotherapy with autologous hematopoietic stem cells (bone marrow transplant) has been tried, but high transplant-related mortality rates have limited its use.

Aggressive Lymphomas

Curative-intent combination chemotherapy should be used in all patients who are able to tolerate it. Cure is possible in a substantial fraction of patients (~30 to 50% in different series). Treatment options for aggressive lymphomas include the following:

- **Systemic chemotherapy:** The most commonly used regimen includes cyclophosphamide, doxorubicin (hydroxydaunorubicin; Adriamycin), vincristine (Oncovin), and prednisone (CHOP). A variety of other regimens have been tried, but none have proved substantially superior in controlled trials.
- **Radiation therapy:** Radiation therapy is useful in patients with localized aggressive lymphomas (in combination with chemotherapy) and may also be useful in patients with bulky disease causing local symptoms.
- **Hematopoietic stem cell transplant:** High-dose chemotherapy with hematopoietic stem cell support (usually autologous peripheral blood progenitor cells harvested by apheresis) has become widely used in patients who have relapsed after conventional combination chemotherapy. There is evidence that *initial* treatment with high-dose chemother-

apy with stem cell support may lead to improved overall survival in patients with adverse risk factors, as defined in the International Prognostic Index.

Patients with localized disease (stage I–II, without a large tumor bulk) have very good survival rates with localized radiation together with an abbreviated course of combination chemotherapy.

HODGKIN'S DISEASE (HODGKIN'S LYMPHOMA)

Hodgkin's disease is dear to the hearts of hematologists and hematopathologists because Thomas Hodgkin's description of seven cases in 1832 was the first description of a distinct disease of hematopoietic or lymphoid tissues. Hodgkin's disease is also historically important in that it was one of the first neoplasms in which a substantial portion of patients could be cured of their disease.

There are important differences in clinical behavior between Hodgkin's disease and NHL (see Table 17–1), and the treatment and prognosis also differ. One of the most important differences is that HD tends to spread in an orderly contiguous fashion (from one lymph node to the next down the path of lymphatic drainage). The widespread dissemination typical of NHL is uncommon in HD.

Hodgkin's disease is characterized by the presence of a very distinctive cell, designated the **Reed-Sternberg (RS) cell** (Figure 17–7). The classic RS cell is large and appears binucleate; each nucleus has a large eosinophilic nucleolus. The nuclei in classic RS cells have been likened to "owl's eyes." There are several described variants of the classic RS cell, and certain variants are associated with specific histologic subtypes of HD. Often the RS cells are greatly outnumbered by the benign background cells (lymphocytes, plasma cells, histiocytes, and eosinophils). *It is important to remember that cells identical in appearance to RS cells can be seen in NHLs, other malignancies, and even benign processes such as infectious mononucleosis.*

➪ Some people prefer the term Hodgkin's *lymphoma* over Hodgkin's *disease*; both are considered acceptable.

Epidemiology

- The incidence of HD is approximately one-fifth that of non-Hodgkin's lymphomas; ~7,500 cases per year in the United States.
- There is a slight overall male predominance.
- There is a bimodal age distribution in United States:
  - The first peak occurs in adolescents and young adults (~15 to 35 years). There is little difference between the sexes, and the most common histologic type is nodular sclerosis HD.

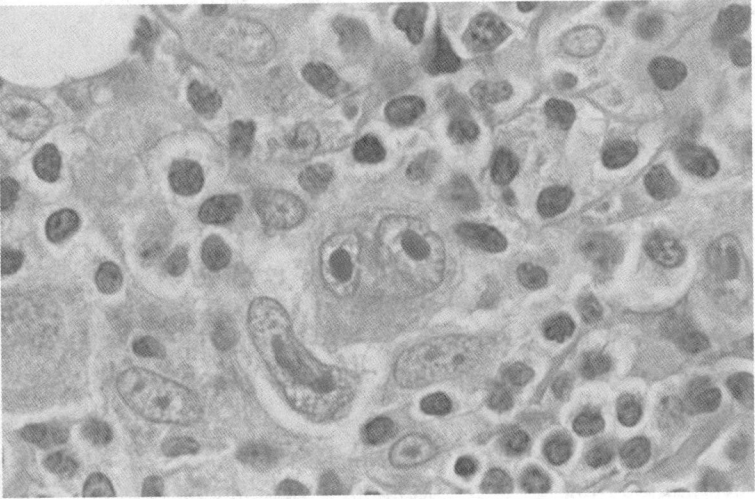

Figure 17–7 Hodgkin's disease: Reed-Sternberg cell. Large binucleate cell with prominent nucleoli in each nucleus.

- The second peak occurs in older adults (>~50 years). There is a male predominance, and the most common histologic type is mixed cellularity. Hodgkin's disease appears to be more aggressive in the older population.

Etiology

- The etiology of HD is largely unknown.
- Genetic factors probably play a role as there is an increased incidence in some families and a high concordance rate in monozygotic twins. There is an association between HD and certain HLA types.
- Epstein-Barr virus has been implicated in HD. There is ~3-fold increase in HD in patients with history of mononucleosis, and the EBV genome can be shown in the malignant cells in ≥50% of cases.
- Interaction between EBV and other factors (possibly genetic, immunologic, or another virus) may be involved.

Cell of Origin

The cell of origin of HD has long been the "Holy Grail" of hematopathology. Nearly every cell that can be found in a lymph node has been suggested as the normal counterpart of the RS cell. Nodular lymphocytic predominance (one HD subtype) is now clearly established to originate from lymphocytes (B cells). The cell of origin of other HD subtypes has not been definitely established, although mounting evidence indicates that they are also derived from B cells.

Pathology and Histologic Classification of Hodgkin's Disease

In contrast to the profusion of histologic types and frequent classification changes of *non*-Hodgkin's lymphomas, the classification of HD is relatively simple and constant. The histologic classification system used for HD since 1966 is the **Rye Classification**, which contains only four histologic subtypes. The classification of HD in the new **WHO classification** is slightly modified from the Rye (Table 17–9). The WHO classification separates nodular lymphocyte predominance HD (NLPHD) from the other types, which are grouped together as classic HD. It also adds another subtype, lymphocyte-rich classic HD. Nodular lymphocyte predominance HD is separate from the other types because it has a B-cell immunophenotype; the other types share a common phenotype that differs from that of NLPHD (Table 17–10).

Pathologic and Clinical Characteristics of Hodgkin's Disease Subtypes

Nodular Lymphocyte Predominance

- Nodular lymphocyte predominance HD is relatively uncommon—only ~2 to 10% of HD cases.
- The key characteristics of NLPHD are rare RS cells and a predominance of background cells (lymphocytes and/or histiocytes), which are presumed to be benign. Nodular lymphocyte predominance HD has a specific RS cell variant called the "popcorn" cell.

Table 17–9
Pathologic Classification of Hodgkin's Disease

Rye Classification	WHO Classification
Lymphocyte predominance	Nodular lymphocyte predominance
Nodular sclerosis	Classic Hodgkin's variants:
Mixed cellularity	Nodular sclerosis
Lymphocyte depletion	Mixed cellularity
	Lymphocyte depletion
	Lymphocyte-rich classic Hodgkin's

Table 17–10
Phenotype of Hodgkin's Disease

Variant	CD45 (LCA)*	CD20 (B-cells)	CD15 (Leu-M1)	CD30 (Ki-1)
Nodular lymphocytic predominance	+	+	−	−
Classic Hodgkin's†	−	−	+ (80%)	+

*LCA = leukocyte common antigen.
†Nodular sclerosis, mixed cellularity, lymphocyte depletion, lymphocyte-rich classic Hodgkin's.

- Nodular lymphocyte predominance HD is most common in young males (below age 35). It often presents as a single lymph node in the cervical, supraclavicular, axillary, or inguinal area.
- The course is generally indolent, with long median survival. Some series have shown late relapses, but this has not occurred in other series. Patients may have long survival despite the occurrence of relapse.
- Three to 10% of NLPHD cases transform into diffuse large cell NHLs. Even after transformation, the clinical course is often indolent, with long survival.

Nodular Sclerosis Hodgkin's Disease

- Nodular sclerosis HD is the most common subtype of HD in United States (~40 to 80% of cases).
- It is most common in young patients (<45 years), with a slight female predominance.
- Patients frequently present with lower cervical or supraclavicular lymphadenopathy; *involvement of the **mediastinum** is characteristic.*
- It is characterized histologically by bands of dense collagen dividing the lymph node into large nodules and by a specific RS cell variant called the "lacunar" cell.
- Patients frequently have limited-stage disease (stage II) at diagnosis and a relatively indolent course.

Mixed Cellularity Hodgkin's Disease

- Mixed cellularity HD is the second most common type in United States (~20 to 40%).
- It is characterized histologically by more frequent RS cells and a variable cellular background, frequently but not invariably including plasma cells and eosinophils.
- Mixed cellularity HD tends to occur at a slightly older age and is more common in men than women.

- The clinical course tends to be more aggressive than NLPHD and nodular sclerosis HD, with more advanced stage at presentation (stage III–IV) and a shorter survival if untreated.

Lymphocyte Depletion Hodgkin's Disease

- Lymphocyte depletion HD is now rare in the United States, ≤5% in most series. Many cases previously diagnosed as lymphocyte depletion HD are now diagnosed as large cell *non*-Hodgkin's lymphomas, other variants of HD, or occasionally as other neoplasms (metastatic carcinoma or melanoma).
- There are two histologic variants: one with a predominance of RS cells and a paucity of benign cells, the other with diffuse fibrosis and only rare RS or benign cells.
- The course is generally aggressive. The patients usually present with advanced-stage disease, and untreated survival is poor.

Lymphocyte-Rich Classic Hodgkin's Disease

- Lymphocyte-rich classic Hodgkin's as a new subtype recognized in the WHO classification. It was not recognized in the Rye Classification.
- The exact incidence is unknown, but it is uncommon. It occurs primarily in males and often presents as localized disease (stage I–II).
- Histologically, it is characterized by a predominance of benign cells and a paucity of RS cells. Unlike NLPHD, it has classic RS cells and the classic HD phenotype.
- The clinical course appears indolent, with good long-term prognosis.

Clinical Evaluation of Hodgkin's Disease

Staging of Hodgkin's Disease

The staging system used for HD is the *Ann Arbor staging system* (the same system used for NHLs; in fact, it was originally designed for HD). The stages are exactly the same, the same systemic systems are considered significant, and the presence or absence of systemic symptoms is designated with the same suffixes used for NHL. There is one significant difference in staging between HD and NHL: staging of HD is subdivided into *clinical stage* and *pathologic stage*, whereas only clinical stage is used for NHL.

- **Clinical stage** is based on history, physical examination, routine laboratory studies, radiographic studies (radiograph and/or CT of chest, CT of the abdomen), and bone marrow biopsy.

- **Pathologic stage** is based on the above, plus *staging laparotomy* with biopsy of multiple intra-abdominal lymph node groups, liver biopsies, and splenectomy.
- Staging laparotomy for pathologic staging is performed if the patient's disease appears to be localized and radiation therapy is being considered as the primary treatment. If the patient appears to have advanced disease, or if chemotherapy is going to be used as primary therapy, a staging laparotomy is not needed.
- A *gallium scan* is used in many centers for staging HD. If the patient's disease shows up on the scan at diagnosis, gallium scans can later be used to follow the disease after therapy. This is particularly useful in patients who have residual masses after completing therapy. If the residual mass is gallium negative, it probably represents a scar rather than residual disease; positivity on gallium scan suggests residual tumor.

Differential Diagnosis of Hodgkin's Disease

- **Benign conditions:** Infectious mononucleosis, other viral infections, and localized infections enter into the differential. Clinically, any cause of lymphadenopathy can raise a question of HD.
- **Non-Hodgkin's lymphoma** is now the most common misdiagnosis of HD.
  - Mistaken diagnosis of NHL as HD is more common in older patients, those with an atypical clinical presentation for HD, and those with a histologic diagnosis of lymphocyte depletion subtype.
  - As noted, cells identical to classic RS cells can be seen in NHL, especially T-cell types.

Treatment of Hodgkin's Disease

The two primary treatments of HD are radiation therapy and combination chemotherapy. **Anatomic stage (spread of disease) is the most important factor in choosing therapy for HD.** In general,

- **Limited disease** (low stage [I–II]; no bulky disease or complicating factors): The treatment of choice is **radiation therapy**.
- **Advanced disease** (stage III–IV, or lower stage with bulky disease, systemic symptoms, or other complicating factors): The treatment of choice is **combination chemotherapy**.
- Both radiation therapy and chemotherapy are used for some patients with bulky advanced disease (*combined modality therapy*).
- Used appropriately, radiation therapy and chemotherapy have equivalent success rates. Primary radiation therapy has an advantage in that

relapses can often be salvaged with chemotherapy. Many patients who relapse after chemotherapy can be salvaged with additional chemotherapy, but the success rate is not as good.

- The current aim of therapy is to maintain the very good cure rates in HD while minimizing side effects of therapy, particularly second malignancies.

Radiation Therapy

Radiation therapy was the first treatment shown to cure patients with HD, and it still has a significant role as primary therapy for HD.

- The aim is to include all known sites of disease, plus one additional lymph node group, above and below, within the radiation field.
- Disease above the diaphragm is often treated with a mantle field, covering the mediastinum and the supraclavicular and cervical lymph nodes. Disease below the diaphragm is often treated with an inverted-Y field, covering the periaortic lymph nodes, the inguinal lymph nodes, and the splenic area.

Chemotherapy

- Chemotherapy is used when all sites of disease cannot be encompassed within a reasonable radiation field. Patients should receive at least six cycles of chemotherapy or treatment to complete response plus two additional cycles.
- The first successful chemotherapy regimen was **MOPP** (mechlorethamine, vincristine [Oncovin], prednisone, and procarbazine). MOPP is successful but is leukemogenic, and therefore other regimens are preferred at many centers.
- Another popular regimen is **ABVD** (doxorubicin [Adriamycin], bleomycin, vinblastine, and dacarbazine), which is less leukemogenic than MOPP. ABVD can be used as the sole regimen or in alternating cycles with MOPP (**MOPP-ABVD**). Many other chemotherapy regimens are also available.

High-Dose Chemotherapy with Hematopoietic Stem Cell Support

- High-dose chemotherapy with hematopoietic stem cell support (usually autologous peripheral blood progenitor cells collected by apheresis) is frequently used in patients who relapse after standard chemotherapy treatment. It can also be used in patients who have not achieved an initial complete response with chemotherapy; this group otherwise has a very poor prognosis.

Side Effects of Therapy

Radiation Therapy

Side effects of radiation therapy are primarily limited to the irradiated field and can include pulmonary fibrosis, premature coronary atherosclerosis, hypothyroidism, and secondary malignancies. Secondary malignancies following radiation are predominantly carcinomas and occur in the radiated field. Examples include carcinomas of the lung, head and neck, stomach, thyroid, and breast carcinoma in women who receive radiation to the breasts while young (teens and twenties). Patients can also get malignant melanomas of the skin and osteosarcomas of bone. The risk of secondary malignancies with radiation therapy increases progressively with time.

Chemotherapy

- There are unique side effects associated with specific drugs. For example, doxorubicin (Adriamycin) can produce a cardiomyopathy, vincristine can cause neurotoxicity (peripheral neuropathies), and bleomycin can produce pulmonary fibrosis.
- Infertility is a problem with certain chemotherapy regimens, particularly in men. Azoospermia occurs in nearly all men who receive six cycles of MOPP. ABVD appears to have less effect on fertility. There is less effect on fertility in women.
- The most feared complication of chemotherapy is **treatment-related acute myeloid** (nonlymphocytic) **leukemia**. This is most strongly related to alkylating agents, such as mechlorethamine and procarbazine (both part of MOPP). Patients treated with MOPP alone have a ~9- to 14-fold increase in the risk of AML (absolute risk ~2 to 4%). The risk begins to increase 2 to 5 years after treatment, peaks at ~5 to 10 years after the start of therapy, and decreases after 10 years. There is often a brief myelodysplastic period preceding the overt leukemia. The leukemia is usually resistant to therapy, and survival is poor.
- The risk of treatment-related AML is dramatically increased in patients who received combined modality therapy of MOPP and radiation therapy, or MOPP as salvage therapy for relapse after primary radiation.

Prognosis

Today the prognosis of patients with HD is very good, with cure obtained in ≥80% of patients overall, and about two-thirds of patients with advanced disease at diagnosis. Important adverse prognostic factors include older age, the presence of systemic symptoms, and involvement of liver or bone marrow (Table 17–11). The histologic subtype does not appear to be prognostically significant in adequately treated patients.

Table 17–11

Adverse Prognostic Factors in Hodgkin's Disease

Age ≥45 years

Male

Involvement of bone marrow, liver, pleura, or multiple extranodal sites

Presence of systemic symptoms

Bulky mediastinal disease

Low serum albumin (<4 g/dL)

Anemia (hemoglobin <10.5 g/dL)

Leukocytosis (>15,000/μL)

Lymphopenia (<600/μL)

Increased erythrocyte sedimentation rate (ESR)

EVALUATING A PATIENT WITH LYMPHADENOPATHY: WHEN AND HOW TO BIOPSY A LYMPH NODE

An important clinical question is how to evaluate a palpable lymph node in a patient: when to biopsy a lymph node and how to do it. There are a variety of causes of lymphadenopathy in addition to malignant lymphoma (Table 17–12). In general, benign causes are far more common than malignant causes. The goal is to recognize causes that require treatment (lymphomas, other malignant neoplasms, and infectious diseases such as tuberculosis) without undue delay, and without biopsying an excessive number of normal or reactive lymph nodes.

Evaluation of Lymphadenopathy

- **Size:** It is not unusual for a careful examiner to palpate small lymph nodes in normal people. **Significant lymphadenopathy** can be defined as **≥1 cm in adults** and **≥2 cm in children**.
- **Age of the patient:** Children tend to have more prominent lymphadenopathy than adolescents or adults; **in general, lymphadenopathy is more concerning in adults than children**. The causes of lymphadenopathy also vary with age. The risk of malignancy is much higher in older adults than children and adolescents; metastatic carcinoma is rare in childhood but is a common cause of lymphadenopathy is adults.
  - In children, lymph node size >2 cm, abnormal chest radiograph, weight loss, or night sweats are indications to consider biopsy. If

Table 17–12
Causes of Lymphadenopathy

Reaction to Infections

Bacteria: localized or systemic infection

Viral: infectious mononucleosis (EBV), cytomegalovirus, HIV, other

Parasites: toxoplasmosis

Direct Infection of the Lymph Node

Bacteria: *Staphylococcus* species, *Pasteurella pestis* (plague)

Cat-scratch disease

Mycobacteria: tuberculosis, atypical mycobacteria

Fungi

Malignancies

Non-Hodgkin's lymphomas

Hodgkin's disease

Metastatic carcinoma

Metastatic melanoma

Others

Miscellaneous

Autoimmune diseases: systemic lupus erythematosus, others

Sarcoidosis

Drug reaction: phenytoin, other hydantoins

Kikuchi-Fujimoto disease (histiocytic necrotizing lymphadenitis)

Other

---

none of these are present, the probability of a serious abnormality in the lymph node is low.

- **Characteristics of the lymph node:** Infected nodes may be tender or fluctuant, and the overlying skin may be inflamed. Reactive lymph nodes may be tender, but other signs of inflammation are usually absent. Lymph nodes with metastatic carcinoma may be hard and fixed to surrounding tissues. Malignant lymphomas may feel firm or rubbery but are usually not rock hard or fixed to surrounding tissues.
- **Site of lymph node:** The significance of lymphadenopathy can vary with the site. Supraclavicular lymphadenopathy is almost always significant; axillary and inguinal lymph nodes are more often reactive; and cervical lymphadenopathy is often reactive but can represent lymphoma or metastatic carcinoma from the head and neck.

- **Persistence or growth:** A lymph node that has been present ≥4 to 6 weeks, or is growing after 2 weeks of observation, should be considered suspicious.
- **Possible localized sources:** Lymph nodes draining a site of infection may be enlarged as a reaction to the infection; therefore, carefully examine the areas draining to the enlarged lymph node.
  - Cervical adenopathy: Scalp, ears, and throat. Sinus infections and dental abscesses can be occult causes of cervical lymphadenopathy.
  - Axillae: Hands and arms
  - Inguinal: Feet and legs, including cutaneous fungal infections (athlete's foot)
- **Evidence of a systemic infection:** Infectious mononucleosis, hepatitis, other systemic infections.
- **Past medical history and medications:** A history of malignant neoplasms, other systemic illnesses, exposure to tuberculosis or other infectious diseases, and medications, particularly phenytoin and other hydantoins.
- **Tests:***
  - Complete blood count and serum chemistries
  - Chest radiograph
  - Serologic studies for EBV, toxoplasmosis, hepatitis, and HIV

Pathologic Evaluation of Lymph Nodes

Once it has been decided that a lymph node requires pathologic evaluation, there are two general ways to proceed: *fine-needle aspirate cytology* and *excisional biopsy*.

Fine-Needle Aspirate Cytology

- Cells from the lymph node are aspirated with a small needle and syringe, smeared out on a slide, stained, and reviewed by a pathologist. The procedure is simple, noninvasive, safe, and (with a little training) can be done in the office. Many pathologists are willing and able to perform the procedure on superficial lymph nodes, and the procedure can also be done on deeper nodes using ultrasonography, CT scan, or other imaging techniques for guidance.
- Fine-needle aspirate (FNA) cytology is an excellent *screening* and *triage* tool for evaluation of lymphadenopathy. It is usually possible to diagnose metastatic carcinoma and sometimes possible to diagnose inflammatory processes. Aspirated material can also be sent for microbial cultures.

---

*The diagnostic evaluation and specific tests ordered will vary depending on history, physical findings, and clinical judgment.

- If the smears show a predominance of lymphocytes, additional aspirates can be obtained and sent for immunophenotyping by flow cytometry. The combination of immunophenotyping and cytologic interpretation by a skilled cytopathologist has good diagnostic accuracy for reactive processes versus NHL. Cytologic interpretation *alone* has lower accuracy.
- Some lymphoma types have characteristic immunophenotypes, and it is possible to make a very specific diagnosis of these lymphomas with the combination of cytology and flow cytometry.
- It is sometimes possible to suggest a diagnosis of HD by FNA cytology by observing RS cells in a background of benign lymphocytes, plasma cells, and eosinophils. However, it is usually recommended that excisional biopsy be performed for definitive diagnosis and classification of HD.
- Fine-needle aspirate cytology can be a good way to look at individual cells. However, you get limited appreciation of *architecture*, which is critical in the diagnosis of some lymphoma types. Therefore, many hematologists and oncologists will not treat a patient for lymphoma based on a cytology specimen alone, even combined with immunophenotyping. Others feel comfortable treating the patient based on FNA without biopsy.
- A common problem with FNA cytology is scanty specimens, with too few cells for diagnosis. Experience on the part of the person doing the FNA, and good coordination with the cytopathologist, can minimize the incidence of inadequate specimens.

Excisional Lymph Node Biopsy

- Excisional biopsy of a lymph node usually provides plenty of tissue for good histology, immunophenotyping, special stains, cultures (if indicated), and other special tests (cytogenetics, antigen gene rearrangement studies). It also allows appreciation of architecture, which can be important for lymphoma diagnosis and classification.
- The *disadvantages* of node biopsy are that it is invasive, more expensive than FNA cytology, and usually must be scheduled in advance.
- For maximum benefit, a lymph node biopsy requires coordination and communication between the clinician, the surgeon, and the pathologist. Ideally, the clinician should discuss the case with the pathologist beforehand, letting him or her know that lymphoma is a possibility and giving any relevant clinical information. The surgeon should also contact the pathologist beforehand, letting him or her know that the biopsy will be done and when the specimen will arrive in the surgical pathology laboratory.
- The lymph node should be removed *intact* as much as possible rather than in fragments. It should be brought to the surgical pathology labo-

ratory *immediately* after removal, and should be brought *fresh*. Moisten the node with *saline*; do **not** put it in formalin or another fixative (flow cytometry and some of the other special tests cannot be done on a specimen that has been put in fixative).

- In the surgical pathology suite, several "touch preparations" should be made by touching the cut surface of the node to a glass slide. A portion should be put in cell culture medium or sent immediately to the flow cytometry laboratory for possible immunophenotyping (preferably at least 0.5 cm^3, or as much as possible). Several thin slices should be put into formalin or other fixative for routine histology. Tissue can be sent for possible cytogenetic analysis and frozen for possible molecular analysis.
  - If cultures are indicated, it is usually preferable that samples be taken in the operating room rather than pathology.
  - If the specimen is small, always submit tissue for *histologic examination **first***; everything else is secondary.

If the original diagnosis (by either FNA cytology or lymph node biopsy) is benign, the patient must be followed to be sure that the lymphadenopathy resolves. Patients with HD, NHL, or metastatic neoplasms can have reactive nodes in the vicinity of neoplastic nodes (or elsewhere), and the important diagnosis might be missed if an uninvolved reactive lymph node is biopsied rather than an involved lymph node. If the lymphadenopathy fails to resolve and no other explanation is known, a repeat FNA cytology or lymph node biopsy should be performed.

18

Multiple Myeloma, Monoclonal Gammopathies, and Other Plasma Cell Dyscrasias

Plasma cell neoplasms have historically been separated from the malignant lymphomas. Plasma cells are the terminal phase of B lymphocytes, and plasma cell neoplasms are grouped with lymphoid neoplasms in the new World Health Organization (WHO) classification. However, there are distinct clinical differences between plasma cell neoplasms and other neoplasms of lymphocytes, and it is useful to consider them separately.

One characteristic of plasma cell neoplasms (also called *plasma cell dyscrasias*) is that they are associated with production of a monoclonal immunoglobulin protein. The monoclonal proteins can be used to diagnose and follow plasma cell neoplasms, and can cause complications by themselves. Monoclonal immunoglobulin proteins can also be produced by other B-cell neoplasms, including non-Hodgkin's lymphomas and chronic lymphocytic leukemia; however, monoclonal proteins are found in a minority of such diseases, and the amount of protein synthesized is usually small (Table 18–1).

There are several neoplasms falling into the general category of plasma cell dyscrasias. The most clinically significant, although not the most common, is **multiple myeloma (MM)**. **Monoclonal gammopathy of undetermined significance** (**MGUS**; previously called *benign monoclonal gammopathy*) is more common than MM, but in most cases it is not clinically significant. The other plasma cell dyscrasias are all relatively uncommon.

Table 18–1
Types of Monoclonal Gammopathies

Multiple myeloma

Myeloma variants:
- Solitary osseous myeloma
- Smoldering or indolent myeloma
- Osteosclerotic myeloma (*POEMS syndrome*: polyneuropathy, organomegaly, endocrinopathy, monoclonal protein, and skin changes)
- Plasma cell leukemia

Monoclonal gammopathy of undetermined significance (MGUS)

Waldenström's macroglobulinemia

Extramedullary plasmacytoma

Primary systemic (AL) amyloidosis

Heavy chain diseases: α, γ, μ

Monoclonal immunoglobulin proteins associated with chronic lymphocytic leukemia or a non-Hodgkin's lymphoma

MULTIPLE MYELOMA

Multiple myeloma is characterized by a triad of abnormalities:
- Accumulation of plasma cells in the bone marrow
- Bone lesions: either discrete lytic bone lesions or diffuse osteopenia
- Production of a monoclonal immunoglobulin (Ig) or Ig fragments

Epidemiology

- Multiple myeloma is the second most common malignancy of lymphoid cells in Caucasians following chronic lymphocytic leukemia (CLL); it is the most common lymphoid malignancy in African Americans.
- It occurs primarily in older populations; the median age is ~70 years at diagnosis. It is more common in men than women.
- The etiology is largely unknown. The incidence is increased in farmers and workers in the petroleum, wood, leather, and asbestos industries, suggesting that chemical exposure is involved.
- Ionizing radiation has been suggested as a predisposing factor; some studies have shown an increased incidence in radiologists and workers in nuclear plants.

Clinical Features

Clinical features include *bone pain* and *fractures, infections, renal insufficiency,* and *hypercalcemia.* Anemia, hyperviscosity, amyloidosis, and neuropathies are less common.

Bone Lesions

Bone lesions are caused by an accumulation of plasma cells in the marrow, with dissolution of the bone.

* **Bone pain** and **pathologic fractures** are the most common presenting complaints.
* The classic bone lesions associated with multiple myeloma are sharp "punched out" osteolytic lesions (Figure 18–1). These are usually multiple and can occur in any bone, but are most common in the vertebral bodies, ribs, skull, pelvis, and femurs.
* The second type of bone lesion seen in MM is diffuse osteoporosis, without discrete osteolytic lesions. This occurs in about 40% of patients. This type of lesion does not show up well on routine skeletal radiographs but may be visualized by magnetic resonance imaging (MRI) scans.
* Bone is eroded due to increased osteoclast activity. The osteoclasts are stimulated by factors produced by plasma cells, generically called **osteoclast activating factors** (**OAF**).

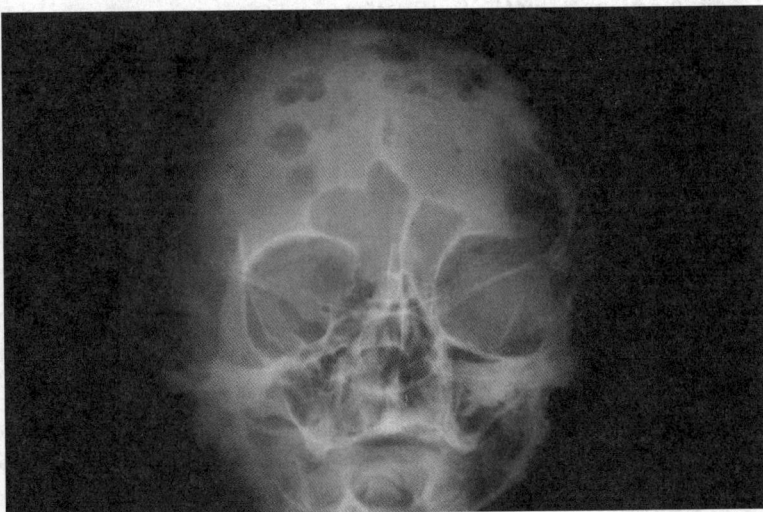

Figure 18–1 Multiple myeloma skull radiograph. Multiple osteolytic lesions are present.

Infections

Infections are the **most common cause of death** in patients with MM.

- Normal immunoglobulin production is suppressed; therefore, patients are particularly susceptible to infections with encapsulated bacteria such as *Streptococcus pneumoniae* (pneumococcus).
- Patients are also susceptible to infections with *Staphylococcus aureus* and gram-negative enteric bacteria such as *Escherichia coli*.
- *Pneumonitis* and *pyelonephritis* are common infections in patients with myeloma.

Renal Disease

Patients with MM are predisposed to several renal complications, including renal failure, proteinuria, renal amyloidosis, kidney stones, and pyelonephritis. Renal disease is the **second most common cause of death** in patients with MM. Examples include the following:

- *Myeloma cast nephropathy*: The monoclonal immunoglobulin may form casts in renal tubules that elicit a phagocytic cellular response.
- Excretion of free immunoglobulin light chains (*Bence Jones proteins*) is toxic to renal tubules.
- Hypercalcemia causes an inability to concentrate the urine (isosthenuria), predisposing to dehydration and prerenal azotemia.
- Hyperuricemia and hypercalcemia can cause kidney stones.
- Some immunoglobulin fragments can precipitate as a β-pleated sheet, resulting in renal amyloidosis (see **Amyloidosis** below).
- Myeloma patients may be predisposed to renal shutdown when given hypertonic x-ray contrast agents for excretory urograms or angiographic studies.
- Proteinuria may be due to excretion of albumin alone, intact Ig or light chain, or albumin with an Ig or light chain. This may present as the nephrotic syndrome.

⇨ *Myeloma is an important diagnostic consideration in any adult presenting with new-onset nephrotic syndrome*

- Renal insufficiency may be due to nephrotoxic medications, particularly nonsteroidal anti-inflammatory agents (NSAIDs) and aminoglycoside antibiotics.
- Renal insufficiency is a significant adverse prognostic feature in patients with myeloma. However, renal insufficiency may be due to reversible causes, such as dehydration, hypercalcemia, or nephrotoxic medications.

Hypercalcemia

Hypercalcemia is common in patients with myeloma, largely due to excess bone resorption. Hypercalcemia can cause confusion, weakness, lethargy, constipation, and loss of renal concentrating ability.

Diagnosis

The diagnosis of MM, and distinguishing MM from other monoclonal gammopathies and plasma cell dyscrasias, requires correlation of several factors (Tables 18–2 and 18–3). In general, the diagnosis depends on the presence of three features: a **monoclonal immunoglobulin protein** in serum and/or urine, **bone lesions**, and **plasmacytosis in the bone marrow**.

- **Monoclonal immunoglobulin protein** (M protein, M component, or M spike):
  - Screening for a monoclonal protein is usually done by *serum protein electrophoresis* (**SPEP**) and *urine protein electrophoresis*. After a monoclonal spike is detected, it should be definitively identified by *immunofixation* or *immunoelectrophoresis* (Figure 18–2).
  - Approximately 99% of patients have a monoclonal immunoglobulin protein in blood, urine, or both; ≤1% of patients lack a monoclonal protein (nonsecretory myeloma).

Table 18–2
Diagnostic Evaluation of Monoclonal Protein or Possible Myeloma

Serum protein electrophoresis and immunofixation; quantitation of monoclonal protein
Urine protein electrophoresis and immunofixation; 24-hour urine collection for quantitation of 24-hour urine monoclonal protein excretion
Complete blood count and differential; examination of blood smear for rouleaux and circulating plasma cells
Serum chemistries, including calcium, serum urea nitrogen (BUN) and creatinine, albumin and total protein, lactic dehydrogenase
Quantitative immunoglobulin levels
Serum β_2-microglobulin
Bone marrow aspirate and biopsy; plasma cell labeling index if available
Skeletal survey; possibly MRI or CT scan
Abdominal fat pad aspiration for Congo red stain if amyloidosis is suspected

Table 18–3
Diagnostic Criteria for Multiple Myeloma

Major Criteria

1. Plasmacytoma on biopsy

2. Marrow plasmacytosis (>30%)

3. M component:
   Serum: IgG > 3.5 g/dL, IgA >2 g/dL
   Urine: ≥1 g/24 hr of kappa or lambda light chain (Bence Jones protein) without amyloidosis

Minor Criteria

1. Marrow plasmacytosis (10 to 30%)

2. M component: present but less than above

3. Lytic bone lesions

4. Reduced normal immunoglobulins (<50% normal):
   IgG <600 mg/dL, IgA <100 mg/dL, IgM <50 mg/dL

The diagnosis of myeloma requires a minimum of one major and one minor criterion or three minor criteria, which must include (1) and (2). These criteria must be present in a symptomatic patient with progressive disease.

Reproduced with permission from Knowles DM, editor. Neoplastic hematopathology. Baltimore, Williams & Wilkins, 1992. p. 1251.

- IgG is the most common (~50% of patients) followed by IgA (~25%). IgM, IgD, and IgE are all rare. Approximately 1 to 2.5% of cases have two clonal immunoglobulins (ie, both an IgG and an IgA immunoglobulin).

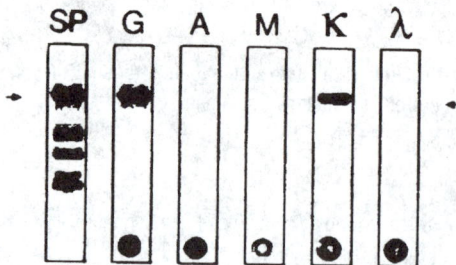

Figure 18–2 Serum protein electrophoresis and immunofixation. The lane on the left is total serum proteins. The dense band at the top is the monoclonal protein. The other lanes are immunofixation for specific immunoglobulin heavy and light chains. The band in the G and in the κ light chain lanes correspond to the band in the SP, indicating a monoclonal IgG-κ protein.

- Kappa (κ) immunoglobulin light chain is more common than lambda (λ) light chain by ~2:1, similar to the ratio of κ to λ in normal immunoglobulins.
- *Light chain only myeloma* makes up ~10 to 25% of cases. This can be missed if only the serum is studied because the monoclonal protein is often found only in the urine. Light chains are small molecules that are filtered through the glomeruli, and therefore they do not accumulate in the serum.

⇨ *Electrophoresis (and/or immunofixation) must be performed on* **both** *serum* **and** *urine if myeloma is suspected.* **The absence of a monoclonal immunoglobulin on serum protein electrophoresis does** <u>not</u> **rule out myeloma.**

- Production of other immunoglobulins is usually suppressed.
- **Bone lesions:** A radiographic skeletal survey may show either multiple sharp (punched out) osteolytic defects *or* diffuse osteoporosis.
  - Nuclear bone scans are less sensitive than skeletal surveys because nuclear scans require an osteoblastic component, which is frequently lacking in MM.
  - Computed tomography (CT) may be more sensitive for vertebral lesions than a routine skeletal survey.
  - Magnetic resonance imaging (MRI) scan may demonstrate myeloma infiltrate in the marrow in cases with diffuse osteoporosis, which may be missed by routine radiologic studies.
- **Bone marrow plasmacytosis:** This is diagnosed by either >10% plasma cells on the bone marrow aspirate *or* by a plasmacytoma on biopsy.
  - The plasma cells may be morphologically unremarkable or may show multinucleation, prominent nucleoli (Figure 18–3), or immature nuclear chromatin.
  - Plasmacytosis in the marrow *alone* is not diagnostic for myeloma; plasma cells may be increased in benign conditions such as chronic inflammatory diseases and human immunodeficiency virus (HIV) infection.

Other Laboratory Findings

- Anemia is very common and is often the presenting feature of myeloma. Leukopenia and thrombocytopenia are less common at diagnosis.
- The blood smear often shows stacked lines of erythrocytes, designated *rouleaux* (Figure 18–4). This may be seen with increased immunoglobulins of any cause but is most characteristic of myeloma and other monoclonal gammopathies.

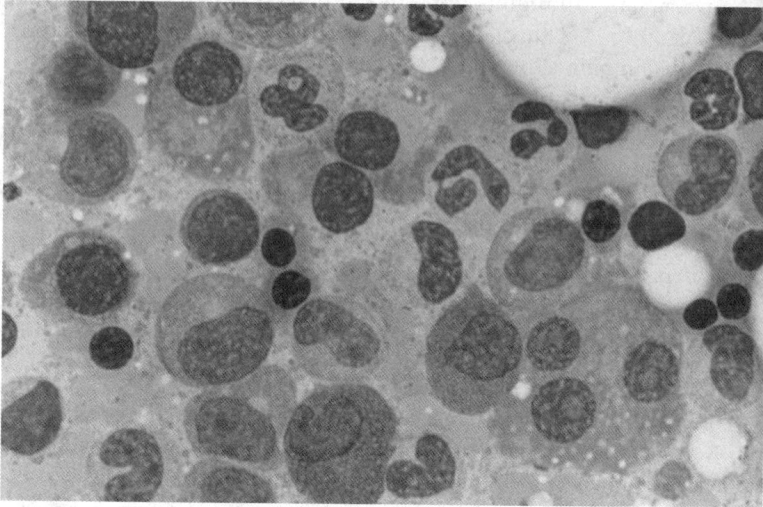

Figure 18–3 Multiple myeloma bone marrow aspirate. Numerous plasma cells, many of which have prominent nucleoli (normal plasma cells lack nucleoli), are present.

- The gamma globulin fraction of serum proteins is often increased (gamma globulin = total protein concentration minus albumin).
- Hypercalcemia is common at diagnosis because of increased bone resorption and decreased calcium excretion by the kidneys due to dehydration.

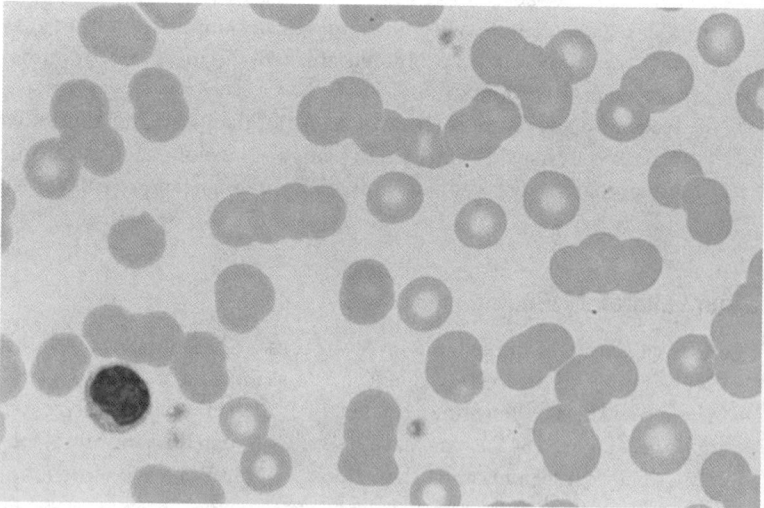

Figure 18–4 Multiple myeloma blood smear. Rouleaux formation.

- Azotemia (increased serum urea nitrogen [BUN] and creatinine) is common.
- The serum level of β_2-*microglobulin* is useful in following patients with multiple myeloma; it appears to be a good reflection of tumor burden. However, it is not useful in patients with impaired renal function because β_2-microglobulin is cleared by glomerular filtration and is elevated with renal insufficiency.

Myeloma Staging (Table 18–4)

- Staging is useful for estimating of prognosis and deciding whether to treat and how to treat the myeloma.
- Staging is based upon the size of the M component and the effects of myeloma, including anemia, renal function, and the presence and number of bone lesions.
- The *plasma cell labeling index* (on a bone marrow aspirate) is a very useful predictor of behavior in MM; however, it is not widely available.

Complications of Multiple Myeloma

In addition to fractures, infections, renal disease, and the other problems listed above, patients may have a variety of other complications.

Table 18–4
Myeloma Staging System

Stage I	1. Low M component levels: IgG <5 g/dL, IgA <3 g/dL; urine Bence Jones proteins <4 g/24 hr
	2. Absent or solitary bone lesions
	3. Normal hemoglobin, serum calcium, and Ig levels (non–M component)
Stage II	Overall values between stages I and III
Stage III	Any one or more of the following:
	1. High M component: IgG >7 g/dL, IgA >5 g/dL; urine Bence Jones proteins ≥12 g/24 h
	2. Advanced multiple lytic bone lesions
	3. Hemoglobin <8.5 g/dL, serum calcium >12 mg/dL

Subclassification: Based on renal function
  A = serum creatinine <2 mg/dL
  B = serum creatinine >2 mg/dL

- **Spinal cord or nerve root compression:** This can occur due to a myeloma tumor in a vertebral body growing into the spinal canal, compressing the spinal cord or a nerve root. *This requires immediate reduction (radiation therapy or surgery) to prevent permanent loss of function.* A high degree of suspicion is required for treatment. The diagnosis can be made by myelogram, CT scan, or MRI of the spinal column.
- **Amyloidosis:** AL (light chain) type amyloidosis occurs in ~10% of patients with MM (see the section on Amyloidosis below).
- **Hyperviscosity syndrome:** Hyperviscosity syndrome is more common in Waldenström's macroglobulinemia (see the section on Waldenström's macroglobulinemia below) but can occur in MM. It is more common with IgA than IgG immunoglobulins.

Treatment of Multiple Myeloma

- Multiple myeloma is considered incurable with conventional therapy, like the indolent non-Hodgkin's lymphomas and CLL.
- Asymptomatic patients and those with indolent or smoldering myeloma are usually not treated initially. There is little evidence that early treatment prolongs survival in these patients.
- Patients with symptomatic disease and multiple bone lesions should be treated at diagnosis. Treatment has been shown to prolong survival in patients who respond.
- The standard chemotherapy has been phenylalanine mustard (**melphalan**) with **prednison**e (**MP**); ~60 to 70% of patients respond to this regimen, although responses are usually partial. It is given orally and is usually well tolerated.
- Combination chemotherapy such as vincristine, doxorubicin (Adriamycin), and dexamethasone (VAD) or one of several other regimens are sometimes used. These regimens have higher *response rates* than MP but have not generally shown significant improvement in *overall survival*. However, they may salvage some patients resistant to MP. The toxicity of such regimens is higher than with MP.
- *Pamidronate* given intravenously is useful to rapidly lower the calcium level in hypercalcemia. Given monthly as an intravenous infusion, it can help prevent or stabilize bone disease due to myeloma.
- Eventually, the disease becomes resistant to chemotherapy, and prognosis and survival thereafter are poor.
- Experimental regimens:
  - Allogeneic bone marrow transplant has been used in a few patients, but the majority of patients with myeloma are too old for allogeneic transplant. Transplant-related mortality has been significant.

- High-dose chemotherapy with autologous peripheral blood progenitor cell support is now often used. It appears to prolong overall survival but does not appear to cure patients with MM.
- Thalidomide has recently been tried and seems to have some activity against myeloma, which has become refractory to conventional chemotherapy.
- Hypercalcemia is treated acutely with saline infusion and diuresis; pamidronate can also be helpful. Calcitonin is also useful to acutely lower the calcium level.

Prognosis and Survival

The course of myeloma is heterogeneous. Some patients have indolent disease with long survival; a few patients have a very aggressive course with short survival. The majority of patients have an intermediate course. Median survival is currently ~3 to 5 years. Patients with renal insufficiency that is not corrected by rehydration, treatment of hypercalcemia, or discontinuation of nephrotoxic drugs have a poor prognosis.

Myeloma Variants

- **Anaplastic myeloma**: Patients with *anaplastic myeloma* (tumors composed of bizarre or immature plasma cells) have an aggressive course with poor survival.
- **Smoldering** and **indolent myeloma**: Patients may have prolonged survival even without treatment (Table 18–5).
- **Solitary osseous myeloma**: Solitary osseous myeloma is defined as a single bone lesion on skeletal survey; a bone marrow aspirate and biopsy taken at another site should be normal. A monoclonal protein may or may not be present in the serum or urine. Approximately half of patients transform to systemic disease with multiple bone lesions within 3 years; however, they may have prolonged survival even after dissemination.
- **Extramedullary plasmacytoma**: Extramedullary plasmacytoma is a plasma cell tumor occurring outside the bone marrow. It is usually solitary. There is either no serum monoclonal protein or only a small amount. The most common location is the upper respiratory tract (~50 to 75% of cases). The majority remain localized, and local therapy (radiation with or without surgery) is frequently curative.
- **Plasma cell leukemia**: Plasma cell leukemia is a rare variant of MM. Approximately half of cases present with plasma cell leukemia as the initial manifestation of myeloma (*primary plasma cell leukemia*). The remaining cases occur as a late terminal event in patients with a previ-

Table 18–5

Diagnostic Criteria for Monoclonal Gammopathy of Undetermined Significance (MGUS), Indolent and Smoldering Myeloma

MGUS

1. M component present, but less than myeloma levels
2. Marrow plasmacytosis <10%
3. **No** lytic bone lesions
4. **No** myeloma-related symptoms

Indolent Myeloma: Same criteria as for myeloma, except:

1. Absent or rare bone lesions (≤3 lytic lesions), without compression fractures
2. M component: IgG <7 g/dL, I gA <5 g/dL
3. Normal hemoglobin, serum calcium, and creatinine
4. No infections

Smoldering Myeloma: Same as indolent, except:

1. No bone lesions
2. Marrow plasmacytosis (10–30%)

Reproduced with permission from Knowles DM, editor. Neoplastic hematology. Baltimore, Williams & Wilkins, 1992. p. 1251.

ous history of myeloma. Survival in either case is usually brief, although patients with primary plasma cell leukemia who respond to aggressive therapy may survive longer.

MONOCLONAL GAMMOPATHY OF UNDETERMINED SIGNIFICANCE (MGUS)

Definition and Epidemiology

Monoclonal gammopathy of undetermined significance (MGUS) is defined by the presence of monoclonal serum immunoglobulin in the absence of signs of multiple myeloma (see Table 18–5). The monoclonal protein in MGUS is relatively small; there are no osteolytic bone lesions, there are <10% plasma cells in bone marrow, other immunoglobulins are not suppressed, and there is no anemia, azotemia, or hypercalcemia.

- It was previously often called *benign monoclonal gammopathy* (BMG). The term *monoclonal gammopathy of undetermined significance* is preferred since the course in an individual patient is unpredictable.
- Monoclonal gammopathy of undetermined significance occurs in older populations and increases with age; such monoclonal proteins have been found in ~3% of people at age 70 years and in ≥10% over 90 years.

- Immunoglobulin G is the most common type (~70%). Immunoglobulin M and IgA are less common.
- A minority of patients with MGUS develop overt MM (~25%), but transformation may not occur for many years (20 years or longer).
  - The median time to transformation to myeloma is 8 to 10 years.
  - Transformation may occur either gradually, with a slow increase in the level of the monoclonal protein, or abruptly.
- It is not possible upon discovery of the monoclonal protein to predict which patients with MGUS will progress to overt myeloma. The serum and urine protein levels, other immunoglobulins, CBC, and routine chemistries should be checked at 3- –6-month intervals for the first year. If stable, they can be rechecked at 6- –12-month intervals thereafter.
- There is no indication for treating MGUS as such. Patients should be monitored for progression of disease and treated for myeloma if progressive disease develops.
- Monoclonal gammopathy of undetermined significance may occasionally be associated with a peripheral neuropathy, due to the antibody reacting with myelin. In rare cases, the antibody has activity against other identifiable antigens, such as erythrocyte antigens, von Willebrand's factor, factor VIII coagulant protein, or others.

WALDENSTRÖM'S MACROGLOBULINEMIA

Definition and Epidemiology

- Waldenström's macroglobulinemia (**WM**) is a proliferation of lymphocytic or plasmacytoid cells that produce a monoclonal IgM protein. It is considerably less common than MM. Like myeloma, it primarily occurs in an older population.
- Waldenström's macroglobulinemia may be seen with non-Hodgkin's lymphomas (characteristically *lymphoplasmacytic lymphoma*) and occasionally with CLL. The characteristic cell of WM is a plasmacytoid lymphocyte.
- Waldenström's macroglobulinemia differs from MM by the absence of discrete osteolytic bone lesions and the presence of frequent involvement of lymph nodes, spleen, and liver, which are usually not involved in MM.
- **Complications of WM** can include the **hyperviscosity syndrome** (see below), **cryoglobulinemia** (proteins that undergo reversible precipitation at low temperatures), **cold agglutinin hemolytic anemia** (due to reactivity against red cell antigens), **peripheral neuropathy** (due to reactivity of the immunoglobulin against myelin), **glomerular disease** (proteinuria), and **amyloidosis**.
- The clinical course is generally indolent, resembling that of CLL or indolent non-Hodgkin's lymphomas. The median survival is ~5 years.

- Treatment includes chemotherapy regimens similar to those for CLL or indolent lymphomas. Nucleoside analogues such as fludarabine or 2-chlorodeoxyadenosine (cladribine) also appear effective.

Hyperviscosity Syndrome

- The hyperviscosity syndrome can complicate any of the monoclonal gammopathies, but is most common in WM.
- It is caused by polymerization of the immunoglobulin in the blood, which increases blood viscosity. It is most common with IgM proteins but also occurs with IgA proteins and occasionally with IgG.
  - The IgM level is usually >3 g/dL, although the level of the monoclonal protein does not correlate perfectly with the occurrence of the hyperviscosity syndrome. The serum viscosity is usually ≥4 times normal viscosity.
- Symptoms include fatigue, dizziness, blurred vision, bleeding from mucous membranes, and difficulty breathing.
- A characteristic physical finding is distended "link sausage" retinal veins on funduscopic examination.
- Plasmapheresis effectively (but transiently) decreases the IgM level and rapidly relieves hyperviscosity.
- Chemotherapy is required to prevent the reaccumulation of the monoclonal protein and should be started concurrently with plasmapheresis. Regimens used are similar to those used for indolent lymphomas or CLL.

AMYLOIDOSIS

Amyloidosis is a heterogeneous group of conditions, with varying severity and causes. **The common feature is precipitation of a protein in a β-*pleated sheet* configuration**. The β-pleated sheet configuration gives the physicochemical properties recognized as amyloid.

The term amyloid (starch-like) denotes a histologic appearance, not a specific protein. A variety of proteins can precipitate as amyloid, including some immunoglobulin light chains, degradation products of a serum protein (serum amyloid-associated protein [SAA]), mutated forms of transthyretin, and a variety of others, including hormones (calcitonin, insulin), β_2-microglobulin, and many more.

Classification of Amyloidosis

Amyloidosis can be classified by the specific protein involved or by the cause or clinical syndrome (Table 18–6).

Table 18–6
Types of Amyloidosis

AL	Immunoglobulin light chain; multiple myeloma and primary systemic amyloidosis
AA	Serum amyloid–associated (SAA) protein; chronic inflammation, malignancies
AF (ATTR)	Familial amyloidosis; mutation in transthyretin (prealbumin) protein
AE	Endocrine: medullary carcinoma of thyroid, pancreatic islet cell tumors, pancreatic islets in non–insulin-dependent diabetes mellitus
AS$_b$	Alzheimer dementia; trisomy 21 (Down syndrome)
Aβ_2M	Hemodialysis associated

AL Type (Primary or Primary Systemic Amyloidosis)

- AL amyloidosis is the deposition of an immunoglobulin light chain or light chain fragment.
- It is a type of monoclonal gammopathy, caused by a plasma cell dyscrasia. Amyloidosis can occur in MM (amyloidosis occurs in ~10% of cases of MM) or with a plasma cell dyscrasia that fails to meet the diagnostic criteria for myeloma.
  - Primary systemic amyloidosis not associated with myeloma has a lower number of plasma cells in the bone marrow, no osteolytic bone lesions, and a smaller monoclonal spike in the serum and urine.
- The light chain is more often lambda (λ) rather than kappa (κ) by ~2 to 4:1. This is the reverse of the normal ratio in plasma immunoglobulins and the ratio in MM. It depends on the specific segments present in the monoclonal protein; some are more "amyloidogenic" than others.
- Rarely, part of an immunoglobulin heavy chain may cause amyloidosis, designated **AH**.

AA Type (Secondary Amyloidosis)

- The AA protein is derived from a serum protein, designated *serum amyloid–associated* (**SAA**) *protein*.
- AA amyloidosis is seen in association with chronic inflammatory conditions or occasionally with malignancies.
- Rheumatoid arthritis is currently the most common cause. Other causes include chronic infections (osteomyelitis, subacute bacterial endocarditis, tuberculosis, malaria), chronic inflammatory bowel disease (Crohn's disease and ulcerative colitis), Sjögren's syndrome, malignan-

cies (renal cell carcinoma, Hodgkin's disease), familial Mediterranean fever, and others.

- The SAA protein acts as an acute-phase reactant; it is increased in acute and chronic inflammation. In some patients, there is defective degradation of the SAA protein, resulting in fragments that precipitate as a β-pleated sheet.
- The combination of chronically increased SAA protein *and* defective degradation of the protein is required to cause amyloid deposition.

AF or ATTR type (Familial Amyloidosis)

- Familial amyloidosis syndromes are usually associated with a mutation in the transthyretin (prealbumin) protein.
- Familial amyloidosis often manifests predominantly as peripheral neuropathy. The prognosis may be better than other forms of amyloidosis.

AE Type (Endocrine)

- Overproduction of several hormones can cause amyloidosis, usually from neoplasms of endocrine cells. Examples include calcitonin in medullary carcinoma of the thyroid and gastrin or other pancreatic hormones in pancreatic islet cell tumors.
- Amyloid deposition can also be seen in pancreatic islets of non–insulin-dependent diabetes mellitus.

Others

- **AS_b:** β-Amyloid accumulates in the plaques and tangles of Alzheimer's disease and in patients with trisomy 21 (Down syndrome).
- **$A\beta_2M$: Hemodialysis-associated** amyloidosis, due to accumulation of β_2-microglobulin. β_2-Microglobulin is derived from class I HLA molecules on cell surfaces, including plasma cells. It is normally excreted renally and accumulates in the serum of patients on hemodialysis. This type of amyloidosis often presents as carpal tunnel syndrome.

Clinical Features

- Amyloidosis usually occurs in an older population and is more common in men than women.
- Symptoms are usually nonspecific; fatigue, weight loss, and light-headedness are the most common.
- Changes on physical examination may include the following:
  - Skin: Purpura or nodules, usually present on the face, neck, and upper chest

- Macroglossia: An enlarged tongue showing impressions of the teeth along the sides. This is the most specific physical sign of amyloidosis but is uncommon.
- Hepatomegaly
- Pseudohypertrophy of skeletal muscles (the "shoulder-pad sign")
- The *four most common presentations of amyloidosis* are
  - Nephrotic-range proteinuria, with or without renal insufficiency
  - Congestive heart failure resulting from restrictive cardiomyopathy
  - Unexplained hepatomegaly
  - Idiopathic peripheral neuropathy

Diagnosis of Amyloidosis

- On routine hematoxylin and eosin stain, amyloid appears as homogeneous eosinophilic material (Figure 18–5). It usually deposits in the walls of blood vessels but can also accumulate in renal glomeruli, the heart, the lamina propria of the gastrointestinal tract, the liver and spleen, and virtually every other organ or tissue in the body.
- **Abdominal fat pad aspiration with staining for amyloid** has become the **diagnostic procedure of choice** to diagnose amyloidosis. Other sites that might be biopsied include skin lesions, the gastrointestinal tract, or other organs that appear involved.

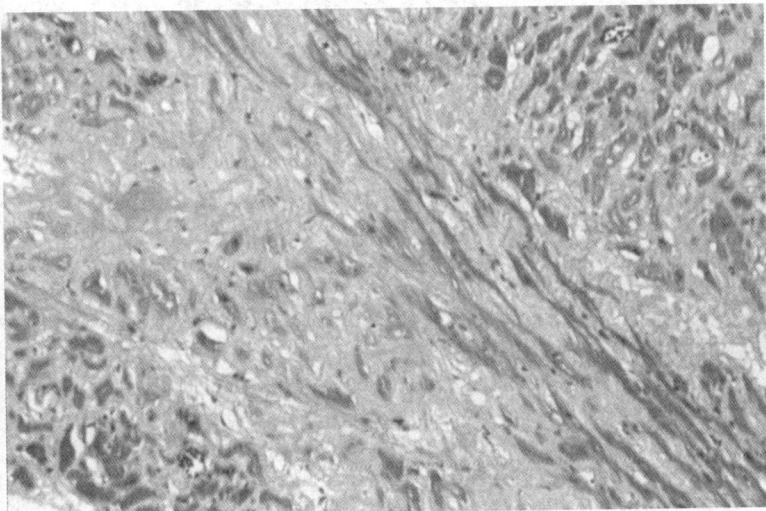

Figure 18–5 Amyloidosis of the myocardium. Amyloidosis due to multiple myeloma. The homogeneous pale material is amyloid.

- The *Congo red* stain is useful in diagnosis of amyloidosis. Amyloid has a characteristic apple-green birefringence when sections stained with Congo red are viewed under polarized light.
- Electron microscopy shows linear non-branching randomly arranged fibrils with a width of ~10 nm; they resemble children's jackstraws or pick-up sticks.
- Once amyloidosis is demonstrated, protein electrophoresis *and* immunofixation should be performed on both serum and urine to look for a monoclonal protein. The monoclonal protein is usually present in low concentration and may be overlooked on routine serum protein electrophoresis if immunofixation is not performed.
- A bone marrow aspirate and biopsy should also be performed. Demonstration of plasma cell expression of κ and λ light chains by immunohistochemistry may be helpful.
- The type of amyloid can be determined by immunohistochemical stains using specific antibodies for the different protein types.
- A Doppler echocardiogram may show a characteristic "granular sparkling" of the myocardium and thickening of the ventricular walls and interventricular septum. Echocardiography is also useful in assessing cardiac status.

Complications of Amyloidosis

In general, the complications of all types of amyloidosis are similar. Familial and hemodialysis-associated amyloidosis often are characterized by peripheral neuropathies (the carpal tunnel syndrome may be the first manifestation), with little involvement of visceral organs. Survival of these types is better than types with visceral involvement.

Complications of amyloidosis include the following:

- **Heart:** Restrictive cardiomyopathy and cardiac arrhythmias. Patients with cardiac involvement have the shortest survival of all patients with amyloidosis.
- **Kidney:** The kidneys are involved in 30 to 50% of patients. Renal amyloidosis causes proteinuria or the nephrotic syndrome, with or without renal insufficiency.
- **Liver:** Hepatomegaly is present in ~25% of patients. The serum alkaline phosphatase level may be elevated; other liver chemistries are usually only mildly abnormal. Ascites may be present, but this is usually due more to the nephrotic syndrome than liver dysfunction.
- **Gastrointestinal tract:** Histologic evidence of gastrointestinal tract involvement is common, but symptoms related to gastrointestinal

involvement are not. Occasional patients may have malabsorption, and ischemic colitis may occur due to involvement of mesenteric vessels.

- **Nerves:** Neuropathy usually presents as symmetric paresthesias in the lower extremities; muscle weakness is frequent. The carpal tunnel syndrome may be the initial feature. The autonomic nervous system may be involved.
- **Hemorrhage:** Cutaneous purpura occur due to increased fragility of blood vessel walls, which are infiltrated by amyloid. The factor X coagulant protein may be decreased due to binding to amyloid protein, causing a coagulopathy.

Treatment and Prognosis

- Survival is heterogeneous, depending on the type of amyloidosis and the specific organs involved, among other factors.
- Patients with cardiac involvement have the worst survival; patients with neuropathy alone have the best survival. Survival of patients with renal disease is intermediate.
- Patients with AL amyloidosis tend to have poor survival. Survival is worse in cases associated with myeloma than in cases not associated with myeloma, but AL amyloidosis has generally dismal survival even in the absence of MM.
- Treatment is directed at the underlying disease; there is no treatment for amyloidosis per se.
- AL type: Standard treatment is chemotherapy as for MM. Survival is improved in patients who have a response.
- AA type: Treatment is directed against the underlying condition. Patients may have good survival if the underlying condition can be treated successfully and the amyloidosis is not advanced.
- Specific treatment is not available for most of the other types.

19

Hematologic Effects of the HIV and AIDS

The human immunodeficiency virus (**HIV**) can affect the hematologic system in many ways (Table 19–1). Patients with HIV may have multiple infections, other complicating illnesses, and poor nutritional status and are often on medications that may have myelosuppressive effects. The virus may have direct effects on the bone marrow by infecting marrow macrophages and other cells and may disrupt production of growth factors and other cytokines. Hematologic complications of HIV can include decreased blood cell production, impaired function of blood cells, immune-mediated destruction of blood cells, and coagulation disorders. The bone marrow can be directly invaded by organisms, including fungi (*Histoplasma*), mycobacteria (*Mycobacterium avium* complex, *M. tuberculosis*), viruses (parvovirus B19, cytomegalovirus), and, rarely, *Pneumocystis carinii*. The bone marrow may also be involved by lymphoma or other malignancies associated with HIV.

Most of the hematologic complications of HIV are infrequent during the initial asymptomatic phase of infection but become more common and severe as the disease progresses to the acquired immune deficiency syndrome (AIDS). However, thrombocytopenia may be the initial symptomatic manifestation of HIV infection and does not necessarily indicate impending progression of HIV infection to AIDS. Patients with advanced AIDS frequently develop refractory pancytopenia. The causes of cytopenia in HIV and AIDS are summarized in Table 19–2.

Table 19–1
Hematologic Effects of HIV

Anemia

Leukopenia

Thrombocytopenia

Dysplastic changes in the bone marrow

Antiphospholipid antibodies

Thrombotic microangiopathy

Patients with HIV may also develop malignancies, the most common being Kaposi's sarcoma and non-Hodgkin's lymphoma. Human immuno-deficiency virus–related lymphomas were discussed in Chapter 17. Kaposi's sarcoma is a non-hematologic neoplasm and will not be discussed further.

Table 19–2
Causes of Cytopenias in HIV and AIDS

Direct effects of HIV on bone marrow
Chronic illness
    Anemia of chronic disease

Myelosuppressive medications
    Zidovudine (AZT)
    Trimethoprim/sulfamethoxazole
    Dapsone
    Pentamidine
    Ganciclovir
    Ribavirin
    Interferon
    Flucytosine
    Many others

Infections
    Mycobacterium avium complex
    Chronic parvovirus B19 infection
    Cytomegalovirus (CMV)
    Others

Autoimmune cytopenias
    Immune thrombocytopenia
    Immune hemolytic anemia

Bone marrow involvement by lymphoma or other malignancy

ANEMIA

Anemia is uncommon in asymptomatic patients with HIV; however, anemia develops in up to 90% of patients with symptomatic AIDS. The anemia is usually normocytic/normochromic, except for patients on zidovudine (AZT) who have macrocytic anemia.

Pathophysiology

Possible causes of anemia in HIV infection include the following:

- **Anemia of chronic disease:** Anemia of chronic disease is due to chronic infections and other medical problems. The serum iron and iron-binding capacity are often both decreased, typical of anemia of chronic disease; the serum ferritin is usually elevated.
- **Defective erythropoietin response:** Patients with AIDS often have decreased erythropoietin levels for the degree of anemia compared to patients without HIV infection.
- *Mycobacterium avium* **complex:** *Mycobacterium avium* complex appears particularly predisposed to cause a selective anemia, with less effect on other cell lines.
- **Parvovirus B19:** Parvovirus B19 causes transient suppression of erythropoiesis in normal individuals and transient aplastic crises in patients with chronic hemolytic anemia. Patients with AIDS (and other immunocompromised patients) may have severe chronic anemia due to parvovirus B19.
- **Medications:** Many medications used in patients with HIV are myelosuppressive. In particular, zidovudine (AZT) is associated with a macrocytic anemia, which can be severe. Trimethoprim/sulfamethoxazole may also be associated with macrocytic anemia.
- **Nutritional deficiency and malabsorption:** Patients with AIDS may be malnourished and have malabsorption. Low cobalamin (vitamin B_{12}) levels have been found in up to 30% of patients with AIDS; however, hypersegmented neutrophils and other changes of megaloblastic anemia are uncommon. Patients usually fail to respond to cobalamin supplementation. Iron stores are usually adequate or increased.
- **Autoimmune hemolytic anemia:** A positive direct antiglobulin test (DAT; Coombs' test) has been reported in up to 8% of asymptomatic HIV-positive individuals and 20 to 40% of patients with AIDS. Actual immune hemolytic anemia is uncommon but has been reported.
- **Pure red cell aplasia:** Pure red cell aplasia has been reported in patients on AZT, with chronic parvovirus B19 infection and without apparent cause.

- **Other:** Patients with HIV may have anemia due to the same conditions that cause anemia in patients without HIV, such as gastrointestinal blood loss.

Evaluation and Treatment

- The **most important consideration** is to **recognize and treat reversible causes**, particularly **infections** and **myelosuppressive medications**.
- *Mycobacterium avium* complex can be diagnosed by blood cultures or cultures and acid-fast bacilli (AFB) stain on the bone marrow.
- Chronic parvovirus B19 can be detected by giant proerythroblasts in the bone marrow or by polymerase chain reaction (PCR). The anemia often responds to intravenous immunoglobulin.
- Myelosuppressive medications, particularly AZT, should be changed or reduced to the minimum necessary dose whenever possible.
- Recombinant erythropoietin may be effective, particularly in patients with low serum erythropoietin levels (<500 IU/L), and may allow continuation of AZT therapy or other necessary medications. The starting dose is 100 U/kg subcutaneously or intravenously three times weekly for 8 weeks. The dose is then increased by 50 U/kg every 4 weeks up to a satisfactory hemoglobin or a maximum dose of 300 U/kg.
- Red cell transfusions may be required for severe symptomatic anemia that does not respond to other measures.
- Supplementation with iron, cobalamin, and/or folate may be tried but is usually ineffective.

LEUKOPENIA

Leukopenia is uncommon in asymptomatic seropositive individuals but becomes frequent with progression to overt AIDS. Both neutropenia and lymphopenia occur. Lymphopenia, particularly a decrease in CD4+ helper T cells, is one of the earliest hematologic manifestations of HIV infection. Neutropenia in patients with HIV predisposes to bacterial infections, in addition to the usual opportunistic infections seen in patients with AIDS. Causes of neutropenia are generally similar to the causes of anemia: infections, myelosuppressive medications, and general effects of HIV on the bone marrow.

Evaluation and Treatment

- Treat any infections.
- Discontinue myelosuppressive medications or decrease to the minimum effective dose.

Dysplastic changes may be present on blood smear (Figure 19–1).

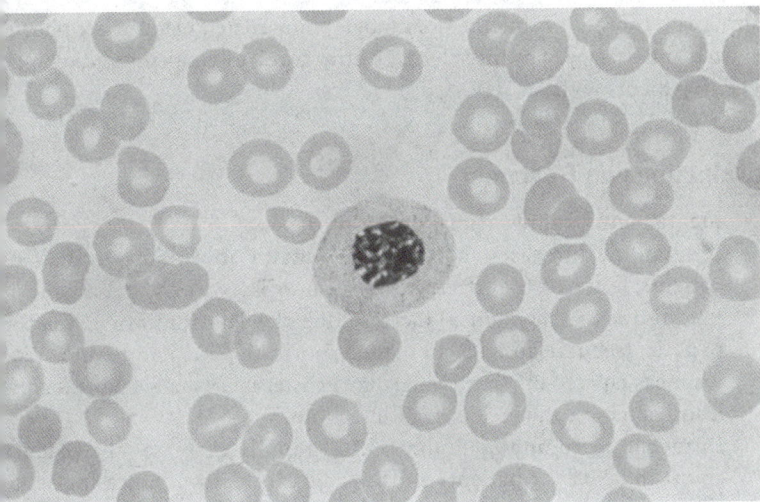

Figure 19–1   Blood. Dysplastic changes. Anisocytosis of erythrocytes, pseudo-Pelger-Huët appearance (hyposegmentation of the nucleus) in neutrophils, and severe thrombocytopenia are seen.

- Granulocyte colony-stimulating factor (G-CSF; *Neupogen*) may be useful. The initial dose is 5 µg/kg/day subcutaneously, which may be increased up to 10 µg/kg/day. Granulocyte-macrophage colony-stimulating factor (GM-CSF; *Leukine*) also appears to be effective. There are concerns that GM-CSF may increase HIV replication, but this appears to be rare.

THROMBOCYTOPENIA

Thrombocytopenia occurs in up to 8% of asymptomatic seropositive individuals and ~30 to 45% of patients with AIDS. In most cases, thrombocytopenia is mild; however, severe thrombocytopenia may occur. Patients may report easy bruising, petechiae, or bleeding, but spontaneous severe bleeding is uncommon unless the platelet count is below 10,000/µL. The risk of serious bleeding due to thrombocytopenia may be higher in HIV-positive hemophiliacs with platelet counts <50,000/µL.

Immune thrombocytopenia resembling idiopathic immune thrombocytopenic purpura (ITP) may be the initial symptomatic manifestation of HIV infection. In this setting, isolated thrombocytopenia does not indicate impending development of AIDS. The mechanism appears to involve both increased platelet destruction and decreased platelet production by the marrow. Antibodies against the viral proteins may cross-react with platelet

surface glycoproteins, and the immunoglobulin-coated platelets are phagocytized and destroyed by the spleen. Treatment resembles that for idiopathic
ITP in patients without HIV.

Evaluation and Treatment

- Identify and treat reversible causes.
- Zidovudine increases the platelet count in approximately half of
  patients; however, the effect takes several weeks.
- Prednisone (~1 mg/kg/day) increases the platelet count in ~60 to 85%
  of patients, but relapses occur in the majority of patients after the prednisone is tapered off. Surprisingly, corticosteroids usually do not significantly increase the incidence of infections.
- Intravenous immunoglobulin (IVIG) rapidly increases the platelet
  count in ~90% of patients and is the treatment of choice for acute
  bleeding due to thrombocytopenia and as supportive therapy for a surgical procedure.
- Anti-Rh$_o$ (D) immunoglobulin may also be effective in Rh-positive
  patients and is less expensive than IVIG.
- Splenectomy results in sustained improvement in the majority of
  patients. Although there are concerns about splenectomy increasing the
  risk of overwhelming infection in these already immunocompromised
  patients, this appears to be uncommon.

ABNORMALITIES OF HEMOSTASIS AND COAGULATION

The most common abnormality of hemostasis and coagulation in patients
with HIV and AIDS is the presence of antiphospholipid antibodies (lupus
anticoagulants). A thrombotic microangiopathy resembling thrombotic
thrombocytopenic purpura (TTP) is uncommon but well described.

Antiphospholipid Antibodies/Lupus Anticoagulants

Antiphospholipid antibodies (**APA**; also known as *anticardiolipin antibodies*) are antibodies directed against phospholipid components or proteins bound to phospholipids. Some antiphospholipid antibodies interfere
with clotting tests, usually the partial thromboplastin time (PTT), and are
called **lupus anticoagulants** (**LA**; discussed further in Chapter 20).
Antiphospholipid antibodies have been found in ~20 to 80% of patients
with HIV. The reason for the high incidence of APA in HIV patients is
unclear but may relate to the polyclonal hypergammaglobulinemia that is
typically present and/or the frequent infections (in some series, the presence
of APA has been linked to infection with *Pneumocystis carinii*, but this has

not been confirmed in other series). In most patients with HIV, the APA are IgM antibodies, not IgG, which are most common in patients without HIV infection.

Antiphospholipid antibodies are usually detected using immunoassays such as enzyme-linked immunosorbent assay (ELISA). Lupus anticoagulants are detected by prolongation of the PTT or the dilute Russell viper venom time.

Antiphospholipid antibodies/lupus anticoagulants are not usually associated with either bleeding or thrombotic complications in patients with HIV, and no specific treatment is required.

Thrombotic Thrombocytopenic Purpura

Patients with HIV may develop a thrombotic microangiopathy similar to **thrombotic thrombocytopenic purpura** (**TTP**). The characteristic features are anemia, schistocytes on the blood smear, and thrombocytopenia. A variable proportion of patients develop fever, neurologic abnormalities, and/or renal insufficiency. The syndrome may occur at any point in the disease, from early HIV infection to overt AIDS. The cause of thrombotic microangiopathy in HIV patients is unknown.

Treatment for TTP in HIV-positive patients is similar to that for TTP in patients without HIV—plasma exchange with plasmapheresis. Approximately 50 to 85% of HIV-positive patients with TTP respond to plasma exchange; corticosteroids or antiplatelet agents can be tried in patients who fail to respond.

BONE MARROW EFFECTS OF HUMAN IMMUNODEFICIENCY VIRUS

Changes in the bone marrow in patients with HIV can include the following:

- **Cellularity:** In most cases, the cellularity in the marrow is normal or increased but may be decreased in the late stages of infection.
- **Dysplastic changes:** Dysplastic changes are common, particularly in erythroid precursors (Figure 19–2). A characteristic feature is multinucleated erythroblasts.
- **Serous atrophy:** Serous atrophy (also known as gelatinous transformation) may occur late in the course of AIDS. It is usually associated with severe pancytopenia and is usually not reversible.
- **Increased plasma cells:** An increase in the number of plasma cells is common and can occasionally be striking. Immunohistochemical stains for kappa and lambda light chains demonstrate mixed immunoglobulin expression.
- **Granulomas:** Granulomas may be present in the marrow and are often poorly formed and indistinct. Granulomas are often associated with the

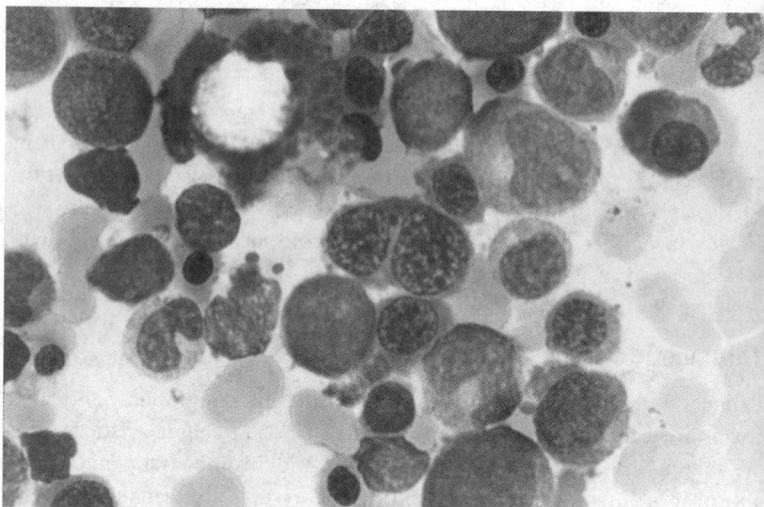

Figure 19–2 Bone marrow. Dyserythropoiesis. Binucleate erythroid precursors are present.

presence of mycobacteria or fungi (Figure 19–3), but in many cases, no organisms are found.

- **Neoplasms:** The bone marrow is often involved in patients with HIV-related non-Hodgkin's lymphoma or Hodgkin's disease. Kaposi's sarcoma has also been found in the marrow.

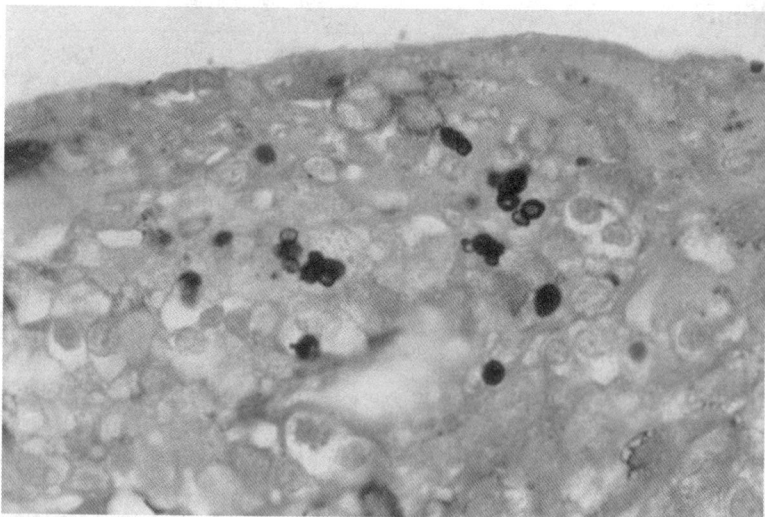

Figure 19–3 Bone marrow biopsy. Fungi. Yeast forms consistent with *Histoplasma* (Gomori-methenamine silver stain). Culture confirmed *Histoplasma capsulatum*.

20

Hemostasis and Thrombosis

The processes of blood coagulation (hemostasis) and clot dissolution (fibrinolysis) are intricate and interrelated. Our concepts of the hemostatic system are constantly evolving and changing. The complexity of the systems, their numerous disorders, and the tests used to investigate them can be mind-boggling. Fortunately, it is possible to have a practical understanding of hemostasis without understanding all of the myriad details, and most coagulation problems can be resolved with a limited number of basic tests.

There are two fundamental properties of the hemostatic system: *exquisite regulation and control* and *surface dependence*.

Regulation and Control Mechanisms

- Each system is balanced by an opposing or inhibiting system
- There are multiple negative feedback loops
- A system and its opposing system are often initiated simultaneously. A system often initiates its own inhibiting system.

Surface Dependence

- Hemostasis is designed to occur on a phospholipid surface. This serves to limit clotting to the sites of tissue injury and prevents clotting from occurring freely in the circulation. *Platelet phospholipid serves as the primary surface for coagulation.*

Calcium dependence is another feature of the coagulation systems. Calcium serves as the link between the platelet phospholipid and the coagulation proteins and is also critical in platelet activation and aggregation. We take advantage of this by using calcium chelators as anticoagulants in our sample tubes (citrate for coagulation studies; ethylenediaminetetraacetic acid [EDTA] for CBCs).

COMPONENTS OF THE HEMOSTATIC SYSTEM

Components of the global hemostatic system include

- Platelets
- von Willebrand's factor (**vWF**)
- Tissue factor, which has a critical role in initiating the coagulation cascade
- Clotting factors (proteins of the coagulation cascade)
- The fibrinolytic system (plasminogen/plasmin, tissue plasminogen activator)
- Anticoagulant proteins (antithrombin, protein C, protein S)
- Endothelial cells, which have an active role in preventing thrombosis

Other less obvious factors are also important in hemostasis. An example is constriction of injured blood vessels (*vasoconstriction*); this decreases blood loss and allows a buildup of activated clotting factors in the injured area. Another overlooked factor is *blood flow*, which helps dilute the activated clotting factors and washes them away from the injured area. This helps to limit clotting to the appropriate area.

ENDOTHELIAL CELLS IN HEMOSTASIS

Endothelial cells are not passive blood vessel wall linings; they are active participants in global hemostasis. Endothelial cells are particularly important in the *prevention* of coagulation.

- **Endothelial cell surface molecules:** Endothelial cells express several molecules on their surface membranes that are important in regulation of coagulation. Examples are **heparan sulfate** and **thrombomodulin**, which activate anticoagulant systems (antithrombin and the protein C-protein S system, respectively).
- **Endothelial cell metabolic products:** Endothelial cells produce a variety of metabolic products that are critical in the prevention of thrombosis, including *tissue plasminogen activator* (**t-PA**), the primary initiator of the fibrinolytic system; *tissue factor pathway inhibitor* (**TFPI**), which inhibits coagulation via the TF-VIIa-Xa complex; and *prostacyclin* (**PGI$_2$**), a potent vasodilator and platelet antagonist. Endothelial cells also produce *nitric oxide* (**NO**; originally called the *endothelial-derived relaxing factor* [EDRF]), which is a potent vasodilator and platelet antagonist, and *endothelin*, which is a potent vasoconstrictor.

DEFECTS IN THE BLOOD VESSEL WALL

Both defects in the blood vessel wall and intravascular processes not directly related to hemostasis can have clinical manifestations resembling coagulaion defects. *In most of these conditions, all of the usual coagulation tests will be normal* (platelet count, prothrombin time [PT], partial thromboplastin time [PTT]). Examples include the following:

- **Hereditary hemorrhagic telangiectasia** (**HHT**; *Osler-Weber-Rendu syndrome*): This is an autosomal dominant syndrome with abnormalities in blood vessel walls, resulting in telangiectasias all over the body. Bleeding from these telangiectasias occurs in the gastrointestinal tract, nose, other mucosal surfaces, and skin. Pulmonary hemorrhage can also be a problem. "Mulberry" lesions on the oral mucosa and cutaneous telangiectasias (particularly on the hands) are characteristic. There is no treatment for HHT as such. Iron supplementation is required to replace the iron lost by the chronic bleeding.
- **Scurvy**: Scurvy (*vitamin C deficiency*) results in weakening of capillary walls, with resultant cutaneous purpuras and mucosal bleeding. "*Corkscrew*" *hairs* and *perifollicular hemorrhages* are characteristic findings on the skin. Scurvy is often seen in malnourished alcoholics. Response to vitamin C supplementation is dramatic.
- **Vasculitis**: A variety of vasculitic processes can result in purpura or petechiae. These include leukocytoclastic (hypersensitivity) vasculitis, allergic reactions to medications (penicillin and others), cryoglobulinemia, Henoch-Schönlein purpura, and others. *Purpura due to vasculitis are often palpable; those due to pure coagulation defects are usually flat (non-palable).*
- **Amyloidosis**: Deposits of amyloid material in cutaneous blood vessels weaken the vessel walls, resulting in purpura.
- **Corticosteroid excess**: Patients with Cushing's syndrome, or on significant doses of corticosteroid medications for a prolonged period of time, develop increased fragility of the skin and blood vessels, resulting in cutaneous purpura.
- **Senile purpura**: Older people have less subcutaneous connective tissue support, with resulting skin fragility and cutaneous purpura.

PRIMARY VERSUS SECONDARY HEMOSTASIS

Coagulation (clotting) is traditionally divided into two systems: **primary hemostasis** and **secondary hemostasis**. This division is artificial, but it helps organize our thinking about hemostasis and corresponds to relatively distinct clinical syndromes. *Recognition of bleeding as involving primary or secondary hemostasis is critical in organizing the diagnostic and therapeutic approach to bleeding disorders.*

Primary Hemostasis

Primary hemostasis primarily involves *platelets* and *vWF* and results in the formation of a platelet plug. If the endothelial injury is small, this may be adequate to stop bleeding. However, if the injury is greater, participation by the coagulation cascade is required. The various causes of defects in the primary hemostasis system are listed in Table 20–1.

Manifestations of Primary Hemostasis Disorders

- *Immediate bleeding* after trauma, cuts, and surgical or dental procedures
- *Mucocutaneous bleeding*: petechia, easy bruising, epistaxis (nosebleeds), gingival bleeding, heme-positive stools, hematuria, and menorrhagia (heavy menstrual bleeding)

Secondary Hemostasis

Secondary hemostasis primarily involves the *coagulation cascade proteins*, which ultimately results in the conversion of fibrinogen to fibrin; fibrin polymerizes to form a clot. The fibrin clot is cross-linked and stabilized by factor XIIIa. The various causes of defects in the secondary hemostasis system are listed in Table 20–2.

Manifestations of Secondary Hemostasis Disorders

- *Delayed bleeding* from cuts or injuries
- *Hemarthroses* and *intramuscular hematomas*
- Deep soft tissue bleeds
- Intracranial hemorrhages
- Menorrhagia

Table 20–1
Causes of Primary Hemostasis Deficiencies

Thrombocytopenia

Inherited disorders of platelet function: Bernard-Soulier syndrome, Glanzmann's thrombasthenia, storage pool deficiency

von Willebrand's disease

Medications: aspirin, ticlopidine, clopidogrel, antibiotics (penicillins, cephalosporins), antihistamines, cough medications (guaifenesin), and many others

Acquired disorders of platelet function: myelodysplasia, increased fibrin degradation products

Table 20–2
Causes of Secondary Hemostasis Disorders

Hemophilias: inherited decrease in clotting factor levels or production of abnormal clotting factors

Decreased fibrinogen

Liver disease

Warfarin drugs: interfere with synthesis of vitamin K–dependent clotting factors

Fibrin degradation products (also interfere with platelet function)

MECHANISMS OF PRIMARY HEMOSTASIS

von Willebrand's Factor

von Willebrand's factor is synthesized by endothelial cells and megakaryocytes. It circulates in plasma complexed with the factor VIII clotting factor. It circulates as multimers of various sizes, with molecular weights up to 20 million daltons. The large multimers are required for normal vWF function; a decrease or absence of the high-molecular-weight multimers results in a bleeding disorder despite the presence of normal levels of *total* vWF (this is characteristic of one form of von Willebrand's disease [vWD]).

Platelets

Platelets are disc-shaped anucleate cells approximately 2 to 3 μm in diameter. The normal platelet number is approximately **150,000 to 350,000/μL** (150 to 350 × 10⁹/L). Platelets contain actin filaments, myosin, and other contractile proteins, which help them retain their shape and allow platelet plugs to contract.

Platelet Receptors

Platelets have a variety of surface glycoproteins, some of which act as receptors for vWF, fibrinogen, or other adhesive proteins. Many platelet receptors consist of complexes of two or more glycoproteins. The most important platelet receptors are the following:

- **GP Ib-IX/V** (previously designated **GP Ib-IX**): The platelet receptor for vWF. Designated **CD42** in the Cluster Designation (CD) system.
- **GP IIb-IIIa**: The platelet receptor for fibrinogen, which also acts as a receptor for vWF, fibronectin, and other adhesive proteins. Designated **CD41/CD61** in the CD system. GP IIb-IIIa exists on the resting platelet in a low-affinity or inactive form. After the platelet is activated by ini-

tial adhesion, the GP IIb-IIIa undergoes a conformational change to a high-affinity form, and additional IIb-IIIa is transferred from the interior to the exterior of the platelet.

Platelet Granules

Platelets contain two specific types of granules, called *alpha granules* and *dense bodies*. Alpha granules contain proteins, such as coagulation factors (fibrinogen, vWF, and factor V), platelet-specific proteins (β-thromboglobulin, platelet factor 4, platelet-derived growth factor), and others. Dense bodies contain small molecules and ions, such as adenosine diphosphate, adenosine triphosphate, calcium, and serotonin. Platelet granule contents are released when platelets are activated, providing an immediate source of clotting factors and platelet agonists, which recruit other platelets into the growing platelet plug.

Platelet Adhesion and Activation

When the endothelial layer of a blood vessel is disrupted, subendothelial collagen is exposed to the circulation. Large vWF multimers bind to subendothelial collagen and GP Ib-IX/V (the vWF receptor) on platelet surfaces, resulting in platelet adhesion and activation. GP IIb/IIIa (the fibrinogen receptor) on the platelet surface is converted from a low-affinity to a high-affinity form, and additional GP IIb/IIIa is brought to the platelet surface. The platelet granule contents are released, which recruit and activate other platelets.

Phospholipase A$_2$ is activated, generating **arachidonic acid** from platelet membrane phospholipids. Arachidonic acid is converted to **thromboxane A$_2$ (TxA$_2$)** by the enzymes **cyclooxygenase** and **thromboxane synthetase**. Thromboxane A$_2$ is a potent vasoconstrictor that stimulates platelet aggregation and causes release of platelet granules. Inhibition of cyclooxygenase (by aspirin and other nonsteroidal anti-inflammatory drugs) blocks the synthesis of thromboxane A$_2$, thus inhibiting platelet aggregation.

- *Inhibition of cyclooxygenase, with subsequent block of TxA$_2$ production, is how aspirin inhibits platelet activation.*
- Note that both prostacyclin (a potent vasodilator and platelet antagonist) and TxA$_2$ (a potent vasoconstrictor and platelet agonist) are derived from arachidonic acid via cyclooxygenase. Endothelial cells predominantly produce prostacyclin, whereas platelets predominantly produce TxA$_2$.

SECONDARY HEMOSTASIS: THE COAGULATION CASCADE

The term coagulation cascade refers to the sequential activation of coagulation factors, resulting in the conversion of fibrinogen to fibrin and the subsequent polymerization of fibrin into a fibrin clot. Most of the coagulation factors are serine proteases. They circulate in the plasma as inactive precursors (*zymogens*), which are converted to the active enzyme by protease cleavage. One coagulation factor cleaves and activates the next factor along the line and so on. Since each active enzyme can activate many molecules of the subsequent factor, there is a geometric increase in the number of molecules activated. Like a small snowball starting at the top of a hill, the end result of the coagulation cascade is an avalanche of activated clotting factors.

The clotting factors are designated by Roman numerals. The inactive precursor is designated by the plain Roman numeral, and the active form is designated by the suffix "a" (for example, factor X is the inactive precursor, factor Xa is the active enzyme form). The clotting factors were also given common names, but most of these are no longer used. Factor VIII is sometimes referred to as the *antihemophilic factor*, and factor IX is occasionally called *Christmas factor*. *Prothrombin* is usually used instead of factor II, *thrombin* instead of IIa, and *fibrinogen* instead of factor I (Table 20–3). A few other proteins involved in laboratory tests of coagulation were not given Roman numerals; examples include **high-molecular-weight kininogen** (**HMWK**) and **prekallikrein** (**PK**).

Table 20–3
Coagulation Factors

Factor	Common Name	Half-life	Other
I	Fibrinogen	3–5 days	
II	Prothrombin	3 days	Vitamin K dependent; active form = thrombin
V		12 hours	
VII		5–8 hours	Vitamin K dependent
VIII	Anti-hemophilia factor	8–12 hours	Circulates bound to vWF
IX	Christmas factor	18–24 hours	Vitamin K dependent
X		36 hours	Vitamin K dependent
XI		3 days	
XII	Hageman factor	48 hours	
XIII		3–5 days	Cross-links polymerized fibrin to form a stable fibrin clot

Factors V and VIII are not enzymes; they are *cofactors*. Factor VIIIa is an essential cofactor for factor IXa in the activation of factor X to Xa, and factor Va is an essential cofactor for factor Xa in the conversion of pro-thrombin to thrombin. Factors V and VIII are converted to Va and VIIIa by thrombin.

Classic Concept of the Coagulation Cascade

The classic concept of the coagulation cascade featured two separate and independent pathways: the **intrinsic pathway** measured by the **partial thromboplastin time** (**PTT**), and the **extrinsic pathway** measured by the **prothrombin time** (**PT**). The two pathways came together at the activation stage of factor X to Xa, and hence the pathway from factor X down to fibrin was called the **common pathway** (Figure 20–1). We now know that there is really only one pathway; the intrinsic pathway is largely a laboratory artifact. However, because we still use the same two main tests to investigate the status of the coagulation cascade, you must understand both pathways in order to interpret the results of laboratory tests of coagulation.

Intrinsic Pathway

The intrinsic pathway (also called the **contact activation pathway**) starts with factor XII coming in contact with a negatively charged surface and

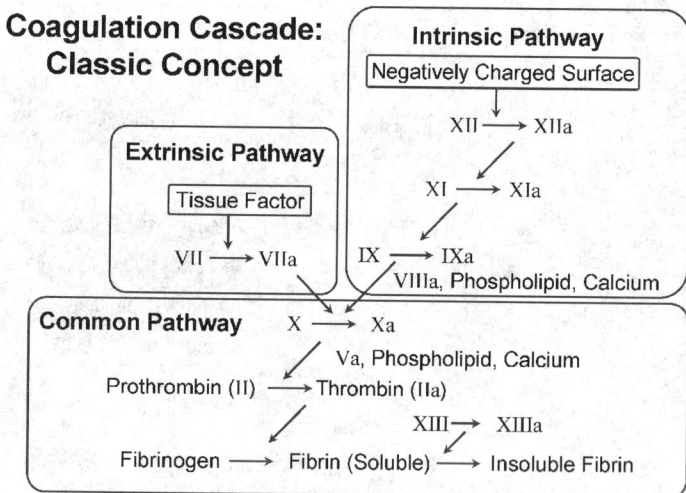

Figure 20–1 Classic concept of the coagulation cascade.

being activated to XIIa. **High-molecular-weight kininogen** and **PK** are required. Factor XIIa then activates XI to XIa, XIa activates IX to IXa, IXa activates X to Xa (in the presence of factor VIIIa, calcium, and phospholipid), and so on. **Deficiencies in any factors involved in the intrinsic pathway result in prolongation of the PTT: factors XII, XI, IX, VIII, and HMWK and PK.** Deficiencies of factors in the common pathway also result in prolongation of the PTT, but the PT is also prolonged.

Extrinsic Pathway

The extrinsic pathway (also called the **tissue factor pathway**) starts with exposure of **tissue factor** (**TF**) to blood. Tissue factor is a transmembrane protein that is highly expressed in the adventitia of blood vessels, the brain, glomeruli, and other tissues. It is not normally present on endothelial surfaces or blood cells. Exposed tissue factor reacts with trace amounts of factor VIIa, which are normally present in the circulation. The TF-factor VIIa complex then activates factor X to Xa, starting the common pathway. **Deficiencies of factor VII result in prolongation of the PT.** Deficiencies of factors in the common pathway also result in prolongation of the PT, but the PTT is also prolonged.

Current Concept of the Coagulation Cascade

In the current concept of the coagulation, *the key initiating step is the exposure of TF to the circulation and reaction of TF with factor VIIa.* The TF-factor VIIa complex can enzymatically activate factor X to Xa, factor IX to IXa, and factor XI to XIa. The initial activation of factor X to Xa may be important in getting the coagulation cascade started; however, a specific inhibitor produced by endothelium called *tissue factor pathway inhibitor* (*TFPI*) rapidly inactivates the TF-VIIa-Xa complex. Therefore, **the major action of the TF-VIIa complex in vivo is the activation of factor IX to IXa, which then activates factor X to Xa.** Activation of factor XI to XIa by the TF-VIIa complex appears to play a relatively minor role in the coagulation cascade (Figure 20–2).

Activation of factor X to Xa and prothrombin (II) to thrombin (IIa) are key steps in the coagulation cascade since both Xa and thrombin have positive feedback activity on earlier steps of the cascade. Factor Xa activates VII to VIIa, increasing the amount of VIIa available to complex with TF. Thrombin converts factor V to Va and factor VIII to VIIIa. It also activates factor XI to XIa and XIII to XIIIa. Thrombin is also a potent platelet agonist. Factor X is activated by a complex of factor IXa, VIIIa, phospholipid, and calcium. Prothrombin is activated by a complex of factor Xa, Va, phospholipid, and calcium.

Coagulation Cascade: Current Concept

Key Initiating Step: Exposure of Tissue Factor on Injured Vessel Wall

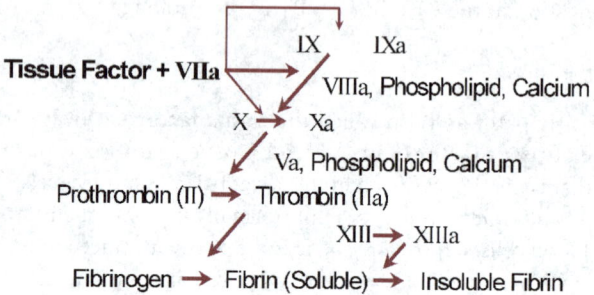

Figure 20–2 Current concept of the coagulation cascade.

Thrombin cleaves off two small peptides from fibrinogen (*fibrinopeptides A and B*), converting fibrinogen to **fibrin monomer**. Fibrin monomer spontaneously polymerizes to form **soluble fibrin polymer**, which is then covalently cross-linked by factor XIIIa, converting it to a stable fibrin clot.

Properties of the Coagulation Factors

Clotting factors are synthesized in the liver. Synthesis of factors II (prothrombin), VII, IX, and X is vitamin K dependent. Vitamin K is required for a reaction that adds an extra carboxyl group to the gamma (γ) position of glutamic acid in a post-translational step, converting it to γ-carboxyglutamate. In the absence of vitamin K, or in the presence of vitamin K antagonists such as warfarin, inactive forms of the precursors are produced and the coagulation cascade is blocked.

Factor VIII circulates bound to vWF. Binding of factor VIII to vWF increases the half-life of factor VIII. A deficiency of vWF, or an abnormal vWF that cannot bind factor VIII, results in decreased plasma factor VIII levels.

⇨ Older terminology for the complex of factor VIII and vWF is confusing. The coagulant component of the complex was formerly designated factor VIII coagulant (factor VIII:C), and vWF was called factor VIII–related antigen (factor VIII:Rag). Current terminology designates the coagulant component as factor VIII and the vWF component as vWF.

Measurement of Clotting Factor Levels

Clotting factor levels can be measured in two main ways: clot-based assays (activity methods) and immunologic methods (enzyme-linked immunosorbent assay [ELISA] or similar immunoassays). Immunoassays give the absolute concentration of the protein (mg/dL); however, they tell you nothing about the *functional* properties of the protein. The clot-based assays tell you how much functional activity of a specific factor is present but may not correlate with the protein concentration. Some patients with hemophilia have mutations that result in the production of a nonfunctional protein, which will be detected by the immunoassay but will show no activity in clot-based assays. The clot-based assays have a wide normal range, typically 50 to 150% or 75 to 150%.

NATURAL INHIBITORS OF THE COAGULATION CASCADE

The rampant amplification of the coagulation cascade must be checked and controlled in order to limit clotting to the area where it is needed. Factors that inhibit coagulation include the following:

- **Blood flow and hepatic degradation of clotting factors:** Normal blood flow dilutes the activated clotting factors below the level required to propagate the cascade. Hepatocytes in the liver digest and destroy the activated clotting factors washed away from the site of clot formation.
- **Antithrombin:** Antithrombin (**AT**; previously called **antithrombin III [AT III]**) is the **most important physiologic inhibitor of activated coagulation factors**. Antithrombin is synthesized in the liver and endothelial cells. It irreversibly binds to and inhibits thrombin, factor Xa, and other activated clotting factors. **Heparin** (or heparan sulfate on endothelial cells) **binds to and activates AT**. By itself, AT has a low affinity for thrombin; however, complexing with heparin increases the activity of AT approximately 1,000-fold.
- **Protein C and protein S:** Proteins C and S are vitamin K–dependent inhibitors of the coagulation cascade that control coagulation by inactivating factors Va and VIIIa. Protein C is activated by the binding of thrombin to **thrombomodulin** on endothelial cell surfaces; therefore, *thrombin, a key mediator of the coagulation cascade, also initiates a key anticoagulant system.* When thrombin binds to thrombomodulin, thrombin is no longer able to convert fibrinogen to fibrin; instead, it enzymatically cleaves and activates protein C. **Activated protein C, in combination with protein S, inactivates factors Va and VIIIa.** Protein

S circulates in two forms: free protein S and protein S complexed with a protein involved in the complement system, the C4b binding protein. Free protein S is active, whereas the bound form is not. Increases in the C4b binding protein (as in acute inflammation) decrease the level of free protein S and can be prothrombotic.

THE FIBRINOLYTIC SYSTEM

Fibrinolysis (clot dissolving) is as important in the global processes of hemostasis as the coagulation cascade. The important players in fibrinolysis are **plasminogen/plasmin** and **t-PA**. There are also plasmin inhibitors, the most important of which is α_2-**antiplasmin**, as well as inhibitors of plasminogen activation.

Plasminogen/Plasmin

Plasmin is the enzyme that digests fibrin and thus dissolves clots. Plasmin circulates as an inactive precursor, *plasminogen*. Plasminogen is activated to plasmin primarily by **t-PA**, which is secreted by endothelial cells. Plasminogen can also be activated by the contact activation pathway (factor XII, HMWK, and PK). This appears to be a minor activator in vivo, but patients with deficiencies of the contact activation pathway may have a slightly increased risk of thrombosis. Plasminogen can also be activated by *urokinase-type plasminogen activator* (**u-PA**), *streptokinase*, and a variety of reptile (snake) venoms. Recombinant t-PA, u-PA, and streptokinase are used therapeutically to dissolve clots (deep venous thrombi, pulmonary emboli, and coronary artery thromboses).

The results of fibrin degradation by plasmin are a variety of **fibrin degradation products** (**FDPs**; sometimes called fibrin split products or FSPs). Fibrin degradation products inhibit coagulation by inserting into the fibrin clot in place of fibrinogen. They also inhibit platelet aggregation. A variety of assays for FDPs are available; most of these detect a miscellaneous mixture of FDPs. Fibrin degradation product assays are not actually specific for *fibrin* degradation; plasmin can also digest fibrinogen, and *fibrinogen* degradation products will also result in a positive test for FDPs. A specific fibrin degradation product is the **D-dimer**; this results from the digestion of fibrin that has been cross-linked by factor XIIIa. Thus, the presence of D-dimer in circulation indicates that thrombin has been activated and has resulted in both fibrin clotting and activation of factor XIII to XIIIa, and that plasminogen has been activated to plasmin with subsequent digestion of the cross-linked fibrin clot.

- Sensitive assays for D-dimer are sometimes used to help exclude deep venous thrombosis or pulmonary emboli. A negative test for D-dimer (using a sensitive assay) is evidence against a significant thrombus.

Plasmin can degrade fibrinogen and other clotting factors as well as fibrin clots, and excessive activity of the fibrinolytic system can result in severe bleeding. Therefore, the fibrinolytic system also needs to be controlled. One important control mechanism is **localization of plasmin activity to the surface of fibrin clots**. Plasminogen is bound into fibrin clots as they are formed. Tissue plasminogen activator has a much higher affinity for plasminogen that is localized on the surface of a fibrin clot than it does for free plasminogen, and this helps to specifically localize fibrinolyis to the clot. There is also a circulating inhibitor of plasmin, α_2-**antiplasmin**, which inactivates any plasmin that is free in circulation. Plasmin bound to fibrin is protected from inhibition by α_2-antiplasmin.

Inhibition of Plasminogen Activation

Just as there are inhibitors to plasmin, there are also inhibitors of plasmin activation. The primary inhibitor of t-PA is **plasminogen activator inhibitor-1** (**PAI-1**). A second inhibitor of plasminogen activation is called **plasminogen activator inhibitor-2** (**PAI-2**). The concentration of PAI-2 is high during pregnancy and is present in high concentration in placental circulation. Otherwise, it plays a relatively minor role.

LABORATORY TESTS OF COAGULATION

There is a huge number of different laboratory tests that can be used to investigate hemostasis and coagulation, ranging from fairly basic (platelet count, PT, PTT, fibrinogen level) to highly exotic. The great majority of hemostasis questions can be resolved with the basic tests, plus a clinical history, physical examination, and a little thought. This discussion will primarily highlight the common, widely available laboratory tests. A few of the more specialized tests will be discussed along with the specific diseases they are used to diagnose. Coagulation textbooks should be consulted for the really exotic tests.

Samples for Coagulation Testing

Nowhere in laboratory medicine is getting a good specimen more important than in coagulation. The only specimen acceptable for routine coagulation testing is blood anticoagulated with **sodium citrate** (the light-blue top tube). It is important that the tube is properly filled (not overfilled and not underfilled). *Blood anticoagulated with EDTA or heparin is unacceptable for most coagulation testing.*

The ratio of plasma to anticoagulant in the sample tube is important; if the tube is inadequately filled, or the patient has a very high hematocrit (over 55%), there will be too much anticoagulant for the amount of plasma and the coagulation tests may be falsely prolonged. Underfilled tubes should be rejected and redrawn. If the patient has a hematocrit over 55%, a small amount of anticoagulant should be withdrawn from the tube prior to drawing the blood sample.

⇨ **Never draw blood for coagulation studies through a running line, especially if heparin is being used to keep the line open.** Even tiny traces of heparin will cause wildy erroneous coagulation tests.

It is important to understand the sensitivities of the tests used for deficiencies in clotting factors. **The PT or PTT will usually be normal with levels of clotting factors above ~30% of normal** (single-factor deficiency). They will also be normal with multiple factor deficiencies if all factors have concentrations above 50% of normal. Some instrument/reagent combinations will give normal results with even lower factor levels. **Therefore, a normal PT or PTT result does *not* reliably exclude a mild or moderate factor deficiency.**

Prothrombin Time

The PT incorporates a source of tissue thromboplastin (TF) such as rabbit brain, which also includes the phospholipid required for clotting. Prewarmed PT reagent suspended in calcium chloride ($CaCl_2$) is added to the test plasma, which is anticoagulated with citrate. The $CaCl_2$ neutralizes the effect of the citrate and initiates clotting. Clotting (fibrin polymerization) can be detected by either photo-optical or mechanical methods. **The PT tests the extrinsic and common pathways; it is prolonged with deficiencies of factor VII and factors in the common pathway** (X, V, prothrombin, fibrinogen) (Figure 20–3). It is also prolonged in liver disease, vitamin K deficiency, therapeutic warfarin and heparin anticoagulation, disseminated intravascular coagulation (DIC), with high levels of FDPs, and occasionally by lupus anticoagulants (lupus anticoagulants typically prolong the PTT; the PT is usually not affected).

The PT is traditionally used to follow anticoagulant therapy with vitamin K antagonists such as warfarin. For monitoring warfarin therapy, the PT is usually reported in terms of the **International Normalized Ratio (INR)**. The INR is the PT adjusted for the sensitivity of the specific thromboplastin reagent to the effect of warfarin, normalized to 1. The **INR = (patient PT ÷ mean normal PT)^{ISI}**, where the ISI (International Sensitivity Index) depends on the sensitivity of the specific thromboplastin to warfarin. The desired INR value depends on the process being treated. The desired INR for treatment of deep vein thrombosis is ~2 to 3. For a patient with a thrombogenic mechanical heart valve, a higher INR is required (~2.5 to 3.5 or 3 to 4.5).

Prothrombin Time

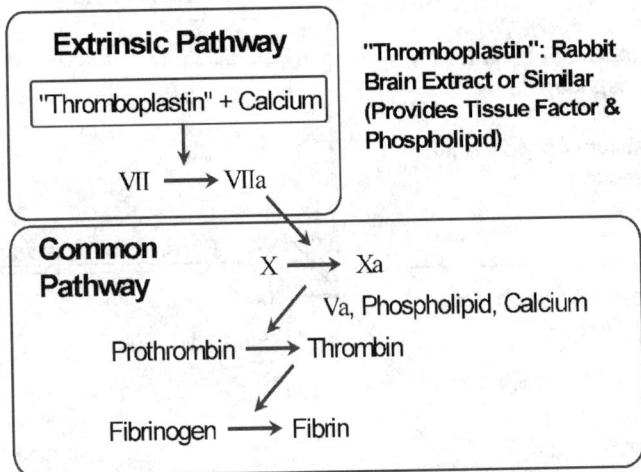

Figure 20–3 Prothrombin time.

A **typical reference range for the PT is ~11 to 13 seconds**. Each laboratory should determine its own reference range for its specific instruments and reagents.

⇨ Some people believe that because we use the PT to follow warfarin therapy and the PTT to follow heparin therapy, the PT is not affected by heparin and the PTT is not affected by warfarin. That is incorrect. The PTT is more sensitive to heparin than the PT, but the PT is also affected by heparin. The PTT is also affected by warfarin, but the PT changes first.

Partial Thromboplastin Time*

The PTT (Figure 20–4) uses phospholipid usually derived from an extract of rabbit or bovine brain tissue (the partial thromboplastin reagent) and an activator of the contact activation system such as silica particles. The anticoagulated test plasma is added to the partial thromboplastin/activator mix and incubated briefly. $CaCl_2$ is added to initiate clotting and clot formation is detected as described above. **The PTT is prolonged with deficiencies of the contact activation pathway** (factors XII, XI, IX, VIII; also HMWK and PK) **and the common pathway** (X, V, prothrombin, fibrinogen). The PTT

---

*The **PTT** is also known as the *activated* partial thromboplastin time (**aPTT**). Activated PTT is technically more correct, but most people use PTT.

Partial Thromboplastin Time

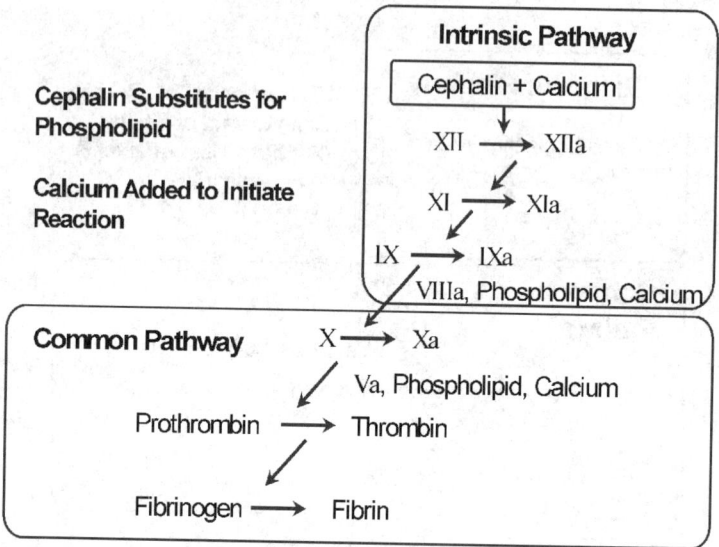

Figure 20–4 Partial thromboplastin time.

will be normal with pure factor VII deficiency. It is prolonged in liver disease, vitamin K deficiency, therapeutic warfarin and heparin anticoagulation, DIC, and with high levels of FDPs. Lupus anticoagulants usually prolong the PTT. **A typical reference range for PTT is ~23 to 35 seconds.** Again, each laboratory should establish its own reference range.

The PTT is traditionally used to monitor therapeutic anticoagulation with regular (unfractionated) heparin. The usual desired therapeutic range is prolongation of the PTT to ~1.5 to 2.5 times the mean normal result. A problem with using the PTT to monitor heparin therapy is that different people have vastly different PTT responses to heparin. The factor Xa inactivation assay is an alternative test to monitor therapy with unfractionated heparin.

Thrombin Time (Sometimes Called Thrombin Clotting Time

The thrombin time (TT) uses exogenous thrombin to convert fibrinogen to fibrin. It is prolonged with decreased fibrinogen, elevated levels of FDPs, dysfibrinogenemias, and heparin. It is not affected by deficiencies in the intrinsic or extrinsic pathways. The TT can be used to monitor heparin therapy, although the PTT is more often used. The TT may be used to monitor heparin therapy in patients with a lupus anticoagulant and a baseline prolonged PTT.

⤳ The **reptilase time** (RT) is similar to the TT. It uses a snake venom that has thrombin-like activity. It is elevated in hypofibrinogenemia, dysfibrinogenemia, and with high levels of FDPs. It is *not* sensitive to heparin. Therefore, the combination of a prolonged TT and a normal RT indicates heparin.

Bleeding Time

The bleeding time (BT) is the *best available* **screening test** of **primary hemostasis**. The BT is performed by placing a blood pressure cuff on the upper arm and inflating it to 40 mm Hg. A small incision is made on the anterior surface of the forearm using a template instrument that makes standardized 3-mm incisions. A piece of filter paper is gently touched to the bleeding spot every 30 seconds until the bleeding stops. The BT tests the function of platelets and vWF. The integrity of blood vessel walls and the skin are also important to the assay. A typical BT range is ~**2.5 to 9 minutes**, but the normal range varies widely.

The **BT is prolonged in thrombocytopenia** (platelet count <100,000/μL), **vWD, inherited or acquired disorders of platelet function** (Bernard-Soulier syndrome or Glanzmann's disease; myelodysplasia), with **antiplatelet agents** (aspirin, ticlopidine), and in **uremia**. The BT is usually normal or minimally prolonged with deficiencies of the coagulation cascade, unless there is some superimposed factor (ie, antiplatelet drugs). The BT may not correlate well with the platelet count in immune thrombocytopenic purpura (ITP); this may be because in ITP many platelets are large and may be more effective in hemostasis.

The BT is most useful in the diagnosis of defects of primary hemostasis, such as vWD. *It is not useful and should* **not** *be ordered in the diagnosis of disorders of* **secondary** *hemostasis, such as hemophilia.* There is usually no reason to do a BT if the patient is thrombocytopenic (<100,000/μL). It is usually not necessary to order a BT if the patient comes in with obvious petechiae or purpura because you can presume that the BT will be prolonged. The BT in children is difficult to interpret since good normal ranges for BT in children have not been established; the BT is often longer than in adults.

The BT is the best *available* screening test of primary hemostasis; however, it is actually not very good. It can be affected by many variables, including the temperature of the room, the person who does the test, a variety of medications, and many others. *If* you carefully standardize the test and have one or two carefully trained people to always perform it, it can be very useful in the work-up of bleeding problems. However, it must be interpreted with caution. Patients with vWD can have variable BT results, and the test may have to be repeated a few times to detect an abnormal result.

⇨ **The BT is *not* useful in predicting the risk of bleeding during surgery or other procedures.** There is a poor correlation between the BT and the occurrence of surgical bleeding.

Mixing Study

Mixing studies are used to distinguish factor deficiencies from factor inhibitors (lupus anticoagulants or specific factor inhibitors such as antibodies directed against factor VIII). Mixing studies take advantage of the fact that factor levels of 50% of normal should give a normal PT or PTT result. If the problem is a simple factor deficiency, mixing the patient plasma 1:1 with plasma that contains 100% of the normal factor level results in a level ≥50% in the mixture (say the patient has an activity of 0%; the average of 100% + 0% = 50%). The PT or PTT will be normal (the mixing study shows correction). However, if there is an inhibitor that inactivates the added clotting factor, the resulting factor level will be low and the clotting test will be prolonged (fails to correct). Therefore, **correction with mixing indicates factor deficiency; failure to correct indicates an inhibitor**. Unfortunately, it is not as simple as that.

Some inhibitors are *time dependent*. In other words, it takes time for the antibody to react with and inactivate the added clotting factor. The clotting test performed immediately after the specimens are mixed may show correction because the antibody has not had time to inactivate the added factor. A test performed after the mixture is incubated for 2 hours at 37°C will show prolongation. Nonspecific inhibitors like the lupus anticoagulant usually are not time dependent; the immediate mixture will show prolongation. Many specific factor inhibitors are time dependent, and the inhibitor will not be detected unless the test is repeated after incubation (factor VIII inhibitors are notorious for this).

Platelet Neutralization Procedure

The platelet neutralization procedure (PNP) is performed to detect phospholipid-dependent inhibitors such as the lupus anticoagulant. These inhibitors tie up the phospholipid added to the reaction cuvette, making it unavailable for the coagulation cascade and thus prolonging the phospholipid-dependent clotting tests (usually the PTT; less often the PT). The PNP incorporates added phospholipid, to overwhelm the inhibitor. The test is performed by adding reagent platelet membranes or other exogenous phospholipid to the patient's plasma and performing the clotting test. Since the phospholipid dilutes the plasma, you must run a parallel mixture to which you add saline, to control for the dilution. If there is a phospholipid-dependent inhibitor, the PNP will usually show at least a 6-second shortening compared to the saline control.

Bethesda Assay

The Bethesda assay is used to measure the strength of inhibitors. One Bethesda unit (BU) is the amount of inhibitor that neutralizes 50% of the factor in the normal plasma. The titer of the inhibitor in BU can be helpful in predicting how the patient will respond to different therapies. If the patient has a low titer of inhibitor (less than about ~3 to 5 BU), you can usually overwhelm the inhibitor by increasing the amount of factor given. If the patient has a high titer (≥10 BU), you will probably need to find some alternative therapy.

Platelet Aggregation Studies

Platelet aggregation studies are used to diagnose disorders of primary hemostasis such as vWD, deficiencies of platelet membrane receptors (Bernard-Soulier syndrome, Glanzmann's thrombasthenia), and platelet storage pool diseases. These are not performed in most community hospitals but may be performed at specialized coagulation laboratories or large medical centers.

INHERITED DISORDERS OF COAGULATION

There are a large number of inherited disorders of coagulation; however, only three are relatively common: **vWD**, **factor VIII deficiency** (**hemophilia A**), and **factor IX deficiency** (**hemophilia B**; **Christmas disease**). All of the others are rare. *It is critical to know the clinical manifestations, inheritance patterns, diagnostic tests, and treatment of these three diseases.*

von Willebrand's Disease

von Willebrand disease is the most common inherited disorder of primary hemostasis. The prevalence of vWD mutations may be as high as 1 to 2% of the population, although many are never diagnosed; the prevalence of *clinically evident* vWD is much lower. *The clinical and laboratory manifestations of vWD are extremely heterogeneous, and diagnosis can sometimes be difficult.*

Three main subtypes of vWD have been defined:

- **Type 1:** This is by far the most common (≥70% of cases of clinical vWD). There is a decrease in the concentration of vWF in the plasma (ie, a **quantitative defect**), but all sizes of multimers, including the very high-molecular-weight multimers, are present. The **inheritance pattern** is **autosomal dominant**.

- **Type 2**: In Type 2 vWD, there is a **qualitative defect** in vWF, not a quantitative defect. Several different subtypes of vWD Type 2 are described. Inheritance is autosomal dominant in most cases, although a few types display autosomal recessive inheritance.
  - **Type 2A**: In Type 2A, there is a deficiency of the high-molecular-weight multimers of vWD, but the absolute level of total vWF is normal. This is the most common variant of vWD Type 2.
  - **Type 2B**: In Type 2B, the vWF appears to have an abnormally increased affinity for the vWF receptor (GP Ib-IX/V) on the platelet surface. Too much vWF is tied up on the platelet surface, rather than being in the plasma, and is therefore not able to bind to subendothelial collagen. The diagnosis of Type 2B vWD is made by demonstrating *increased* platelet agglutination with ristocetin rather than decreased ristocetin agglutination, as seen in the other types of vWD. Mild thrombocytopenia is common.
  - **Type 2M**: In Type 2M vWD, there is a mutation that affects some important functional domains of the protein (think "**M**" for **M**utation). A variety of mutations in different regions of the protein have been described.
  - **Type 2N (vWD Normandy)**: In Type 2N, there is a deficiency of the binding site for factor VIII on the vWF, so it cannot act as a chaperone for factor VIII. Consequently, the factor VIII half-life and plasma levels are decreased, and the patients *clinically* resemble mild hemophilia A. von Willebrand's disease Type 2N should be suspected when the family history does not fit the typical X-linked recessive inheritance pattern in a patient who otherwise appears to have hemophilia A. The diagnosis is established by demonstrating decreased affinity of vWF for factor VIII.
- **Type 3**: In Type 3 vWD, there is a **total or near-total absence of vWF** in the plasma. Type 3 vWD is rare. The patients have markedly decreased factor VIII levels (since they have no vWF to act as chaperone for factor VIII), and thus they may have bleeding manifestations resembling hemophilia. The inheritance pattern is autosomal recessive; some cases appear to represent homozygous Type 1 vWD.

⇨ *This classification system for vWD is simplified and relatively new. Older textbooks and articles use a different, more complicated classification with many more subtypes (Type IID, IIE, and so on). These have mostly been combined together in the present Type 2A category. Types 1, 2B, and 3 are pretty much the same in the new and old classifications.*

Clinical Manifestations of von Willebrand's Disease

Most cases of vWD present with the typical picture of a **primary hemostatic defect**: mucocutaneous bleeding (epistaxis, bleeding gums), easy bruising, and immediate bleeding from cuts, incisions, and dental extractions. Most patients have a mild to moderate bleeding tendency. *The severity of illness in different patients is highly variable*, and *it can also vary over time in individual patients*. The clinical phenotype can vary between different members of the same family. Many patients have relatively minor bleeding, and it is common for Type 1 vWD not to be diagnosed until the patient has a major hemostatic challenge as an adult, such as a dental extraction. The laboratory manifestations of vWD can also be highly variable; sometimes laboratory tests must be repeated several times to make a firm diagnosis. As noted, **the inheritance pattern of most cases of vWD is *autosomal dominant***.

Type 3 vWD presents with a mixed picture. Since the factor VIII levels are low, the patients may have hemarthroses, muscle hematomas, and other manifestations of defects of secondary hemostasis in addition to mucocutaneous bleeding.

Laboratory Diagnosis of von Willebrand's Disease

The most important diagnostic tests for vWD are the *bleeding time, ristocetin cofactor assay*, a *quantitative assay of vWF concentration* (ELISA or Laurell rocket immunoelectrophoresis), *ristocetin-induced platelet aggregation*, and *agarose gel electrophoresis* to determine whether the high-molecular-weight multimers are present or absent. Not all of these tests may be needed in every case.

- von Willebrand's factor levels vary over time in a given individual; they are increased with estrogen, during stress, and with liver disease. These levels also increase dramatically during pregnancy (as does the level of the factor VIII coagulant protein). If you strongly suspect vWD but the assay shows a normal level, consider repeating the test at another time. If the patient is a pregnant woman, repeat the work-up after she has delivered (several weeks after, to allow time for the vWF level to decrease).
- von Willebrand's factor levels vary with the blood group; they are lowest in patients with blood group O, higher in patients with groups A, B, or AB. Always be a little suspicious of the diagnosis of vWD in people with blood group O.

In vWD Type 1, the BT will usually be prolonged. The PTT may also be slightly prolonged due to decreased factor VIII concentration. The absolute level of vWF is decreased; the vWF multimer pattern is normal (the high-molecular-weight multimers are present, but the concentration of all sizes

of multimers is decreased). Platelet aggregation with ristocetin and the ris
tocetin cofactor activity are decreased; platelet aggregation with other
agents is usually normal. Addition of normal plasma to platelets from
patients with vWD corrects the aggregation deficiency, confirming that the
deficiency is in the plasma, not the platelets.

Type 2A is diagnosed by demonstrating an absence of the high-molecular-weight multimers by agarose gel electrophoresis. The absolute concentration of vWF is usually normal.

Type 2B is diagnosed by demonstrating *increased* platelet agglutination
with ristocetin. Plasma from patients with Type 2B will agglutinate platelets
at very low ristocetin concentrations, which will not induce agglutination
in normal people. The absolute level of vWF is decreased; agarose gel electrophoresis demonstrates a decrease in high-molecular-weight multimers
(because they are all stuck on the platelets). Mild thrombocytopenia is
common.

Diagnosis of Type 2M requires sophisticated techniques, which are not
widely available; therefore, specimens must usually be sent to reference laboratories that specialize in coagulation. Diagnosis of Type 2N may be suspected from the clinical history (resembling a mild or moderate case of
hemophilia) and inheritance pattern (autosomal, not X-linked). Definitive
diagnosis of Type 2N requires an assay of the affinity of vWF for factor VIII
(available in some specialized reference laboratories).

Type 3 is diagnosed by demonstrating a total or near-total absence of
vWF in the plasma.

Treatment of von Willebrand's Disease

Most cases of vWD Type 1 can be very successfully treated with *desmopressin acetate* (**DDAVP**), which causes release of preformed vWD from
endothelial cells. Desmopressin acetate is cheap, is safe, and has no infectious risk. It can be administered either intravenously or intranasally; the
advantage of the intranasal method is that patients can easily treat themselves. *Desmopressin acetate has been considered contraindicated in vWD
Type 2B since it may induce thrombocytopenia.*

⇨ There are two types of DDAVP nasal sprays: one for diabetes insipidus
and one for vWD. *The preparation for vWD is 10 times more concentrated
than the one for diabetes insipidus, so be sure your patient gets the correct
one.*

Other types of vWD, or a patient with Type 1 requiring major surgery,
may need replacement therapy. There are no commercially available vWF
concentrate preparations, but some factor VIII concentrate preparations
contain enough vWF to be effective. However, not all factor VIII concen-

rates contain significant amounts of vWF, and the high-molecular-weight multimers may be lacking. Humate-P has been recommended as having the most normal distribution of multimer sizes, but some other brands of factor VIII also contain significant amounts of vWF. Check the package insert, which should state the amount of vWF contained.

⇨ *Recombinant* factor VIII has *no* vWF and would not be useful in patients with vWD.

⇨ The treatment of choice *used to be* cryoprecipitate since it is high in the vWF/factor VIII complex. However, there is no way to sterilize cryoprecipitate, unlike factor VIII concentrates, which are intensively treated. **Factor VIII concentrates have therefore replaced cryoprecipitate as the treatment of choice for vWD requiring factor replacement**.

Other Inherited Disorders of Primary Hemostasis

Other inherited disorders of primary hemostasis include Bernard-Soulier syndrome and Glanzmann's thrombasthenia, which are deficiencies of the GP Ib-IX/V and IIb/IIa receptors on the platelet surface, respectively. A deficiency of platelet granules may also occur (*platelet storage disease*). These are all rare. Bernard-Soulier and Glanzmann's thrombasthenia can be diagnosed by flow cytometry, using antibodies against the platelet glycoproteins (available in reference flow cytometry laboratories). Storage pool disease is diagnosed by electron microscopy of platelets, demonstrating an absence of granules.

The Hemophilias

The hemophilias are *inherited disorders of the coagulation cascade*. Deficiency of **factor VIII** (**hemophilia A**) is by far the most common (~85% of cases). **Factor IX** deficiency (**hemophilia B**) is second (~15%), and all others are rare. The incidence of hemophilia A is estimated at 1 per 5,000 to 10,000 male births in the United States; the incidence of hemophilia B is approximately 1 in 30,000 male births. **Hemophilia A and B** are both inherited as **X-linked recessive**: women are carriers, men develop the disease. All of the other factor deficiencies are inherited as autosomal recessive. **Factor XI** deficiency (sometimes called **hemophilia C**) is the third most common inherited disorder of coagulation factors but is much less common than deficiency of factors VIII or IX. In the United States, factor XI deficiency is most often seen in Ashkenazi Jews (origin from Eastern Europe).

• It is important to remember that not all clotting factor deficiencies result in clinical bleeding. Deficiency of factor XII, for example, results in dramatic prolongation of the PTT but no bleeding tendency. Deficiency of factor XI is associated with a bleeding tendency in about half of cases. The best guide to the likelihood of bleeding in such patients is the history. Factor V deficiency results in a bleeding deficiency, which is often surprisingly mild. Deficiencies of the other clotting factors result in a bleeding tendency.

Hemophilia A and Hemophilia B

Clinical Features

The clinical features of hemophilia A and B are identical. The manifestations are those of deficiencies of secondary hemostasis: **hemarthroses, muscle hematomas, soft tissue bleeding, and delayed but prolonged bleeding from cuts or incisions**. Recurrent hemarthroses result in joint destruction and can be disabling. Bleeding into muscle or soft tissue can result in a compartment syndrome, with compression of nerves and blood vessels; this may require fasciotomy for relief. **Intracranial bleeding** is an especially serious complication, and even minor head trauma in a severe hemophiliac should be treated with factor replacement. *There is no such thing as minor head trauma in a severe hemophiliac.* Another potentially lethal complication is bleeding into the soft tissues of the oropharynx; dissection of the hematoma into the trachea can result in airway occlusion and asphyxiation.

Children with severe hemophilia usually begin to have problems at about 9 to 12 months of age, at about the time they begin to walk. Some will come to medical attention earlier due to prolonged bleeding after circumcision or other surgery. Mild or moderate cases may not have problems until they undergo a severe challenge to hemostasis, such as a dental extraction, major surgery, or severe injury.

The severity of bleeding depends on the level of the deficient factor (Table 20–4). It is not uncommon for patients with a mild deficiency to go undiagnosed until adulthood, even if they have played football or other contact sports. Approximately half of hemophilia A cases have severe disease, with a total absence of detectable factor activity.

Most patients will have a family history of pathologic bleeding on the maternal side, including maternal brothers, uncles, and other male relatives. A history of bleeding on the paternal side, or a history of bleeding in female relatives, suggests vWD or another clotting factor deficiency. The severity of bleeding tends to run true within the family: patients with severe disease tend to have relatives with severe disease, and patients with mild disease have relatives with mild disease (this is not true with vWD).

Table 20–4
Hemophilia: Factor Level versus Severity*

Severity	Factor Level	Manifestations
Severe:	<1%	Spontaneous bleeding; bleeding with minor surgery or trauma
Moderate:	1–5%	Spontaneous bleeding uncommon; may bleed with surgery or trauma
Mild:	5–20%	No spontaneous bleeding; may bleed with major trauma or surgery

*Generally applies to both factor VIII and factor IX deficiencies; may not apply to deficiency of other factors.

⇨ *A relatively high proportion of cases of factor VIII deficiency (~20 to 30%) represent **new mutations**; therefore, these patients will **not** have a family history of bleeding.*

Laboratory Diagnosis

The PTT is prolonged; the PT is normal. Mixing studies show correction of the PTT with normal plasma. Specific diagnosis and distinction of factor VIII deficiency from factor IX deficiency require assay of the factor levels and demonstration of a deficiency. **It is critical to distinguish factor VIII deficiency from factor IX deficiency because the treatment is completely different.** Remember, it is impossible to distinguish hemophilia A from hemophilia B based on clinical or family history. Clotting factor assays also allow you to predict clinical severity if it is not obvious from the history.

Treatment

Treatment depends on which factor is deficient, the severity of the deficiency, and the nature of the bleeding, injury, or planned surgery. Various highly purified preparations of factors VIII and IX are available. These have been intensively treated to prevent infection, and are generally very safe. Recombinant forms of both are also available.

Always be sure to determine which factor the patient is deficient in before you start replacement therapy.

For severe bleeding or major surgery, it is desirable to achieve peak factor levels of 100% and maintain trough levels >50%. For minor bleeding or surgery, aim for peak levels of ~50% and trough levels ≥25%. A variety of different formulas are available for dosing factor concentrates (Tables 20–5 and 20–6).

Table 20–5
Treatment of Hemophilias

Factor VIII Deficiency (Hemophilia A)

Dose per % increase
1 unit of factor VIII per kilogram body weight will raise the factor VIII concentration ~**2%**.

Formula
The dose of factor VIII needed to raise the factor VIII level to any desired concentration can be estimated by the following formula:

$$\text{Units of factor VIII needed} = \frac{[(\text{Desired concentration} - \text{Initial concentration}) \times \text{body weight (kg)}]}{2}$$

Sample Calculation
Example: 72-kg patient with severe hemophilia A (factor VIII level <1%); desired factor VIII level 50%

$$\text{Units needed} = \frac{(50 - 0) \times 72}{2} = 1{,}800 \text{ units}$$

Administration
One half of the initial dose will need to be repeated every 8 to 12 hours to maintain a therapeutic level. It is preferable to follow factor VIII levels after infusion to be sure that the desired concentration is achieved and maintained.

Alternatively, the factor concentrates can be given as a continuous infusion. Give an initial bolus as above (to attain therapeutic level rapidly), then give a continuous infusion at approximately 3 U/kg/hr. Check factor VIII levels and adjust as necessary.

Factor IX Deficiency (Hemophilia B)

Dose per % increase
1 unit of factor IX per kilogram body weight will raise the factor IX level by **1%**.

Formula
One half of the initial dose of factor IX needed can be estimated as follows:

$$\text{Units of factor IX needed} = [(\text{Desired concentration} - \text{Initial concentration}) \times \text{body weight (kg)}]$$

Administration
The dose will need to be repeated every 12 to 24 hours. Check peak and trough levels and adjust the dose and dosing interval as necessary.

Because the factor concentrates are derived from pooled plasma from thousands of donors, many hemophiliacs treated with factor concentrates before 1985 became infected with the HIV, hepatitis C virus, and/or hepa-

Table 20–6
Guidelines for Factor Replacement in Hemophilia A and B

Site of Bleed	Hemostatic Level	Hemophilia A	Hemophilia B
Joint	30–50%	20–40 U/kg/day until healed	30–40 U/kg every other day until healed
Muscle	40–50	20–40 U/kg/day until healed	40–60 U/kg then 20–30 U/Kg every other day until healed
Gastro-intestinal, genitourinary	Initially 100%, then 30% until healed	50 U/kg, then 30–40 U/kg per day	100 U/kg then 30–40 U/kg per day
CNS	Initially 100%, then 50–100% for 14 days	50 U/kg then 25 U/kg every 12 hours	100 U/kg then 50 U/kg daily
Surgery or trauma	Initially 100%, then 50% until wound healing begins, then 30% until suture removal	50 U/kg then 25 U/kg every 12 hours adjusted according to healing	100 U/kg then 50 U/kg daily adjusted according to healing

CNS = central nervous system.
Adapted from DeLoughery TG. Hemostasis & thrombosis. In: Austin , Landes, editors. Bioscience. Georgetown (TX): 1999. p. 36.

titis B virus. Current factor concentrates are intensively treated to destroy these viruses and are much safer. However, it is not possible to completely eliminate virus transmission by factor concentrates. Recombinant forms of both factors are available and have essentially no infectious risk.

Desmopressin acetate can be a useful adjunct to treatment of mild or moderate hemophilia A. It induces release of vWF and factor VIII from endothelial cells and can temporarily raise the factor VIII level. **It is *not* effective for patients with *severe* hemophilia A** because they are unable to synthesize any factor VIII, and DDAVP will have no effect. It is also not helpful in the treatment of hemophilia B. **Antifibrinolytic agents** such as ε-aminocaproic acid (EACA; Amicar) or tranexamic acid can also be helpful, particularly in dental procedures such as tooth extraction. The mouth is very rich in fibrinolytic activity, and any clot that is formed will be dissolved unless fibrinolysis is inhibited. A dose of the factor is given before the extraction is performed and the antifibrinolytic is started afterward. This prevents the clot from dissolving, and often no additional factor replacement is needed.

Approximately 5 to 20% of patients with severe hemophilia A develop antibodies (inhibitors) against the factor. The presence of an inhibitor results in resistance to factor replacement therapy. Inhibitors are detected in the laboratory by failure of a mixing study to correct the PTT. Once an inhibitor is detected, a Bethesda assay should be done to determine the titer of the inhibitor. In children and sometimes adults, it is possible to induce immunologic tolerance to the protein by giving frequent large doses of the the factor. If this is not successful, therapy is based upon the titer of the inhibitor and the patient's response to receiving factor. If the titer of inhibitor is low (≤3 to 5 BU) and the patient does not respond with a big increase in titer (*low responder*), then the inhibitor can usually be overcome by giving a higher dose of the factor and/or by using a continuous infusion. If the titer is higher, or the patient responds with a big increase in inhibitor titer (*high responder*), an alternative therapy will be required. Porcine factor VIII (Hyate-C) is successful in many cases because the inhibitor is less active against porcine than human factor VIII. However, some patients will also develop high titer inhibitors against porcine factor VIII. In this case, prothrombin complex concentrates that bypass the inhibitor may be helpful (available preparations include Autoplex and FEIBA). A recent therapy for hemophilia A patients with inhibitors is **recombinant factor VIIa**; by combining with TF, the increased VIIa can drive the conversion of IX to IXa and thus bypass the inhibitor. However, this treatment is expensive and requires frequent administration (the half-life of VIIa is very short).

Patients with mild or moderate hemophilia A seldom develop inhibitors. Patients with factor IX deficiency, even severe cases, also tend not to develop inhibitors.

Spontaneous Factor VIII Inhibitors

Some people who are not factor VIII deficient can spontaneously develop factor VIII inhibitors. This can occur in autoimmune diseases such as systemic lupus, with pregnancy, with malignancies, with monoclonal immunoglobulins, and also for no apparent reason. Idiopathic inhibitors cause severe bleeding, resembling that of typical hemophilia. Immediate therapy is similar to hemophiliac patients with inhibitors. Prednisone can decrease or eliminate the inhibitor in these patients.

Diagnosis of Female Hemophilia Carriers

The normal range for factor activities is extremely wide: a typical range is 50 to 150%. It is therefore not possible to diagnose carriers based solely on factor activity levels (a woman with 50% activity may be a heterozygous carrier or may simply be at the bottom of the normal range). Another way of dentifying hemophilia A carriers is to measure simultaneous vWF and factor VIII levels. The normal ratio of vWF to factor VIII activity ranges from 0.74 to 2.2; the ratio in carriers is ~0.18 to 0.9. Genetic tests are also available, which can definitively diagnose female carriers.

Other Clotting Factor Deficiencies

Deficiencies of other clotting factors occur and can be associated with significant bleeding, but they are rare. The clinical severity of bleeding is not always easy to predict from the type of deficient factor and the level of factor present. For example, it would *seem* that a deficiency in factor V should result in a severe bleeding tendency, similar to that seen with deficiencies in factors VIII or IX. In fact, factor V deficiency usually results in only a mild or moderate bleeding disorder.

ACQUIRED BLEEDING DISORDERS

Acquired bleeding disorders are more common than inherited disorders. Acquired disorders can be of the primary hemostatic system or the secondary hemostatic system, or involve both systems. Unlike the inherited disorders of coagulation, which typically involve an abnormality in one factor or system, acquired bleeding disorders are often complex and involve multiple factors or systems.

Acquired Disorders of Primary Hemostasis

Antiplatelet Drugs

Probably the most common acquired deficiency of platelet function is antiplatelet drugs. We tend to think primarily of aspirin and other nonsteroidal anti-inflammatory drugs, which interfere with platelet function by inhibiting the enzyme cyclooxygenase. However, there is a long list of other drugs that can inhibit platelet function including antibiotics (penicillins, cephalosporins), antihistamines, cough medications (guaifenesin), and many others.

Uremia

Uremia causes platelet dysfunction, resulting in a prolonged BT. Anemia is part of the problem; abnormalities in prostaglandin metabolism may also be involved. Correction of anemia to a hemoglobin of ~10 to 11 g/dL with erythropoietin results in improvement in the BT. Desmopressin acetate, cryoprecipitate, and dialysis also improve the BT.

Miscellaneous

Platelet dysfunction may also be present in **liver disease**. The etiology is probably multifactorial. Patients who have been on **cardiopulmonary bypass** also have dysfunctional platelets; the platelets are partially activated and release their granules as they pass through the bypass pump, and are thus exhausted or spent. This lasts for about 2 to 3 days after surgery. Platelet transfusions should be given if significant bleeding develops in this setting.

Acquired Disorders of Secondary Hemostasis

Liver Disease

Liver disease is a common cause of coagulopathy. The etiology is multifactorial: decreased synthesis of clotting factors, anticoagulants, and plasminogen; impaired clearance of activated clotting factors; gastroesophageal varices; thrombocytopenia; malabsorption of vitamin K; and others. The PT and PTT will both be elevated; the PT is one of the most sensitive measures of hepatic synthetic function. Replacement of clotting factors with fresh frozen plasma and cryoprecipitate, and platelet transfusions for thrombocytopenia, may temporarily improve the situation. Administration of vitamin K occasionally helps. The ultimate therapy is to treat the liver disease; if you cannot fix the liver, you will not be able to fix the coagulopathy.

Disseminated Intravascular Coagulation

Disseminated intravascular coagulation, also known as *consumptive coagulopathy* or *defibrination syndrome*, is a common cause of coagulopathy in hospitalized patients. Disseminated intravascular coagulation is heterogeneous in etiology, pathophysiology, and clinical manifestations. The clinical spectrum ranges from asymptomatic, to florid bleeding from every orifice, to large and/or small vessel thrombosis, to a mixed picture that can include any or all of the above. In DIC, there is pathologic activation of both the coagulation cascade (thrombin conversion of fibrinogen to fibrin) and fibrinolysis (plasminogen activation to plasmin with digestion of fibrin, fibrinogen, and other clotting factors). The regulatory controls of coagulation and fibrinolysis are overwhelmed, and the coagulation process is freed from its normal surface dependence. The exact manifestations of DIC depend on the balance between coagulation/thrombosis and fibrinolysis in the individual patient. The best way to conceptualize DIC is to divide it into two main types: *acute* (*uncompensated*) and *chronic* (*compensated*).

In **acute** (**uncompensated**) **DIC**, there is activation of both the coagulation cascade and the fibrinolytic system. The liver is unable to compensate for consumption of coagulation, anticoagulation, and fibrinolytic factors; the levels of fibrinogen, other clotting factors, antithrombin, proteins C and S, plasminogen, and α_2-antiplasmin all decrease. Platelets are consumed, with resulting thrombocytopenia. Disseminated fibrin thrombi occur in the microvasculature all over the body. Plasmin digestion of fibrin results in the accumulation of FDPs, which interfere with both fibrin polymerization and platelet aggregation, further aggravating the coagulopathy. The primary event underlying most cases of acute DIC is endothelial injury and/or tissue necrosis, with release of TF into the circulation. Inflammatory cytokines, particularly interleukin-6, also appear to be critical. Ischemia resulting from microvasculature thrombosis or hypotension result in further tissue injury, with resulting acidosis and release of additional TF into the circulation. A vicious circle develops, with the complications of DIC further contributing to the underlying mechanisms causing DIC. *Infections, particularly bacterial sepsis, are the most common causes of acute DIC* (Table 20–7).

In **chronic (compensated) DIC**, there is low-grade activation of the coagulation and fibrinolytic systems; the liver is able to compensate for the degradation of clotting factors. **The primary manifestation of chronic DIC is thrombosis or thromboembolism**; hemorrhage is uncommon. Malignancies are a common cause of chronic DIC. The association of migratory

Table 20–7
Causes of Disseminated Intravascular Coagulation (DIC)

Acute DIC

Bacteremia: gram-negative and gram-positive bacteria

Sepsis with other organisms: fungi, mycobacteria, rickettsias, some viruses

Obstetric accidents: retained products of conception, placental abruption, amnionic fluid embolism

Severe trauma, especially head trauma

Burns

Shock or acidosis of any cause

Surgery

Acute hemolytic transfusion reaction

Malignancies: acute leukemia (especially acute promyelocytic leukemia); some carcinomas (especially mucin-producing carcinomas like gastric, prostatic, pancreatic)

Chronic DIC

Malignancies: carcinomas, particularly gastric and pancreatic thrombophlebitis with visceral malignancies (often gastric or pancreatic adenocarcinoma) has been designated *Trousseau's syndrome*. Deep vein thrombosis with resulting pulmonary embolism is a common cause of death in cancer patients.

Diagnosis of Disseminated Intravascular Coagulation

The keys to making the diagnosis of DIC are (1) *recognize the existence of an underlying predisposing condition*, and (2) *remember the protean clinical manifestations* of DIC. When you recognize a possible clinical feature of DIC, and note the existence of a predisposing cause, you can then initiate the appropriate diagnostic workup in a timely fashion. A relatively simple battery of tests should confirm or exclude the diagnosis of DIC in most cases. However, you must remember that DIC is an evolving, changing process; a set of laboratory tests done at a single time point may be misleading, and serial observation of some laboratories may be required.

Diagnosis of Acute Disseminated Intravascular Coagulation

A basic screen for acute DIC includes a PT and PTT, platelet count, fibrinogen level, and an assay of FDPs (FDP assay and/or D-dimer assay). A blood smear should be checked for the presence of schistocytes. **The PT, PTT, platelet count, and fibrinogen level can all be *completely* normal in a patient with DIC.** The PT and PTT may actually be shorter than normal, and the fibrinogen level may be normal or increased. The PT is said to be more sensitive than the PTT for acute DIC. If the original tests are normal or borderline in a patient who is strongly suspected of having DIC, repeat values after a few hours may show a drop in fibrinogen or platelet count, or a prolongation of the PT or PTT.

More exotic tests are available but are not needed in the average case. These include antithrombin, protein C and plasminogen levels, thrombin-antithrombin complexes, and plasmin-α_2-antiplasmin complexes. Protein C and antithrombin levels may have prognostic value; a decrease in the levels of these proteins suggests a worse prognosis. Clotting factor assays are often done but are of limited utility; it is important to remember that the factor VIII level is often normal and may be increased. Activation of prothrombin to thrombin can be measured by the prothrombin activation peptide $F_{1.2}$ ($F_{1.2}$ is released by proteolytic cleavage when prothrombin is activated to thrombin). Activation of fibrinogen to fibrin can be measured by assays for fibrinopeptides A and B.

Diagnosis of Chronic Disseminated Intravascular Coagulation

The basic assays for chronic DIC are the FDP and/or D-dimer tests. The PT and PTT tests are usually normal or may even be shortened. The fibrinogen level and platelet count are usually normal or increased.

Treatment of Acute Disseminated Intravascular Coagulation

The fundamental principle of treatment of DIC is to treat the underlying cause. Other than that, there is no consensus on treatment of acute DIC. Success at treating DIC depends primarily on the ability to treat the underlying cause. Mortality in patients with DIC is often due to the underlying condition rather than the DIC itself, although DIC may be a contributing factor.

- **Heparin:** Heparin can be used to shut off thrombin activity, thereby preventing conversion of fibrinogen to fibrin. This stops the coagulation cascade, prevents further depletion of fibrinogen, and prevents the deposition of fibrin thrombi in blood vessels. The use of heparin is controversial. Some experts believe that heparin is essential in the treatment of acute DIC, whereas others believe that heparin is almost never indicated. I believe the use of heparin should be on an individual basis. For example, heparin should be used in a patient who is having obvious thrombotic complications (gangrene of skin or digits) but should be avoided in patients with primarily bleeding problems. When used, heparin is generally given as a low-dose continuous infusion (~500 to 600 units/hour).

- **Transfusion of clotting factors**: Transfusion of clotting factors (fresh frozen plasma or cryoprecipitate) has generally been avoided in acute DIC for fear of "adding fuel to the fire" by increasing the formation of fibrin clots in blood vessels and increasing tissue ischemia and breakdown. However, some experts advocate giving cryoprecipitate to patients with severe hypofibrinogenemia and fresh frozen plasma to patients with decreased levels of other clotting factors. Again, use should be determined on an individual basis.

- **Platelet transfusions**: Platelet transfusions have usually been avoided, for the same reasons that clotting factors have. However, some experts suggest giving platelets to patients with severe thrombocytopenia.

- **Antithrombin concentrates**: Antithrombin is consumed in acute DIC. Antithrombin concentrates have become available and have shown benefit in animal models of DIC and small series of patients with DIC.

- **Protein C concentrates**: Protein C concentrates are available. Like AT concentrates, they have appeared beneficial in small series, but large controlled trials are lacking.

- **Antifibrinolytic agents**: Antifibrinolytic agents such as ε-aminocaproic acid (Amicar) have generally been avoided, for fear that they would result in florid intravascular thrombosis. They may be beneficial in patients who have primarily fibrinolysis and hemorrhage.

- **Miscellaneous**: Acute DIC associated with **acute promyelocytic leukemia** (APL; FAB-M3) usually responds quickly to treatment with all-*trans*-retinoic acid (ATRA). Low-dose heparin is also used in this condition.

Treatment of Chronic Disseminated Intravascular Coagulation

Again, the first principle is to **treat the underlying cause**. Chronic DIC with thromboemboli due to metastatic carcinoma is usually treated with low-dose heparin; warfarin is usually unsuccessful and may aggravate the situation.

HYPERCOAGULABLE STATES (THROMBOPHILIA)

Thrombophilia is the technical term for hypercoagulable states. Virchow originally defined the conditions that predispose to thrombosis as (1) **abnormalities in the blood vessel wall**, (2) **abnormalities in the blood**, and (3) **abnormalities of blood flow** (stasis). His definition remains valid today.

Thrombophilia can be either *inherited* or *acquired*. Suggestions of an inherited thrombophilia include **thrombosis without any predisposing condition** (ie, no surgery, injury, prolonged inactivity), **thrombosis at a young age** (less than about 40 to 45), **thrombosis in unusual sites** (upper extremities, mesenteric vessels, hepatic or portal veins, cerebral veins), and a **family history of thrombosis**. We now know that many individuals with thromboemboli who appear to have an obvious predisposing factor for thrombosis (ie, recent surgery) also have an inherited thrombophilia.

Inherited Hypercoagulable States

Inherited thrombophilic states can be due to a deficiency of a natural anticoagulant, such as antithrombin or protein C; a mutation in a clotting factor, making it resistant to inhibition (factor V Leiden); or resistance to fibrinolysis. Most of the inherited deficiencies of natural anticoagulants (AT, proteins C and S) are inherited in an **autosomal dominant fashion**. Infants who are homozygous for a deficiency of one of these factors die shortly after childbirth due to overwhelming systemic thrombosis, with necrosis of skin and other tissues (*neonatal purpura fulminans*). Resistance to activated protein C (factor V Leiden) is inherited as an autosomal trait with variable penetrance in heterozygotes (Table 20–8).

Many people (probably the majority) who are heterozygous for a deficiency in one of these natural anticoagulants *never* have an episode of thrombosis, and there is currently no way to predict which individuals will be affected. There is no reason to prophylactically anticoagulate these patients on a routine basis. However, if a person known to have an inherited thrombophilia is to undergo major surgery or some other situation that would increase the risk of thrombosis, it might be reasonable to anticoagulate them during the period of increased risk. In addition, if someone is

Table 20–8
Inherited Hypercoagulable States

Syndrome	Inheritance	Frequency*
APC resistance (factor V Leiden)	Autosomal; variable penetrance	2–7%
Protein C deficiency	Autosomal dominant	1:200–300
Protein S deficiency	Autosomal dominant	Unknown
Antithrombin deficiency	Autosomal dominant	1:2,000–5,000
Prothrombin G20210A	Autosomal dominant	1–3%

*US and Europe.
APC = activated protein C resistance.

known to have an inherited thrombophilia, it would be wise to avoid or minimize factors that would add to the risk of thrombosis (ie, oral contraceptives).

Antithrombin Deficiency

Antithrombin is the most important inhibitor of activated coagulation factors. A deficiency of AT is responsible for ~1 to 2% of cases of thrombosis in patients, with an apparent inherited thrombophilia in the United States. Patients with AT deficiency usually suffer from deep venous thrombosis in the lower extremities.

Protein C Deficiency

Protein C deficiency is found in ~2 to 5% of patients with thrombosis and a probable inherited thrombophilia. The prevalence of deficiency in the general population is approximately 1:200 to 1:700. Like AT deficiency, the majority of thromboses are venous, predominantly in the lower extremities.

Protein S Deficiency

Protein S deficiency is found in ~2 to 3% of patients with thrombosis and probable inherited thrombophilia. The frequency of protein S deficiency in the general population is unknown. Protein S deficiency may be associated with arterial as well as venous thrombosis.

Activated Protein C Resistance (Factor V Leiden)

Resistance to activated protein C is the most common inherited thrombophilia in the United States and Europe. Most cases result from a mutation in the factor V gene resulting in a substitution of glycine for arginine at position 506, called **factor V Leiden**, which makes the factor Va protein resistant to inactivation by activated protein C (APC). The estimated prevalence of this mutation is ~2 to 7% in the general population of the United States and Europe, and it is believed to be responsible for approximately 20 to 50% of cases of thrombosis in patients with presumed inherited thrombophilia. The mutation is uncommon in Africa and Asia. Activated protein C resistance is inherited as an autosomal trait with variable expression in heterozygotes. The homozygous state is not lethal, but homozygotes do have a higher rate of thrombosis than heterozygotes. Heterozygotes are thought to have ~5- to 10-fold increase in risk of thrombosis; homozygotes have a 50- to 100-fold increase in risk. The primary manifestation is deep venous thrombosis. Possession of the gene for APC can interact with other thrombophilic conditions, such as protein C or S deficiency, or oral contraceptives. The condition can be diagnosed using either a clot-based assay or by a molecular genetic test.

⇨ The clot-based test for APC resistance cannot be performed on a patient who is on warfarin; the molecular test can.

Prothrombin G20210A

In 1996, a mutation in the prothrombin gene was described that appears to be associated with thrombophilia. The prevalence of the mutation in United States and Europe is similar to that of factor V Leiden; it also appears to be uncommon in Africa and Asia. The prothrombin G20210A mutation appears to be associated with arterial as well as venous thrombosis. There appears to be a particular association with cerebral vein thrombosis, especially in women taking oral contraceptives. Many patients with the prothrombin G20210A mutation have increased levels of prothrombin, and this has been the suggested mechanism for thrombophilia with this mutation. However, there is overlap in the prothrombin level between patients with this mutation and the normal population lacking the mutation.

Hyperhomocysteinemia

It has recently been shown that hyperhomocysteinemia is a risk factor for thrombosis, both arterial and venous. Hyperhomocysteinemia can be inherited or acquired. Acquired causes include deficiencies in cobalamin, folate, or pyridoxine. Animal models suggest that hyperhomocysteinemia is toxic to endothelial cells and has a variety of other effects that may increase the risk of thrombosis. Hyperhomocysteinemia appears to be a risk factor for stroke, myocardial infarction, peripheral arterial disease, extracranial carotid artery stenosis, and recurrent venous thrombosis in the lower extremities.

Miscellaneous

A variety of other inherited thrombophilic states have been described, including abnormal fibrinogen molecules (*dysfibrinogenemia*), deficiency of heparin cofactor II, defects in the fibrinolytic system, and others. All of these are quite rare.

Screening for Inherited Thrombophilias

Screening for an inherited thrombophilia should be considered in patients with thrombosis and a family history of thrombosis, thrombosis in unusual sites, thrombosis at an early age (less than ~40 to 45 years), or thrombosis without an obvious predisposing cause. The testing protocol would depend on the ethnic background of the patient, the particular thrombotic manifestation, and whether a specific inherited thrombophilia has been identified in relatives. As a general rule, tests should include an assay for APC resistance, AT and protein C and S levels, and possibly an assay for the prothrombin G20210A mutation. Acquired thrombophilic conditions, such as a lupus anticoagulant, should also be considered.

Some people have advocated that *all* women who are going to be put on oral contraceptives or post-menopausal estrogen replacement should be screened for inherited thrombophilia. The cost of this per episode of thrombosis prevented would probably be excessive, and it is not currently standard practice to screen for thrombophilia before prescribing oral contraceptives or estrogens. However, if the woman has a family history that suggests the presence of an inherited thrombophilia, it might be prudent to consider such screening.

Acquired Hypercoagulable States

Lupus Anticoagulant/Antiphospholipid Antibody Syndrome

Lupus anticoagulants are antibodies directed against proteins bound to phospholipids, which interfere with clotting assays. A closely related but not synonymous term is *antiphospholipid antibodies* (also called *anticardiolipin antibodies*). Lupus anticoagulants interfere with phospholipid-dependent clotting assays, usually the PTT. Occasionally, both the PTT and PT are prolonged and, rarely, just the PT. The term lupus anticoagulant derived from the fact that the antibodies were first described in two women who had systemic lupus erythematosus and a coagulopathy. It is now known that lupus anticoagulants are found in many patients who do not have lupus and in the majority of cases are associated with little risk of bleeding. In fact, lupus anticoagulants are associated with a significant risk of thrombosis, including thrombi in deep veins of the lower extremities, arteries, cerebral vessels, and unusual sites such as the mesenteric vessels and the portal or hepatic veins.

Lupus anticoagulants appear to be a subset of antiphospholipid antibodies (APAs). Not all APAs interfere with phospholipid-dependent clotting tests; those that do are lupus anticoagulants. Antiphospholipid antibodies are usually detected by immunologic methods, such as an ELISA. Lupus anticoagulants are detected by clot-based tests such as the PTT, dilute Russell viper venom time, or a variety of others. *Nearly all patients with lupus anticoagulants have a positive assay for APA* ($\geq 90\%$); however, *many patients with a positive APA do not have lupus anticoagulants*. There is not a good correlation between the titer of APA and the strength of the lupus anticoagulant in the individual case (ie, the patient may have a low titer APA by ELISA but striking prolongation of the PTT, or vice versa). The APA is actually directed against a protein stuck on the phospholipid rather than the phospholipid itself; probably the most common protein is the β_2-glycoprotein I (also called apolipoprotein H). Antibodies may also be directed against prothrombin, protein C or S, and others.

Lupus anticoagulants/APAs are seen in some patients with lupus (often patients with a "biologic false-positive" VDRL test), in patients with other autoimmune diseases, with a variety of infections, with certain medications (antiarrhythmic drugs such as quinidine and procainamide, psychiatric drugs such as phenothiazines, and others), with HIV infection, and also for no apparent reason (idiopathic).

Pathologic bleeding in people with lupus anticoagulants is uncommon; however, some patients also have a decrease in the prothrombin level, and these patients may have bleeding problems. **Thrombosis is a much greater risk**. In many cases, the lupus anticoagulant is detected by a PTT ordered as a preoperative screen, in which case it is more a nuisance than anything else (the surgeon has to hold the procedure until you can work up the coagulopathy).

The **APA syndrome** includes a lupus anticoagulant or moderate- to high-titer APA together with some combination of venous and/or arterial thrombosis, central nervous system events (transient ischemic attacks, strokes, amaurosis fugax, others), thrombocytopenia, recurrent fetal loss, cardiac valvular abnormalities (nonbacterial vegetations on valves, most often the mitral valve), and livedo reticularis.

It used to be believed that patients with lupus anticoagulants due to a medication or infection did not have a significantly increased risk of thrombosis; unfortunately, this may not be absolutely true. However, it is important to remember that many (possibly most) patients with lupus anticoagulant do not have thrombotic episodes.

Screening tests for detection of lupus anticoagulants include the PTT, dilute PTT, dilute Russell viper venom time, kaolin clotting time, and others. Several tests are available to confirm the phospholipid dependence of the inhibitor; one is the **platelet neutralization procedure** (**PNP**). In this test, exogenous phospholipid (such as reagent platelet membrane phospholipid) is added to the clotting test to overwhelm the antibody. The result of the plasma plus phospholipid mixture is compared to a plasma plus saline mixture (the saline is added to control for the dilutional effect of the extra reagent phospholipid). If the plasma plus phospholipid mixture shortens the clotting test significantly, the test is positive for a lupus anticoagulant. If the test used is the PTT, shortening by more than 6 seconds compared to the plasma plus saline control is usually considered positive.

Malignancies

Many malignancies are associated with thrombophilia. Patients with malignancies may have several predisposing factors for thrombosis, including chronic DIC, debilitation and inactivity, medications, frequent surgical procedures, and abnormal blood vessel walls. Evidence of chronic DIC has been found in up to 50% of patients with metastatic carcinomas. As described above, thrombosis is the primary complication of chronic DIC. Patients may also have abnormalities of procoagulant and/or anticoagulant factors in the blood, such as increased fibrinogen or decreased protein C levels.

Oral Contraceptives

The relationship of oral contraceptives to thrombosis has become a big issue of late. Women taking oral contraceptives appear to have ~3- to 4-fold increased risk of thrombosis (primarily deep venous thrombosis in the lower extremities) compared to women not taking oral contraceptives. The risk is lower in young women with no other risk factors for thrombosis, higher in older women or women with other risk factors. Oral contraceptives can interact with inherited thrombophilia, notably factor V Leiden. Women who are heterozygous for the mutation and take oral contraceptives have a ~30-fold increase in risk of deep venous thrombosis compared to women without the mutation and not taking oral contraceptives. Women who are homozygous for the mutation and take oral contraceptives have a several hundred-fold increase in risk of thrombosis.

Heparin-Induced Thrombocytopenia/Thrombosis

Heparin-induced thrombocytopenia/thrombosis was discussed in Chapter 11.

Miscellaneous

A variety of other conditions confer an increased risk of thrombosis, including pregnancy, surgery, sepsis, the nephrotic syndrome, and many others. In pregnancy, the blood levels of many clotting factors are increased. Women may be less active or confined to bed rest, and the gravid uterus presses on the veins from the lower extremities, predisposing to stasis. A "dead fetus syndrome" may induce a chronic DIC state. Surgery increases the risk of thrombosis by several means. The risk is particularly high with hip replacements and other orthopedic surgeries. Sepsis can be thrombogenic due to decreased levels of protein C and free protein S. The nephrotic syndrome may be thrombogenic because of loss of antithrombin in the urine.

Anticoagulation

There are several types of anticoagulation therapy. The main choices are heparin for immediate use, vitamin K inhibitors like warfarin, and antiplatelet agents like aspirin or ticlopidine. In addition to anticoagulants, fibrinolytic agents (plasminogen activators) have become widely used for the treatment of acute myocardial ischemia, pulmonary embolus, or deep vein thrombosis.

- **Heparin:** Heparin is the drug of choice for *immediate* anticoagulation, such as an acute pulmonary embolus. It is also used for prophylaxis against thrombosis. It must be administered parenterally (intravenously or subcutaneously). Heparin works by activating antithrombin, which then inactivates thrombin, factor Xa, and other activated clotting factors. Heparin is available in two main forms: **unfractionated heparin** (Table 20–9) and **low-molecular-weight heparin** (Table 20–10). Unfractionated heparin is a mix of miscellaneous sizes and varies from company to company and batch to batch. It binds to a variety of plasma proteins; the degree of binding varies between individuals, which makes unfractionated heparin a pharmacologic nightmare. Use of unfractionated heparin is traditionally monitored using the PTT; probably a better test is the factor Xa inactivation assay. Low-molecular-weight heparin has many advantages over unfractionated heparin. Low-molecular-weight heparin does not bind to plasma proteins significantly and is therefore much more pharmacologically predictable. It is given on a milligram per kilogram basis and usually does not require monitoring. However, low-molecular-weight heparin preparations are expensive.
- **Warfarin:** Coumarin drugs block the synthesis of the vitamin K–dependent clotting factors (II, VII, IX, X); they also block the synthesis of the vitamin K–dependent *inhibitors* of coagulation, proteins C and S. Warfarin is the most commonly used form in the United States.

Table 20–9
Anticoagulation with Unfractionated Heparin

Treatment of Deep Venous Thrombosis or Thromboembolism

Unfractionated heparin used therapeutically is usually given as a continuous intravenous infusion. PT, PTT, and platelet count should be obtained prior to initiation of heparin therapy. The platelet count should be checked every 2 to 3 days during heparin therapy.

- **Bolus: 5,000 units** (U) intravenously (up to 10,000 U for large thrombi or pulmonary embolus).
- **Infusion:** A continuous intravenous infusion of **~1,200 to 1,400 U/hr** is started after the initial bolus. The intravenous infusion is adjusted based on PTT or factor Xa inactivation tests.
- **Monitoring heparin administration:** Check the PTT or factor Xa inactivation level approximately 6 hours after the infusion is begun. The test should be repeated two or three times daily until the heparin infusion is stabilized and then daily thereafter while the patient is on heparin.

Goals:

- PTT ~ 1.5–2.5 times control level
- Factor Xa inactivation level of 0.3-0.7 U/mL
- **Duration of therapy:** Heparin is usually continued for approximately 5 days or for at least 24 hours after the PT is therapeutic on warfarin.

If the PTT becomes excessively prolonged (or the factor Xa inactivation level becomes supratherapeutic), stop heparin for a few hours and recheck. Restart the infusion at a reduced dose after the laboratory test reaches the desired range.

Prophylaxis Against Thromboembolism

- **5,000–6,000 U subcutaneously twice daily** is often used as prophylaxis against deep venous thrombosis in hospitalized patients or temporarily in patients at high risk for thrombosis.
- It is usually not necessary to monitor low-dose heparin given subcutaneously as prophylaxis.

It is given orally and takes 4 to 5 days to take effect. Since factor VII has the shortest half-life of the vitamin K–dependent clotting factors, the PT is affected before the PTT, and the PT has traditionally been used for monitoring warfarin therapy. Different PT reagents have different sensitivities to warfarin; therefore, the **INR** has become the standard way to monitor warfarin therapy (Table 20–11).

- Protein C has about the same half-life as factor VII. If the person is protein C deficient, the level of protein C can drop below the effec-

Table 20–10

Anticoagulation with Low-Molecular-Weight Heparin

Treatment of Deep Venous Thrombosis or Thromboembolism

Two low-molecular-weight heparin preparations are currently available: **dalteparin** and **enoxaparin**. Low-molecular-weight heparins are much more pharmacologically predictable than standard heparin and are dosed based on body weight. They are often used subcutaneously rather than intravenously, and patients are now being treated for deep venous thrombosis of the lower extremities on an outpatient basis.

- **Dose:**
  - **Dalteparin:** 100 U/kg every 12 hours
  - **Enoxaparin:** 1 mg/kg every 12 hours

- **Monitoring:** Laboratory monitoring of low-molecular-weight heparin is usually not necessary. Monitoring should be considered in patients who are very obese, those with heart failure or liver disease, pregnant women, or patients on long-term therapy. The factor Xa inactivation level should be used; the PTT is relatively unaffected by low-molecular-weight heparins.

- **Goal:** 0.7–1.2 anti-Xa units; the level should be drawn approximately 4 hours after injection.

Prophylaxis Against Thromboembolism

- Dalteparin: 2,500 U/day for low-risk patients; 5,000 U/day for high-risk patients
- Enoxaparin: 40 mg/day or 30 mg/day every 12 hours (orthopedic use)

tive anticoagulant level before the patient is effectively anticoagulated. Therefore, you have induced an iatrogenic state of protein C deficiency, and the patient could develop **warfarin-induced skin necrosis** (similar to *neonatal purpura fulminans* in infants homozygous for protein C deficiency). This is usually prevented if the patient is anticoagulated with heparin while warfarin is started. By the time heparin is stopped, the factor VII level has dropped below the effective range, and the patient is effectively anticoagulated. If you do encounter warfarin-induced skin necrosis, immediately administer protein C concentrates or fresh frozen plasma.

- **Warfarin is contraindicated during pregnancy** because it is teratogenic. Heparin should be used for women who require anticoagulation during pregnancy.
- Many medications can interact with warfarin. Table 20–12 provides a summary of such drugs.
- **Aspirin:** Aspirin (acetylsalicylic acid) is the traditional antiplatelet agent. Aspirin irreversibly inhibits cyclooxygenase, which prevents synthesis of TxA_2 (a potent vasoconstrictor and platelet agonist). The effect

Table 20–11
Anticoagulation with Warfarin

Warfarin is used for long-term oral anticoagulation. The majority of warfarin in circulation is bound to albumin; the unbound active form is only ~3% of the total. Warfarin is metabolized in the liver, and there is marked variability in the rate of warfarin metabolism in different patients. Many drugs either displace warfarin from albumin, thus increasing the effect, or alter hepatic metabolism (either increasing or decreasing metabolism). *It is critical that the INR be monitored closely after changes in medications.*

Warfarin is usually begun while the patient is being anticoagulated with heparin. The therapeutic effect of warfarin lags behind the INR; heparin must be continued until the INR has been in the therapeutic range for at least 2 days.

Beginning warfarin therapy

- **Initial dose:** The usual starting dose is **5 mg/day** for average adults; older or smaller patients can be started on 2.5 mg/day. Children can be started on 0.2 mg/kg. The dose is then adjusted based on the INR. Loading doses (10 mg for the first dose) are unnecessary and may lead to overshooting the desired INR.
- **Monitoring warfarin administration:** Warfarin is monitored using the INR (International Normalized Ratio), which is the prothrombin time (PT) adjusted for the specific PT reagent used. The INR should be checked 2 to 3 times weekly while the proper dose is being established, weekly for several weeks afterward until the INR is stable on a fixed dose of warfarin, and then every 3 to 4 weeks thereafter as long as the patient is on warfarin.
  - The INR should be checked weekly for several weeks after any medication is added or discontinued.
- **INR Goals:**
  - 2.0–3.0: Deep venous thrombosis, pulmonary embolism, atrial fibrillation.
  - 2.5–3.5 (3.0–4.5): Mechanical heart valve, antiphospholipid antibody syndrome.

Reversing warfarin therapy

- The effect of warfarin can be reversed by holding warfarin for a few days, administration of vitamin K, or, in urgent situations, by administering fresh frozen plasma.
- Treatment for a high INR depends on the INR level and the clinical status of the patient.
  - **INR 3–5:** If the patient is stable and not bleeding, either hold warfarin for a few days and restart at a lower dose or continue warfarin at a decreased dose. Recheck the INR in a few days.
  - **INR 5–10:** If the patient is stable, either hold warfarin for a few days or give vitamin K (1–2 mg orally or subcutaneously, or 1 mg intravenously). Do not give a high dose of vitamin K; this will make the patient resistant to warfarin, and reinstitution of warfarin will be difficult.

Continued

Table 20–11
Anticoagulation with Warfarin—Continued

- **INR >10:** Vitamin K as above and fresh frozen plasma (2–4 units) if bleeding.
- **Minor bleeding with any INR:** Vitamin K 2 to 5 mg orally, subcutaneously, or intravenously. Recheck the INR in 6 to 12 hours. The INR should decrease within 12 hours.
- **Life-threatening bleeding with any INR:** Give 2 to 4 units of fresh frozen plasma plus 2 to 5 mg of vitamin K subcutaneously or intravenously.
- **Surgery:** If a patient is scheduled for surgery, warfarin should be discontinued approximately 1 week prior to the date of surgery. The patient should be maintained on low-dose subcutaneous heparin until just before the surgery. Warfarin can be re-started after the procedure.

Table 20–12
Medications That May Interact with Warfarin

Increased Warfarin Effect

Acetaminophen	**Fluconazole***	Quinidine*
Allopurinol	Furosemide	Quinine*
Amiodarone*	Gemfibrozil	Quinolones
Anabolic steroids	Isoniazid	Serotonin uptake inhibitors
Aspirin*	**Itraconazole***	**Sulfinpyrazone***
Cephalosporin antibiotics	**Ketoconazole***	Sulfonylureas*
Cimetidine*	**Metronidazole***	Tamoxifen*
Clofibrate*	**Micronase***	Tetracycline*
Cyclophosphamide	Omeprazole	**Thyroid hormones***
Disulfiram	**Propafenone**	Triyclic antidepressants
Erythromycin*	Propranolol	Vitamin E*

Decreased Warfarin Effect

Alcohol	**Phenytoin**	Rifampin
Barbiturates*	**Cholestyramine**	Sucralfate
Carbamazepine	Estrogens	Vitamin K
Corticosteroids	**Griseofulvin**	

*Major effect.
Most commonly implicated drugs are indicated in boldface.
Reproduced with permission from DeLoughery TG. Hemostasis & thrombosis. In: Austin, Landes, editors. Bioscience. Georgetown (TX): 1999. p. 176.

lasts the lifetime of the poisoned platelet. Aspirin also blocks the synthesis of PGI_2 by endothelial cells; however, unlike platelets, the endothelial cells are able to make more cyclooxygenase. So, low-dose aspirin given once a day establishes a favorable ratio of PGI_2 to TxA_2, inhibiting platelet aggregation. Aspirin is considered only a moderately strong platelet antagonist.

⇨ *Aspirin is contained in a host of over-the-counter medications; therefore, always ask about **all** medications that the patient is taking.*

- **Ticlopidine (Ticlid) and Clopidogrel (Plavix):** Ticlopidine and clopidogrel are new antiplatelet agents that work by inducing a functional deficiency of GP IIb/IIIa on the platelet surface. They are potent antiplatelet agents but have significant side effects. A particularly devastating side effect is a microangiopathic hemolytic anemia resembling thrombotic thrombocytopenic purpura-hemolytic uremic syndrome (TTP-HUS). Ticlopidine can also cause pancytopenia.
- **ReoPro:** ReoPro is a monoclonal antibody against the GP IIb/IIIa complex on platelet surfaces. It is widely used during coronary angioplasty to prevent re-stenosis.

APPROACH TO THE PATIENT WITH POSSIBLE DISORDERS OF HEMOSTASIS

It is impossible to describe a single approach that is appropriate for *all* patients who may have a possible disorder of hemostasis. What follows is a general approach, which should get you started in most cases (Table 20–13). The results of history, physical examination, and initial tests will allow you to alter the approach for each specific patient.

⇨ **Always remember that a good history is the most specific and most sensitive diagnostic test for a patient with a possible hemostatic disorder. Doing laboratory tests does NOT substitute for a good history and physical.**

Questions to Ask

⇨ **Does the patient have a bleeding disorder, or is it just an abnormal laboratory test?** Not every patient with an abnormal laboratory test has a significant bleeding disorder. For example, people with a deficiency of factor XII, PK, or HMWK have strikingly high PTTs but no increased risk of bleeding.

⇨ **Has the patient ever had a serious challenge to hemostasis? Ask about** *specific circumstances*, like circumcision, previous surgeries, and den-

Table 20–13
Approach to the Patient with Possible Disorders of Hemostasis

History

Physical examination

Basic laboratory tests
    PT, PTT
    Fibrinogen level
    CBC with platelet count
    Examination of blood smear

Additional laboratory tests*
    Bleeding time
    Mixing study for prolonged PT or PTT
    Fibrinogen degradation products or D-dimer

Possible hemophilia: factor assays, beginning with factors VIII and IX

Possible von Willebrand's disease: quantitative assay of vWF, ristocetin co-factor activity, ristocetin-induced platelet aggregation, vWF multimer analysis

*Additional tests performed selectively, based on results of history, physical examination, and initial laboratory tests.

tal extractions. Questions like "Do you bruise easily?" or "Do you have heavy menstrual periods?" are useless. Many normal people will say they bruise easily, and one woman's heavy period might be another woman's light day (ask how many pads or tampons she uses per day, and how many per average menstrual period).

⇨ **Does the patient have a vascular disorder that could cause bleeding?** Consider hereditary hemorrhagic telangiectasia, scurvy, and senile purpura. Look for mulberry lesions on the oral mucosa and telangiectasias on the hands and other sites.

⇨ **If the patient has had surgery, could it be surgical bleeding rather than a coagulation disorder per se?** For example, a vessel that was not tied off.

⇨ **If the patient does appear to have a disorder of hemostasis, is it in the *primary* or *secondary* system?** If the defect appears to be in the primary system, you would worry about thrombocytopenia, platelet defects, vWD, and drugs that interfere with platelet function. If the defect is in secondary hemostasis, you would be interested in factor deficiencies, warfarin ingestion, or liver disease.

⇨ **Does the patient have a *family history* of increased or abnormal bleeding? If so, what is the inheritance pattern? Is it in the primary system or the secondary system?** A pattern of bleeding in male relatives on the maternal side would suggest an X-linked disorder such as hemophilia A or B. A pattern of bleeding in every generation would suggest an autosomal dominant disorder such as vWD. A history of consanguinity would raise the possibility of a rare bleeding disorder such as vWD Type 3, factor XI deficiency (common in Ashkenazi Jews), or one of the other factor deficiencies. Be aware, however, that a significant number of cases of factor VIII deficiency (hemophilia A) represent new mutations, and the family history will be negative. Primary hemostasis-type bleeding would suggest vWD; and less often Bernard-Soulier syndrome, Glanzmann's thrombasthenia, or one of the other rare inherited platelet disorders. Secondary hemostasis-type bleeding would suggest some type of hemophilia.

⇨ **Is the patient on any medications?** Ask about *all* medications that the patient might be taking, both prescription and over the counter; get the patient or relative to bring in all the pill bottles in the medicine cabinet. Many medications can interfere with platelet function; some antibiotics can induce a coagulation factor deficiency. Remember that innumerable over-the-counter medications include aspirin (acetylsalicylic acid), and remember to ask about vitamins, herbal supplements, and herbal teas. Something to think about, particularly in medical personnel, is surreptitious ingestion of warfarin (a Munchausen syndrome).

⇨ **What is the platelet count? What do platelets look like on the blood smear?** A low platelet count would start a search for causes of thrombocytopenia. A high platelet count would raise the possibility of primary thrombocythemia or one of the other myeloproliferative disorders (although reactive thrombocytosis is far more common than primary thrombocythemia). Platelets may be large and look abnormal in the Bernard-Soulier syndrome; platelets may appear agranular in the gray platelet syndrome. The combination of thrombocytopenia and small platelets raises the possibility of Wiskott-Aldrich syndrome. If the patient has bleeding suggesting a defect in primary hemostasis and the platelet count is normal, you would consider doing a BT, assays for vWD (ristocetin cofactor activity, ristocetin-induced platelet aggregation, quantitative analysis of vWF, vWF multimer analysis), and platelet aggregation studies.

⇨ **Does the patient have evidence of liver disease?** Check the liver function tests (albumin, aspartate transaminase, alanine transaminase, bilirubin).

⇨ **Does the patient have any evidence of DIC?** Does the patient have any illness or condition that would predispose him or her to DIC? Are there any schistocytes on the smear?

INVESTIGATING AN ABNORMAL COAGULATION TEST (PT OR PTT) RESULT

A common problem is an unexplained increase in the PT and/or PTT (Figure 20–5 and Table 20–14). **The first thing to do is get a fresh sample and rerun the test. Another consideraton is *heparin*.** It is possible that the blood sample was mistakenly drawn though a running line. Interference by heparin can be detected by absorbing the heparin with a resin ("Heparsorb") or by using an enzyme to digest the heparin ("Hepzyme"). Also, *check the history*: Is the patient on any anticoagulants? Does the patient have liver disease? Provided that the abnormal result is reproduced on a good specimen and there is no obvious explanation from the history, the next thing to do is a *mixing study*. If the mixing study shows correction and no prolongation with incubation, you will need to do factor assays to look for factor deficiency: start with VIII and IX since they are the most common deficiencies. It is useful to do a few vitamin K–dependent and a few non-vitamin K–dependent factors to be sure that the problem is not accidental or surreptitious warfarin ingestion.

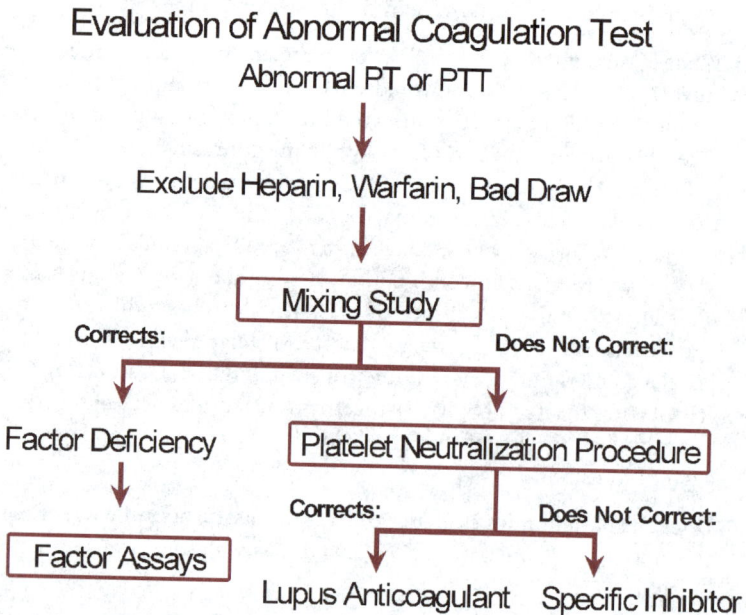

Figure 20–5 Evaluation of an abnormal coagulation test.

Table 20–14
Interpreting PTT or PT Mixing Studies

Specimen	Immediate	Post-Incubation
Patient	___	___
1:1 Mix	A	C
Control	B	___
1:1 Mix (incubated separately)	N/A	D

Interpretation

1) Compare the immediate 1:1 mix (A) to the control (B):

   ⇨ If the immediate mix is prolonged (greater than the normal range) report as "**Failure to correct with mixing; consistent with inhibitor.**" It is not necessary to perform the post-incubation studies if the immediate 1:1 mix shows significant prolongation.

   ⇨ If the immediate 1:1 mix shows correction into the normal range, continue with the post-incubation studies (see 2 below).

   ⇨ If the initial patient value is markedly prolonged *and* the immediate 1:1 mix shows marked correction (to within a few seconds of the normal range), continue with the post-incubation studies (see 2 below).

2) Compare the incubated 1:1 mix (C) to the 1:1 mix after separate incubation (D):

   ⇨ If the incubated 1:1 mix (C) shows minimal prolongation compared to the 1:1 mix after separate incubation (D), report as "**Correction with mixing; consistent with factor deficiency.**"

   ⇨ If the post-incubation mix (C) shows more than a few seconds prolongation compared to the 1:1 mix after separate incubation (D), report as "**Failure to correct with mixing; consistent with time dependent inhibitor.**"

If the mixing study fails to correct, then you need to think about an inhibitor. The most common inhibitor is a nonspecific inhibitor such as a lupus anticoagulant. Perform a test to demonstrate a phospholipid-dependent antibody, such as a platelet neutralization procedure. Spontaneous specific inhibitors against clotting factors occur (ie, not in hemophiliacs), most often against factor VIII. This can occur in patients with systemic lupus, monoclonal gammopathies, other malignancies, during pregnancy, and for no apparent reason (idiopathic). These patients can have devastating bleeding. The thing to do is identify the specific factor involved and find out how high the titer is. If the patient has a low titer inhibitor, try to overwhelm it with high doses of the factor. If the patient has a high titer antibody against factor VIII, try porcine factor VIII or prothrombin complex concentrates to stop the bleeding. Prednisone will often lower the titer over time. Intravenous immunoglobulin has been reported to also help (however, IVIG does not seem to work for hemophiliacs with an inhibitor).

Index